T0203258

Rett Syndrome

Rett Syndrome

Edited by

WALTER E KAUFMANN
Greenwood Genetic Centre
Greenwood, SC, USA

with
ALAN K PERCY
University of Alabama School of Medicine, Birmingham, AL, USA

ANGUS CLARKE
School of Medicine, Cardiff University,
Wales, UK

HELEN LEONARD
Telethon Kids Institute
The University of Western Australia
Crawley, Australia

SAKKUBAI NAIDU
Johns Hopkins University
School of Medicine, Baltimore, MD, USA

2017
Mac Keith Press

© 2017 Mac Keith Press
6 Market Road, London, N7 9PW

Managing Director: Ann-Marie Halligan
Commissioning Editor/Production Manager: Udoka Ohuonu
Project Management: Riverside Solutions Ltd

First published in this edition in 2017

British Library Cataloguing-in-Publication data
A catalogue record for this book is available from the British Library

Cover image: Sydney Crandall, a patient of Prof Kaufmann. Cover design: Hannah Rogers

ISBN: 978-1-909962-83-5

Printing managed by Jellyfish Solutions Ltd

Mac Keith Press is supported by Scope

CONTENTS

Contents

AUTHORS' APPOINTMENTS

Hayley Archer

Former Consultant Clinical Geneticist, All Wales Medical Genetics Service, University Hospital of Wales, Cardiff, UK

Gordon Baikie

Honorary Research Fellow, Murdoch Childrens Research Institute; Honorary Clinical Senior Lecturer, Department of Paediatrics, University of Melbourne, Australia

Bruria Ben-Zeev

Head of Pediatric Neurology Unit & National Rett Clinic, Safra Children Hospital, Sheba Medical Center, Tel Ha Shomer, Sackler School of Medicine, Tel Aviv University, Israel

Mary E Blue

Associate Professor of Neurology and Neuroscience, Hugo W Moser Research Institute at Kennedy Krieger, Inc., and Johns Hopkins University School of Medicine, Baltimore, MD, USA

Sonia Brower

Senior Technical Writer, ATCC Federal Solutions, Manassas, VA, USA

Sarojini Budden

Emeritus Associate Professor, Department of Pediatrics, Oregon Health and Sciences University Portland, OR, USA

John Christodoulou

Head, Neurodevelopmental Genomics Research Group, Murdoch Children's Research Institute; Chair of Genomic Medicine, Department of Pediatrics, University of Melbourne, Melbourne, Australia

Angus Clarke

Professor of Clinical Genetics, School of Medicine, Cardiff University, Wales, UK

Leopold MG Curfs

Professor and Director Governor Kremers Center and Head, Rett Expertise Center Netherlands, Maastricht University Medical Center, Maastricht, the Netherlands

Jenny Downs

Co-Head, Child Disability and Senior Research Fellow, Telethon Kids Institute, Perth, Australia

Carolyn Ellaway Associate Professor, Clinical Geneticist, Genetic Metabolic Disorders Service, Sydney Children's Hospital Network, Sydney University, Australia

James H Eubanks Senior Scientist, Krembil Research Institute, University Health Network, Toronto, Ontario, Canada

Rosa Angela Fabio Professor of Experimental Psychology, Department of Cognitive Science, Psychological, Pedagogical and Cultural Studies, University of Messina, Italy

Daniel G Glaze Professor, Departments of Pediatrics and Neurology; Medical Director, The Blue Bird Circle Rett Center, Baylor College of Medicine, Houston, TX, USA

Wendy A Gold Senior Lecturer, Kids Research Institute, The Children's Hospital at Westmead, University of Sydney, Australia

Michael L Gonzales Senior Scientist, Fluidigm Corporation, Biotechnology Company, San Francisco, CA, USA

Bengt Hagberg Emeritus Professor of Pediatrics, University of Gothenburg, Sweden

Kathy Hunter Founder, International Rett Syndrome Association, Fort Washington, MD, USA

Michael V Johnston Chief Medical Officer and Blum Moser Endowed Chair for Pediatric Neurology, Kennedy Krieger Institute; Professor of Neurology, Pediatrics and Physical Medicine and Rehabilitation, Johns Hopkins University School of Medicine, Baltimore, MD, USA

Water E Kaufmann Ravenel Boykin Curry Chair in Genetic Therapeutics, Professor of Neurology, Greenwood Genetic Center; Research Professor of Pediatrics, University of South Carolina School of Medicine; Adjunct Professor of Human Genetics, Emory University School of Medicine, Atlanta GA, USA

Alison Kerr Honorary Clinical Senior Lecturer (Retired), Institute of Health and Wellbeing, University of Glasgow, Scotland, UK

Janine M LaSalle
Professor, Medical Microbiology and Immunology, School of Medicine, University of California, Davis, CA, USA

Helen Leonard
Associate Professor, NHMRC Senior Research Fellow, Principal Research Fellow, Telethon Kids Institute, The University of Western Australia, Crawley, Australia

Francesca Mari
Associate Professor, Medical Genetics Unit, Policlinico S. Maria alle Scotte, Siena, Italy

Peter B Marschik
Head of Interdisciplinary Developmental Neuroscience; Associate Professor, Department of Phoniatrics, Medical University of Graz, Austria; Associate Professor, Karolinska Institutet, Center of Neurodevelopmental Disorders (KIND), Department of Women's and Children's Health, Stockholm, Sweden

Kathleen J Motil
Professor of Pediatrics, Baylor College of Medicine, Section of Gastroenterology, Hepatology, & Nutrition, Texas Children's Hospital, Houston, TX, USA

SakkuBai Naidu
Professor, Departments of Neurology and Pediatrics, Johns Hopkins University School of Medicine; Research Scientist, Department of Neurogenetics Kennedy Krieger Institute, Baltimore, MD, USA

Jeffrey L Neul
Professor and Chief of Division of Child Neurology, Department of Neurosciences, University of California, San Diego, La Jolla, CA, USA

Andreea Nissenkorn
Head of Rare Diseases Service, Pediatric Neurology Unit, Safra Children Hospital, Sheba Medical Center, Tel Ha Shomer, Sackler School of Medicine, Tel Aviv University, Israel

Yoshiko Nomura
Director, Yoshiko Nomura Neurological Clinic for Children, Tokyo, Japan

Alan K Percy
Professor, Pediatrics, Neurology, Neurobiology, Genetics, and Psychology, University of Alabama at Birmingham School of Medicine, Birmingham, AL, USA

Maria Pintaudi Child Neuropsychiatrist, Department of Neuroscience Rehabilitation, Opthalmology, Genetics and Maternal-Infant Sciences, University of Genoa, Italy

Jan Marino Ramirez Professor of Neurological Surgery and Pediatrics, University of Washington School of Medicine; Director, Center for Integrative Brain Research, Seattle Children's Hospital, Seattle, WA, USA

Alessandra Renieri Professor, Department of Medical Biotechnology, University of Siena, Italy

David P Roye Jr Professor of Clinical Pediatric Orthopedic Surgery, Columbia University Medical Center, New York, NY, USA

Jeff Sigafoos Professor, School of Education, Victoria University of Wellington, Wellington, New Zealand

Teresa Temudo Pediatric Neurologist, Serviço de Neuropediatria, Centro Hospitalar do Porto, Porto, Portugal

Gillian S Townend Researcher, Rett Expertise Centre-GKC, Maastricht University Medical Centre, Maastricht, The Netherlands

Christopher S Ward Preclinical Studies Manager; Research Associate, Jan and Dan Duncan Neurological Research Institute, Baylor College of Medicine, Houston, Texas USA

Brendan A Williams Chief Resident in Orthopedics, University of Florida, Gainesville, FL, USA

FOREWORD

Rett syndrome is an important disorder to a great many people. This is not so much because it affects several thousand individuals worldwide (it is a *rare* disease), or that it results in substantial disability but because the recognition of its complexity has paralleled fundamental developments in pediatric neurology, neurogenetics, and neurodisability. It has become impossible to make sense of any neurodevelopmental disorder without a thorough multi-dimensional perspective, which is ably demonstrated in this book. In addition to accurate, up-to-date information about every aspect of Rett syndrome, regarding both basic understanding and clinical management, this timely volume provides messages that may serve as guiding principles across a wide array of neurological conditions.

As described in the Prologue, the characterisation of Rett syndrome originated in self-confident, clinical observation: Andreas Rett observed facts (i.e. empirical data) and in the face of incomplete knowledge, made a situational judgement that the girls he had observed who showed stereotypical hand movements and other signs shared a specific syndrome that had not been described previously. This approach remains at the core of all good medical practice.

The same scenario was repeated by other clinicians in Japan, Sweden and elsewhere until the syndrome gained wide recognition in the medical world. The phenotype of Rett syndrome was refined to suggest diagnostic criteria, update them based on better observation, and pave the way to the discovery of its biological basis. A breakthrough in this process was the demonstration of *MECP2* mutations, with crucial implications for diagnosis and new questions on pathophysiology, many of them still unanswered. Thus, Rett syndrome became the first neurodevelopmental disorder related to defective transcription of methylated DNA.

Importantly, those clinicians recognised the value of behavioural manifestations by characterising the association of the cognitive, language, social skills, and motor control features that constitute the behavioural phenotype of Rett syndrome. The behavioural phenotype of conditions that were described around the time of Andreas Rett's first observations (e.g. Williams syndrome [1961], Lesch–Nyhan syndrome [1964], or Angelman syndrome [1965]), remain highly relevant to current clinical practice, in particular with regard to diagnosis, management, and outcome measures.

Yet the clinical course of Rett syndrome poses a challenge to the classic distinction between neurodevelopmental disorders, in which a brain defects cause symptoms from birth, and neurodegenerative disorders in which progressive, life-limiting changes induce the gradual loss of acquired skills. In Rett syndrome, most infants do not show any obvious developmental problems. After a few months, however, severe regression occurs, together with a delay in acquiring new skills, emergence of autistic features, loss of purposeful manipulation skills replaced by stereotyped hand movements, ataxia and apraxia, while no neuronal degeneration explains the change. This has led clinicians to consider development and neurodevelopmental disorders in a more complex way than the linear approach that has long prevailed in the field. Several models have been suggested to explain the 'natural history' of Rett syndrome, from arrested development to stage systems, though the current trend tends to focus on individual developmental trajectories, activities of daily living, quality of life, and specifically tailored objectives. Thus, there is slowly increasing knowledge about how to select realistic and meaningful management objectives, how to pursue them and evaluate outcomes—from promoting physical activity and appropriate nutrition, to therapy and surgical interventions.

Tremendous hope has also been fostered by findings in animal models and the development of targeted therapy aimed at the *MECP2* gene and its expression or downstream factors, such as neurotransmitters or neurotrophic factors. As discussed in Chapter 14 several clinical trials are currently being carried out, with some promising early results.

Finally, the history of Rett syndrome also exemplifies the power of family support groups. It shows how collaboration between clinicians, researchers and support groups can contribute to the improvement of knowledge, and the development of appropriate information for patients, health professionals and the general public, as well as promote access to screening and diagnostic testing. Many of the experts who authored chapters for this book have long been proactively involved in family support programs. Although this book is intended primarily for clinicians and scientists, it is likely to serve as a rich resource for families striving to improve the quality of life of their children.

Rett Syndrome is a momentous book; it is comprehensive, well organized and well written and will be very useful to many.

Bernard Dan
Professor of Neurophysiology and Developmental Neurology,
Université libre de Bruxelles, and Director of Rehabilitation at
Inkendaal Hospital, Brussels, Belgium.

BENGT HAGBERG: LEADING THE WAY TO RETT SYNDROME TODAY

A tribute by Dr Alan K Percy

Bengt Hagberg (1923–2015) was a significant medical figure in Sweden, regarded as the father of child neurology there. As an exceptional physician and clinical scientist and a leading proponent of a pan-European organization of child neurologists, he broached the subject of an unusual disorder he had been observing since the late 1950's and early 1960's throughout Sweden. Unlike Andy Rett, he did not write about these findings, simply collecting the clinical data. He was aware of Andy Rett's work, but was at first skeptical of a connection as he had not identified hyperammonemia in his patients in contradistinction to Andy. When he found out that this finding was in question, he presented his collected data at a meeting of European child neurologists in the late 1970's and was joined subsequently by Jean Aicardi, also recently deceased, in preparing a manuscript for publication. Subsequently, a chance meeting with Andy led Bengt to term the disorder Rett syndrome and with this single publication in the *Annals of Neurology* in 1983, a literal explosion of reports emerged from throughout the world heralding this heretofore unknown and unrecognized disorder. Bengt then encouraged a number of important efforts to standardize consensus diagnostic criteria, provide initial staging criteria, and recognize variant features that are well-engrained today.

Andy and Bengt started a movement that has created a groundswell in clinical and laboratory investigations leading to the present state of knowledge and underscoring the importance of discovery and perseverance in tracking down the causal factor of the syndrome, understanding its natural history, and stimulation of translational studies.

Bengt was a true pioneer in the burgeoning field of child neurology. He made key advances in teaching, training, and clinical discovery. His history of key advances in diverse disorders affecting the nervous system is astonishing. These included a long series of critical descriptions on the changing patterns of the cerebral palsies over many years, and important observations on the sphingolipidoses, notably Krabbe disease and metachromatic leukodystrophy as well as other lysosomal storage diseases such as the infantile form of neuronal ceroid lipofuscinosis predominantly present in the Finnish population. His vision had seemingly limitless breadth and depth.

Bengt had a keen mind that could understand clearly the difference between real and imagined advances, regardless of the subject, always pointing to the potential point of concern in a line of reasoning. I know that Bengt, in his typically modest response, would deflect attention to the many individuals throughout the world who have contributed to the present understanding of Rett syndrome and its related disorders. Nevertheless, we know the great and lasting impact of his incisive and insightful diagnostic acumen, his recognition of solid conclusions, and his ability to synthesize the landmark advances that place us now on the verge of effective disease-modifying treatment.

PREFACE

This volume comes to light at the time in which we are commemorating more than 50 years since Andreas Rett's initial publication describing the syndrome carrying his name. In these five decades we have acquired a remarkable amount of information about the clinical features of the disorder, its etiology, and its pathophysiology. Much less progress has been made in terms of interventions, although some recommendations for specific management are available and the number of ongoing and planned clinical trials is increasing.

Fifty years is a relatively short period in the 'life' of a disorder. The remarkable accomplishments in the Rett syndrome (RTT) field were jump started by the first publication in the English-speaking medical literature in 1983 by Bengt Hagberg and colleagues. Bengt's generosity in acknowledging the pioneer work of Andreas Rett, by naming the disorder after Rett, and his subsequent contributions in many areas are an example of the best of scholarship and collegiality. For this reason, we dedicate this volume to Bengt Hagberg.

The first section of the book deals with fundamental clinical issues, diagnostic criteria and evolution, including the challenging issues we are experiencing these days with expanding genotypes and phenotypes. This is followed by a section expanding on the genetic aspects of RTT already addressed in the chapter on diagnosis, also covering genotype–phenotype correlations. The third section is the central component of the book, addressing the main clinical features of RTT and their management. The fourth section, brief by design, intends to provide a basic foundation of molecular and neurobiological aspects of RTT with a focus on their clinical application. An in-depth review of the neurobiology of *MECP2* and RTT, a field rich in literature, is beyond the scope of this clinically oriented volume. The book properly closes with a section on general drug management and rehabilitation, including an overview of treatments under development.

Editing a medical book in the 21st century presents the obvious dilemma of obsolescence. Devoting this volume to the commemoration of the 50 years of RTT helps us to understand that this is only a blueprint or outline for approaching this complex and still novel disorder. For those facing RTT for the first time, the book is a roadmap for understanding afflicted individuals. For those knowledgeable about the disorder, we hope the book will help to find new viewpoints about key aspects as well as historical perspectives that may generate new ways to think about RTT.

I am certain that Andreas Rett never foresaw the revolution he started, with great help from Bengt Hagberg, by identifying the first affected individuals. RTT is now not only a disorder but a field, a model neurological disease, and a gene (*MECP2*) that plays a crucial role in synaptic development and function.

I am grateful to Alan Percy, Angus Clarke, Helen Leonard, and SakkuBai Naidu, leaders in the Rett syndrome field, who served as associate editors. I thank Dr. Dawna Armstrong for enlightening discussions about RTT neuropathology. I am also indebted to the team at Mac Keith Press, particularly Udoka Ohuonu and Ann-Marie Halligan, for their support and patience that made possible the successful conclusion of this project.

Walter E. Kaufmann
Greenville, South Carolina, USA
July 2017

PROLOGUE:
PERSONAL PERSPECTIVES

My 'Rett' Story

Bengt Hagberg[†]

I am extremely happy to see this new book on Rett syndrome. I believe I am now the oldest living person who has the possibility of following the progress in delineating and under-standing the syndrome in terms of clinics, genetics, and therapy through the last 50 years.

In 1960 as an Associate Professor in child neurology in Uppsala, Sweden, I met an 18-month-old girl with a deviating development I had never seen before. From having been quite normal, she had developed an autism-like condition with ataxia, loss of hand function, and the appearance of stereotypic hand wringing. Her father insisted that all efforts should be made to discover the cause of the disease. Everything was shown to be completely typical, even the findings of a brain biopsy from the frontal lobe. By 1980, I had met another 15 girls with the same peculiar, and for me unknown, disorder. I took the files to a meeting of the board of the European Federation of Child Neurology Societies (EFNS) in Manchester, UK, asking the participants if they had seen similar patients. I found that they had, and that all their patients were girls like ours. Together with Drs Jean Aicardi and Ovidio Ramos from Paris and Dr Karin Diaz from Lisbon, we sent in a paper for publication in the *Annals of Neurology*, titled 'A progressive syndrome of autism, dementia and loss of purposeful hand use in girls: Rett's syndrome, a report of 35 cases' (Hagberg et al. 1983).

During the process of writing our paper, Dr Francoise Goutières in Paris had accidentally found a photo under the heading 'Hyperammonemia', illustrating peculiar hand-washing movement by a young girl, reported by Dr Andreas Rett from Vienna, Austria; however, we discounted it because Dr Rett's patients were reported to have elevated blood ammonia levels and ours did not.

In 1981, I was invited to a congress in Toronto to lecture on known causes of intellectual disability. As I spoke about the 'hand-wringing' syndrome, a loud voice from the back of the room was heard. Dr Andreas Rett, who was attending the congress, ran down the aisle toward me, excitingly saying 'Ich bin Rett' (I am Rett). In 1966, Dr Andreas Rett had observed two preschool-aged girls who sat next to each other in his waiting room, both making the same peculiar hand-washing movements. He recalled having seen other similar patients over the years and made a film of four girls and brought it to medical meetings all over Europe, asking if the syndrome had been seen elsewhere. Over the following years, he published several papers (Rett 1966, 1977) on the condition, but they had been written in German and their distribution was limited. Following a discussion, I learned that the elevated ammonia levels found earlier were later attributed to invalid laboratory errors. It was quite clear that Dr Rett and I were investigating the same condition. I then recalled the manuscript from *Annals of Neurology* to name the syndrome 'Rett syndrome' in honor of the physician who was the first to discover it.

Dr Rett invited me, together with a small group of experienced neuropediatricians of my choice, to a workshop in Vienna. This was held in 1982 and became the important start of the first more organized Rett conferences in Vienna. This first workshop also became the background to important contacts with Japanese researchers, who had been aware of the condition since 1978, and also with the US, in particular with Professor Hugo Moser from Baltimore. I had a most productive dialogue about Rett syndrome with him. Diagnostic clinical criteria were established in the second workshop. In Sweden, intensive investigations were started in terms of understanding genetics, clinics, and potential trials for treatment.

In 1983, our paper (Hagberg et al. 1983) appeared in the *Annals of Neurology* as the first English paper on the syndrome, and the syndrome became recognized worldwide. A large international symposium was organized in Baltimore in 1985, with the participation of an impressive number of families with Rett syndrome. That opened the door to a rapidly-extended international scientific and multi-professional network in Sweden as well as in many other European countries, USA, Japan, and Australia. An internationally-focused family organization was started by Mrs Kathy Hunter and collaborators, and the disease could be shown to exist all over the world.

In 1999, there came the important breakthrough in genetics when Amir et al. (1999) (USA), found mutations in the X-linked *MECP2* gene. However, it turned out that although some 80% of females with classic Rett syndrome had the mutation, it was found also in variants, in males, as well as in healthy individuals. Thus, it could not be used as a diagnostic criterion of Rett syndrome, which still was considered to be a clinically diagnosed condition, as established in Baden-Baden (Hagberg et al. 2002).

Since then, the efforts to characterize Rett syndrome and its variants have expanded yet more, as you will learn from this book. I really hope that in the near future a disorder clarification and a cure and/or treatment for these patients will be found.

---

†Professor Bengt Hagberg passed away on April 12 2015.

REFERENCES

Amir RE, Van den Veyver IB, Wan M, Tran CQ, Francke U, Zoghbi HY (1999) Rett syndrome is caused by mutations in X-linked MECP2, encoding methyl-CpG-binding protein 2. *Nat Genet* 23(2): 185–188.

Hagberg B, Aicardi J, Dias K, Ramos O (1983) A progressive syndrome of autism, dementia, ataxia, and loss of purposeful hand use in girls: Rett's syndrome: report of 35 cases. *Ann Neurol* 14(4): 471–479.

Hagberg B, Hanefeld F, Percy A, Skjeldal O (2002) An update on clinically applicable diagnostic criteria in Rett syndrome. Comments to Rett Syndrome Clinical Criteria Consensus Panel Satellite to European Paediatric Neurology Society Meeting, Baden Baden, Germany, 11 September 2001. *Eur J Paediatr Neurol* 6(5): 293–297.

Rett A (1966) On an unusual brain atrophy syndrome in hyperammonemia in childhood. *Wien Med Wochenschr* 116(37): 723–726.

Rett A (1977) Cerebral atrophy associated with hyperammonaemia. In: Vinken PJ, Bruyn GW, editors. *Handbook of Clinical Neurology*, Vol. 29, Amsterdam: North Holland, 305–329.

A Mother's Journey

Kathy Hunter

When I started on the Rett journey more than 35 years ago, I was simply the mother of a precious baby girl, Stacie. She had developed as typically as her two older brothers until at 18 months she had become withdrawn and irritable. When she began to lose skills without explanation, there was no place to turn, not even in the medical community. She was described as 'one of a kind' and a 'medical enigma'. There was no one to help, and there were no answers for the myriad of questions about what had gone wrong, and why. A lonely, frustrating decade ensued, with visits to several specialists who said with regret that we would probably never have answers. One doctor even dared to suggest that her autistic-like behavior and regression must be my fault, due to an outdated Bruno Bettelheim 'refrigerator mother' theory. From that day forward, I referred to the day of diagnosis as D-Day.

By the time Stacie was 9 years old in the spring of 1983, she had a diagnosis of severe-to-profound intellectual disability. She was ambulatory but nonverbal and she cried a lot for unknown reasons. Her hands were in continual motion, which seemed an insignificant factor considering the totality of her disabilities. She had lost the ability to use her hands and needed help for every aspect of daily living. Yet, she was as beautiful as a porcelain doll and her eyes were bright and searching. We had begun to believe the prediction that we would never know what had gone wrong, when out of the blue, we received a call from Dr Mary Coleman at the Children's Brain Research Clinic in Washington, DC. Dr Coleman had been following Stacie since she was 2 years old, ruling out the most common neurological disorders, and even testing her for the rarest of syndromes, always passionately committed to finding a diagnosis. Attending Grand Rounds at a pediatric hospital in France, she had listened acutely as Dr Jean Aicardi presented a paper on newly discovered disorder, Rett syndrome, about to be published in the *Annals of Neurology*. Dr Coleman described it as a 'eureka moment' as she instantly recognized all of Stacie's symptoms. We anxiously awaited the publication of the first English-language paper (Hagberg et al. 1983) several months later, and when it arrived, we read it in near disbelief at the likeness of photographs and the precise description of our child's deviation in development. We rejoiced in odd celebration for finally, a diagnosis. And while the devastating diagnosis brought more questions than answers, it was at last a comfort to know that Stacie was not 'one of a kind' and that we were no longer alone. Stacie had been, *all at the same time*, my deepest despair and the height of my greatest joy. Her courage and her sweet spirit inspired me to reach out to others and try to make a difference.

I founded the International Rett Syndrome Association (IRSA) in early 1984 as an organization dedicated to our slogan to 'Care Today … Cure Tomorrow'. IRSA was The Club You Never Wanted to Join, a fraternity of parents who were united in pain and anguish, denial, anger, despair, frustration, bewilderment, and fear. It was created as a place where a confused parent could reach out for immediate answers and resources that increase their knowledge and show them how to lessen the physical challenges and minimize the emotional burdens that come with having a child with special needs. Our first family conference took place in conjunction with the 1985 International Symposium and 35 families from the USA and Canada traveled to Baltimore to meet Dr Andreas Rett and the conference sponsor, Dr Hugo Moser. As families gathered at the hotel that first night, we were completely awed as one by one, girls were wheeled in the door demonstrating the same hallmark hand-wringing movements that before had seemed trivial. The bond which parents felt was magical and healing; just to know that we had each other and some kind of hope for answers. We quickly formed a shared commitment to work together to make better lives for our beloved daughters. Without really recognizing it, we were following the sage advice of St Francis of Assisi: 'Start by doing what is necessary, then do what is possible, and suddenly you are doing the impossible.'

At that historic meeting in Baltimore, not all of the medical community accepted Rett syndrome as a distinct clinical entity. It would take some years of persistence, medical and public awareness campaigns, and the information and data provided by the National Institutes of Health (NIH)-sponsored Natural History Study (Amir et al. 1999) before Rett syndrome gradually became universally recognized.

The IRSA's development of the first patient database and maintenance of a strong liaison with researchers were crucial factors in keeping the Rett syndrome movement alive and in convincing scientists to devote energy and funds to a little-known rare disorder. Guidance and support from Maryland Congressman, Steny Hoyer, was pivotal in bringing attention to the need for research funding to the US Congress, and from this resulted the appropriation of several million dollars each year in support to research studies through the NIH. In 1991, the IRSA was proud to make its own first research grant, which would be followed by dozens of additional grants over the next decade. By 1999, the researchers had narrowed down the certainty of a genetic cause for Rett syndrome. To boost the chance of discovery, IRSA gave small grants of US$10000 to several of the labs leading the genetic search to allow them to recruit full-time lab assistants. Within months, the announcement of the finding of the *MECP2* mutation by one of the sponsored researchers, Dr Ruthie Amir, in the lab of Dr Huda Zoghbi at Baylor College of Medicine, was made. The elation of families resounded throughout the world as word of the exciting finding made its way across the globe.

Following the genetic discovery, medical research skyrocketed as animal models came to fruition, increasing the possibility of treatments and cures that had never been possible before. At the same time, researchers in the field of education and communication pushed forward with much greater understanding of the potential for learning. Today, we are rewriting the history of Rett syndrome! No longer are girls sentenced to languish without education, relegated to wheelchairs without the benefit of therapy. No longer are they expected to remain silent with no means of communication. And for the very first time, there is real hope, not just for those born today, but even for those born long ago; hope that the disabling and painful symptoms of Rett syndrome can be not only ameliorated, but possibly eradicated.

As I look forward to the promise of a better tomorrow for my daughter, Stacie, I realize how very much I owe her. She has given me strength I never knew I had, but more importantly, she has shown me how to turn tragedy into triumph. While others may remark on my patience, I remind them that Stacie is the one who eats when I think she is hungry, goes to bed when I think she is tired, and continually endures my clumsy attempts to figure out by trial-and-error what hurts her. I look at her with eyes of love and see the power of her powerlessness, the strength and courage of the life she lives without the value of one spoken word. And then I realize that she is who she is, and that she touches others in a miraculous way, not by what she can do, but by what she cannot. I find myself stronger, richer, fuller, and so much more appreciative because she has taught me to recognize the smallest gifts that others take so easily for granted. Beyond all of this, Stacie and others like her deserve better lives and I know that they all join me in looking forward to changing the sentence that once defined us, 'What is Rett syndrome?' to 'What *was* Rett syndrome?'

REFERENCES

Amir RE, Van den Veyver IB, Wan M, Tran CQ, Francke U, Zoghbi HY (1999) Rett syndrome is caused by mutations in X-linked MECP2, encoding methyl-CpG-binding protein 2. *Nat Genet* 23(2): 185–188.

Hagberg B, Aicardi J, Dias K, Ramos O (1983) A progressive syndrome of autism, dementia, ataxia, and loss of purposeful hand use in girls: Rett's syndrome: report of 35 cases. *Ann Neurol* 14(4): 471–479.

A Perspective from the British Isles

Alison Kerr

That Britain was involved in Rett syndrome research in as early as 1982 was due to careful observations and recordings made by John Stephenson at the Royal Hospital for Sick Children in Glasgow. At a pediatric meeting in Oxford, Bengt Hagberg had just demonstrated the hand movements typical of the disorder and described Andreas Rett's research and Dr Stephenson realized that cases he had recorded over 12 years fitted that description.

Our first task in 1982 was, therefore, to review these patients and to discover the incidence of the condition. We were able to publish our observations on 19 girls and to provide a minimum incidence in the study area of 1 in 10 000 female births (Kerr and Stephenson 1985). We observed that the girls, although severely disabled, were sociable and ranged in age from early childhood to adulthood without apparent deterioration. Developmental histories indicated that movement and cognition had been affected before the regression event. Although all displayed the same clinical signs, severity varied, even between identical twins.

Further research was greatly assisted when Yvonne Milne and Isobel Allan founded the two British Rett syndrome associations supporting both families and research. They invited Andreas Rett to visit Britain and together in 1986 we organized a weekend meeting and clinic at the Children's Hospital in Glasgow, involving over 50 girls, their parents, many British pediatricians, and Andreas Rett. Research in Britain thus began and has continued to rely upon clinical observation and a series of collaborations, mainly on a voluntary basis, with colleagues from a wide variety of disciplines.

I was invited to base the research at Quarrier's Epilepsy Centre near Glasgow where, with the expert encephalographer Pat Amos and respiratory physician David Southall, we developed a technique for simultaneous monitoring of behavior, respiration, and blood gases. We demonstrated how the extreme respiratory abnormality affected the blood gases and led to non-epileptic vacant spells.

Collaboration with Swedish colleagues and support from the British Paediatric Surveillance Unit led to development of the British Isles Survey for Rett Syndrome. Two-day advice clinics planned throughout the British Isles by the Rett syndrome associations made it possible for me to examine hundreds of girls and women, many repeatedly, and to develop a longitudinal health database. This store of clinical data served a large series of research studies, all now published and readily accessible through the medical databases and from the Rett syndrome associations. Here, I will briefly reflect on some of our major research themes.

First, and still under scrutiny, were the intermittent disturbances of breathing, behavior, and electrical activity in the brain. Our first studies in 1986 had indicated that this abnormality must involve the cardiorespiratory centers in the brainstem. In 1996, I was invited to join the Glasgow University Department of Psychological Medicine at Gartnavel Hospital and was able to collaborate with Peter Julu who, through his diabetes research, had already developed a non-invasive technique for accurate monitoring of brainstem activity. Putting together all our monitoring equipment and with able support from electro-encephalographer Flora Apartopoulos and medical physicist Stig Hansen, we achieved continuous recording and were able to characterize the brainstem abnormality and the resulting patterns of behavior (Julu et al. 2001).

Our findings agreed with earlier suggestion from Masaya Segawa and Yoshiko Nomura (Nomura et al. 1985) that an early adrenergic abnormality underlay the syndrome and the conclusions from neuropathological studies by Dawna Armstrong (1995) that implicated the brainstem cardiorespiratory nuclei. In 1998, in collaboration with Ingegerd Witt Engerstrom, we arranged an Autonomic Workshop at the Swedish Rett Centre, bringing together brainstem researchers in Rett syndrome. In 1999 came the discovery in Huda Zoghbi's Texas laboratory of the mutated gene (Amir et al. 1999). The textbook, *Rett Disorder and the Developing Brain* was commissioned by Oxford University Press (Kerr and Witt Engerstrom 2001). In Edinburgh, Adrian Bird's department where the *MECP2* gene had already been discovered, achieved development of the first mouse model; another major breakthrough for Rett research (Guy et al. 2001).

When the genetic defects underlying the disorder became known, our British colleagues, Angus Clarke and Hayley Archer in Cardiff and later Mark Bailey in Glasgow set up a service to find the specific mutations in the British cases identified through the survey. The clinically 'classic' cases were almost invariably found to have *MECP2* mutations and we began to distinguish the several other diseases whose clinical problems, atypical for Rett, had led to their being referred to the Rett clinics.

With the clinical signs now characterized and the genetic diagnosis available, we found it best to describe each case in both genetic and clinical terms, providing the diagnosis of Rett disorder for individuals with both the genetic and clinical abnormality. Thus, pairs of twins could be described as each having the Rett disorder, even when the level of severity differed. A presumptive diagnosis of Rett disorder was made when the signs were clear but a mutation was not identified. Individuals without the constellation of clinical signs were regarded as awaiting a final diagnosis and kept under review. It has been in the study of such people that awareness of CDKL5 and other neurodevelopmental disorders, quite distinct from Rett disorder, is now emerging. In 2001, in a 21-author paper, we proposed guidelines for the description of published cases, in order to encourage clear and full reporting of clinical details along with the genetic data (Kerr et al. 2001).

Another early and continuing concern was with the period from birth to regression. The prevailing view had been that the infant was normal until the onset of regression, but our detailed developmental histories suggested much earlier involvement. In 1985, I began to study family videos recorded by parents, right from the child's birth. These were strongly suggestive of early cognitive and motor difficulties; however, it was in collaboration with the psychologist and movement therapist Bronwen Burford in 2003, and with physiologists Heinz Prechtl and Christa Einspieler in 2004, that detailed analysis of the early video material provided the indubitable evidence.

Using our wealth of longitudinal clinical data and working with the orthopedic surgeon Peter Webb we were able to review the results of scoliosis surgery. With geneticist Hayley Archer (Kerr and Archer 2005) we reviewed the precise mutations and clinical characteristics of the people with retained speech. We noticed short fourth metatarsals in many cases, recognizing a further sign of developmental significance. With Janet Eyre, in Newcastle, a week's investigation of nine girls using nuclear magnetic resonance demonstrated, for the first time, prompt conduction in the long motor axons and suggested central processing delays. In 2005, with statistical support from Robin Prescott (Kerr and Prescott 2005) at Edinburgh University and using longitudinal health and severity data for 1159 cases, we were able to chart the long-term clinical course in groups of people with differing levels of severity.

From our experience in the UK, what can we share with the new generation of Rett researchers? The most important factor in all our studies has undoubtedly been direct and long-term clinical observation, extended with video recordings. Collaboration with colleagues from different disciplines has brought valuable fresh light, as well as enlarged technical expertise to the solution of clinical problems. In general, for clinical studies, we have worked with minimal or no official funding and for us this has had advantages. We have attracted only the most strongly motivated, energetic, well-organized, and reliable co-researchers, prepared to work at all hours and for many years, while simultaneously fulfilling the obligations of another salaried post. Relatively free from the constraints of grant application and obligations we have thus been able to spend more time in service and research. Of course, that freedom is not always possible in the organizing of large trials of medication or laboratory studies; however, lack of funding should not discourage well-informed and motivated research.

I feel tremendously privileged to have had the opportunity to spend more than 23 years in research into Rett syndrome and in service for the families. The work has been endlessly fascinating, the contact with families and colleagues delightful, and now that my contribution is finished (Kerr 2006), there is great satisfaction in seeing how the work we began is being carried forward by younger, able, and enthusiastic colleagues.

REFERENCES

Amir RE, Van den Veyver IB, Wan M, Tran CQ, Franke U, Zoghbi HY (1999) Rett syndrome is caused by mutations in x-linked MECP2, encoding methyl-CpG-binding protein 2. *Nat Genet* 23: 185–188.
Armstrong DD (1995) The Neuropathology of Rett Syndrome – overview 1994. *Neuropediatrics* 26: 100–104.
Guy J, Hendrich B, Holmes M, Martin JE, Bird A (2001), A mouse Mecp2-null mutation causes neurological symptoms that mimic Rett syndrome. *Nat Genet* 27(3): 322–326.
Julu PO, Ker AM, Apartopoulos F et al. (2001) Characterisation of breathing and associated autonomic dysfunction in the Rett Disorder. *Arch Dis Child* 85: 29–37.

Kerr AM (2006) A critical account of clinical and physiological studies in Rett syndrome. Doctoral Thesis, Edinburgh University.

Kerr AM, Stephenson JPB (1985) Rett's Syndrome in the West of Scotland. *Br Med J (Clin Res Ed)* 291: 579–582.

Kerr AM, Archer HL (2005) People with MECP2 mutation-positive Rett disorder who converse. *J Intellect Disabil Res* 50(Pt 5): 386–394.

Kerr AM, Prescott R (2005) Predictive value of the early clinical signs in Rett Disorder. *Brain Dev* 27: S20–S24.

Kerr AM, Nomura Y, Armstrong D et al. (2001) Guidelines for reporting clinical features in cases with MECP2 mutations. *Brain Dev* 23(4): 208–211.

Nomura Y, Segawa M, Higurashi M (1985) Rett Syndrome: An early catecholamine and indolamine deficient disorder? *Brain Dev* (Tokyo) 21: 377–341.

1
THE DIAGNOSIS OF RETT SYNDROME

Walter E Kaufmann and Jeffrey L Neul

Introduction

Diagnostic criteria of a disorder are its defining features, reflecting in many instances the etiology, pathophysiology, and evolution. This is the case of Rett syndrome (RTT), with a history of diagnostic criteria tracing the trajectory of our knowledge on the disorder. Our current view is that RTT is a neurodevelopmental disorder, and not a degenerative one, despite its temporal dynamics that includes periods of loss of function and, in many individuals, decline in abilities after childhood. During the 50 years since the initial description of RTT (Rett 1966), there has been an extraordinary gain in knowledge and awareness despite the relatively low prevalence of the disorder (Kaufmann et al. 2016; Percy 2016; Leonard et al. 2017). A major milestone was reached in 1999, with the report of the association between the majority of cases of RTT and mutations in *MECP2* (Amir et al. 1999), the gene encoding the transcriptional regulator methyl-CpG-binding protein 2 (MeCP2) (Kaufmann et al. 2005). Despite this major achievement, the diagnosis of RTT remains a clinical one due to the imperfect correlation between genotype and phenotype (Neul et al. 2010). Identification of other genes as closely associated with some variations in RTT's clinical presentation (Neul et al. 2010; Olson et al. 2015; Sajan et al. 2017), as well as the report of a wide variety of neuropsychiatric symptomatology in individuals with *MECP2* mutations (Suter et al. 2014; Lombardi et al. 2015), have increased the complexity of the diagnostic criteria and classification of the disorder. The following sections cover key issues related to RTT's diagnosis, classification, and evolution. Detailed information about symptomatology and genetic testing is provided in the respective chapters.

Overview of the clinical features of Rett syndrome

RTT is a complex, primarily neurological disorder. Its complexity derives from its wide range of neurological, behavioral, and systemic impairments and their dynamic evolution. Although developmental delay is usually the earliest abnormal feature in RTT, developmental regression (i.e. loss of acquired skills) is the defining feature (Hagberg et al. 1983, 1985, 2002; The Rett Syndrome Diagnostic Criteria Work Group 1988; Kerr et al. 2001a; Neul et al. 2010). The current diagnostic criteria specify and require the loss of expressive language and fine motor (i.e. hand) skills (Neul et al. 2010). Impairment in ambulation, another major diagnostic criterion, could also include the loss of this function (Foley et al. 2011). Decline in neurological function led to the label of dementia in the initial English literature description of the disorder (Hagberg et al. 1983); however, the course of RTT is not progressive and irreversible. Indeed, variable and usually incomplete recovery of lost abilities is also a characteristic feature of the disorder (Neul et al. 2014). While standard medical histories reveal relatively typical development during the first 6 months of life (Neul et al. 2010), research studies using more sensitive methods demonstrate that deviation from typical trajectory may be present earlier (Marschik et al. 2013).

In addition to abnormal developmental trajectories of motor and language function, presence of hand stereotypies is a hallmark feature of RTT (Carter et al. 2010) and, as such, it is included in the core diagnostic criteria (Neul et al. 2010). As in other neurodevelopmental disorders, the prevalence of seizures is high and, as for most features of RTT, their frequency and severity are quite variable (Nissenkorn et al. 2015; Tarquinio et al. 2017). Autistic behavior was one of the first identified features of RTT, highlighted in Hagberg and colleagues' (1983) publication. Nonetheless, severe autistic features are not clearly present in every affected individual and, if identified, they tend to be restricted to the period of regression (Mount et al. 2003; Kaufmann et al. 2012). On the other hand, other behavioral abnormalities such as anxiety and mood instability seem to be common and present throughout the individual's life (Mount et al. 2002a, b; Anderson et al. 2014; Barnes et al. 2015; Cianfaglione et al. 2015). At present, inappropriate laughing/screaming spells is the only behavior considered a supportive diagnostic criterion for atypical RTT. A variety of other neurological features are highly prevalent and a cause of concern in RTT. These include breathing abnormalities and bruxism mainly when awake, peripheral autonomic (vasomotor) disturbances, sleep problems, diminished response to pain, and abnormal muscle tone; all of these features are also included as supportive diagnostic criteria for atypical RTT (Neul et al. 2010).

In addition to the neurological and behavioral features listed above, systemic abnormalities are almost invariably present in RTT with the consequent substantial impact on functioning and quality of life. Some of these systemic features appear to be the result of primary neurological abnormalities, such as orthopedic problems secondary to abnormal muscle tone (e.g. scoliosis, kyphosis, contractures, and foot deformities). Other manifestations seem to represent autonomic nervous system abnormalities. Examples of these include gastroesophageal reflux, constipation, and cardiac rhythm disturbances (e.g. long QT interval) (McCauley et al. 2011; Motil et al. 2012; Baikie et al. 2014). The role of MeCP2 in non-neurological function is exemplified by the high prevalence of osteopenia/osteoporosis in RTT (Jefferson et al. 2016). Indeed, MeCP2 seems to be involved in bone turnover (Blue et al. 2015; Ross et al. 2016), although nutritional status, decreased mobility, and use of antiseizure medications could also play a role in the development of abnormal bone density in individuals with RTT.

Finally, RTT is a growth disorder. Deceleration of head growth after the neonatal period, which results in average head circumference reduction of 20–25%, was recognized in the first descriptions of RTT (Nomura et al. 1984) and incorporated into its diagnostic criteria (The Rett Syndrome Diagnostic Criteria Work Group 1988). Nevertheless, growth disturbances are more global and include weight, height, and hand and feet size (Tarquinio et al. 2012). The latter abnormality is most likely to be also influenced by peripheral vascular abnormalities. Orthopedic and growth abnormalities are included among the supportive diagnostic criteria for atypical RTT (Neul et al. 2010).

In summary, RTT is a complex neurodevelopmental disorder with a wide range of manifestations and high variability in clinical severity. Chapter 2 presents an overview of RTT in the context of the Natural History of the disorder. Other chapters in the Clinical section of the book cover in detail specific features of RTT and their management. The subsequent sections address how the intricate clinical picture of RTT has led to the current diagnostic criteria and how these may evolve in the next decades.

Evolution of diagnostic criteria

The history of the diagnostic criteria of RTT is illustrative of our evolving perspectives about the disorder. Initial descriptions already reported elements of current diagnostic criteria, such as developmental regression involving language and hand use, gait abnormalities (apraxia, ataxia) as well as hand stereotypies, but also included autistic behavior, acquired microcephaly, vasomotor disturbances, and seizures (Rett 1966; Hagberg et al. 1983). Efforts at developing formal clinical criteria 'for research purposes' began shortly after that. In 1985, Hagberg and colleagues published inclusion and exclusion criteria that began with the recognition of the almost exclusive female presentation of the disorder. Some concepts that emerged at this time and extended until recently included a typical pre- and perinatal period, typical head circumference at birth followed by early deceleration of head growth, and exclusion of individuals with perinatally acquired brain impairment. For the first time, loss of communication abilities and purposeful hand use along with gait abnormalities were required for the diagnosis (Hagberg et al. 1985). The 1988 revision of criteria did not introduce major conceptual changes, but relabeled the inclusion criteria as necessary diagnostic criteria and expanded the exclusion criteria. The only noticeable difference was the delineation of supportive criteria representing common but not obligatory features that could assist in the diagnosis (The Rett Syndrome Diagnostic Criteria Work Group 1988). Two more updates, one focused on case reporting and genetic testing (Kerr et al. 2001a) and the other a formal revision of diagnostic criteria (Hagberg et al. 2002) attempted to address the recent identification of *MECP2* mutations in a substantial proportion of patients with RTT. The 2002 criteria continued to emphasize that the diagnosis of RTT is clinical and made minor changes to the criteria (e.g. delayed psychomotor development as an option under necessary criteria) for the common cases, termed classic or typical. A unique contribution of this publication was the acknowledgement of uncommon presentations, termed variants or atypical. It refined early attempts at delineating this type of RTT (Hagberg and Skjeldal 1994) by defining combinations of six main and 11 supportive criteria (Hagberg et al. 2002). The 2010 revision or current criteria built upon these valuable initial efforts, attempted to increase reliability and provide empirical evidence of its adequacy (Neul et al. 2010; Percy et al. 2010).

Current diagnostic criteria of Rett syndrome

As mentioned above, the diagnosis of RTT continues to be clinical and based on consensus statements. Despite the changes in criteria over the years (Hagberg et al. 1983, 1985, 2002;

The Rett Syndrome Diagnostic Criteria Work Group 1988; Neul et al. 2010), many concepts have remained. The first is that developmental regression is a key feature, required (i.e. obligatory) in the current diagnostic criteria. The second is that there is a broad range of clinical severity that results in some individuals not displaying all the core features of RTT. Thus, two main clinical presentations are recognized: typical or classic, displaying all the core features; and atypical or variant, presenting some but not all the key features of the disorder. The current criteria, published in 2010 (Neul et al. 2010), is a simplified version of the previous one (Hagberg et al. 2002) and, in contrast to earlier diagnostic revisions, it was validated on a large cohort (Percy et al. 2010). It retains the concepts of necessary and supportive criteria, which are helpful for delineating all forms of RTT from other neurodevelopmental disorders. Its simplified scheme intended to facilitate a broader application, beyond neurologists and other specialists.

TYPICAL RETT SYNDROME

The diagnosis of typical RTT requires the common necessary criterion, presence of regression, plus four main criteria derived from the natural history of most individuals with the disorder: (1) regression of purposeful hand use; (2) regression of spoken language; (3) gait abnormalities; and (4) hand stereotypies (Neul et al. 2010; Table 1.1). Because the course of RTT is dynamic, including stabilization and potentially partial recovery of skills after the period of regression, a careful developmental history needs to be obtained.

With our increasing knowledge of the evolution of RTT, it has become clear that postnatal deceleration in head growth is not found in all individuals with typical course (Tarquinio et al. 2012). Therefore, this is no longer a necessary criterion. Nevertheless, as stated in the 2010 publication, it is a clinical feature that can alert a clinician to the potential diagnosis. Exclusion criteria were also simplified in the 2010 revision to any other primary cause of neurological dysfunction, either genetic or acquired. While individuals with pathogenic *MECP2* mutations can also have a concurrent genetic disorder (e.g. trisomy 21, pathogenic mutations in the *NF-1* gene), they do not present the typical evolution of RTT or that of the second entity. Consequently, they should be labeled as having atypical RTT if they meet the respective criteria. A second exclusion criterion for typical RTT remains and that is the presence of major deviations in typical development in the first 6 months of life. This does not exclude minor developmental abnormalities during this period, as retrospective use of videos and other approaches have revealed relatively common early mild deviations in communication or motor development (Einspieler et al. 2005; Marschik et al. 2013). As emphasized in the 2010 guidelines, this distinction is important since one of the atypical forms of RTT, termed congenital variant, is characterized by grossly atypical development from birth.

Sex is not an exclusion criterion for typical RTT, as a few males meet all criteria (Christen and Hanefeld 1995). Similarly, absence of *MECP2* mutation or abnormality in another gene are not exclusionary criteria considering that there is still a small percentage of individuals with RTT who do not present with *MECP2* mutations (e.g. 2.2% in Neul et al. 2014), and new sequencing techniques reveal other genes associated with typical RTT (Sajan et al. 2017). This issue is discussed in the 'Genotype–Phenotype' section below and in Chapter 3 on the Clinical Genetics of RTT.

4

TABLE 1.1
Current diagnostic criteria of typical and atypical Rett syndrome (RTT)

Revised diagnostic criteria for RTT (Neul et al. 2010)

Consider diagnosis when postnatal deceleration of head growth observed.

Required for typical or classic RTT

1. A period of regression followed by recovery or stabilization
2. All main criteria and all exclusion criteria
3. Supportive criteria are not required, although often present in typical RTT

Required for atypical or variant RTT

1. A period of regression followed by recovery or stabilization
2. At least two out of the four main criteria
3. Five out of 11 supportive criteria

Main criteria

1. Partial or complete loss of acquired purposeful hand skills.
2. Partial or complete loss of acquired spoken language (best acquired spoken language skill, not strictly the acquisition of distinct words or higher language skills).
3. Gait abnormalities: impaired (dyspraxic) or absence of ability.
4. Stereotypic hand movements such as hand wringing/squeezing, clapping/tapping, mouthing, and washing/rubbing automatisms.

Exclusion criteria for typical RTT

1. Brain injury secondary to trauma (peri- or postnatally), neurometabolic disease, or severe infection that causes neurological problems with clear evidence (neurological or ophthalmological examination and MRI/CT) that the presumed insult directly resulted in neurological dysfunction.
2. Grossly abnormal psychomotor development in first 6 months of life to the point that normal milestones (acquiring head control, swallowing, developing social smile) are not met.

Supportive criteria for atypical RTT (counted if an individual has or ever had a clinical feature listed)

1. Breathing disturbances when awake
2. Bruxism when awake
3. Impaired sleep pattern
4. Abnormal muscle tone
5. Peripheral vasomotor disturbances
6. Scoliosis/kyphosis
7. Growth retardation
8. Small, cold hands and feet
9. Inappropriate laughing/screaming spells
10. Diminished response to pain
11. Intense eye communication – "eye pointing"

The current diagnostic guidelines eliminated the use of supportive criteria for the diagnosis of typical RTT because, as demonstrated by the large-scale validation study (Percy et al. 2010), they are not necessary. On the other hand, recognition of features commonly present in individuals with RTT is helpful in cases that do not follow the typical trajectory, as reported by the same study (Percy et al. 2010).

ATYPICAL RETT SYNDROME

Increased awareness about RTT and greater availability of genetic testing for *MECP2* muta-tions have emphasized the need for a clear delineation of the boundaries of the disorder. Diagnosing atypical or variant RTT has always been challenging. The 2010 revised criteria attempted to simplify the process and, at the same time, to add precision (Neul et al. 2010). The current guidelines use the same main criteria applied to typical RTT but with a lower threshold (i.e. developmental regression plus two or three of the four main criteria). This is complemented by supportive criteria that increase the certainty of a RTT profile. Evaluating loss of skills in individuals with limited or protracted early neurological development could be very difficult. This is further complicated by the presence, in some individuals of seizures since the first few months of life that make the differentiation between primary regression and post-epileptic changes very difficult. Despite all these issues, it is important to make the distinction between RTT, which is associated with developmental regression, and other disorders that have a relentless neurodegenerative course, or from other forms of intellectual disability. Nonetheless, these diagnostic challenges, in conjunction with the genetic diver-sity of atypical RTT, have raised the possibility of removing some subgroups of atypical RTT from the disorder's spectrum.

Supportive criteria are helpful in the diagnosis of atypical RTT, but only as a group of features since individual symptoms could be present in either other neurodevelopmental disorders (e.g. diminished pain response, seen also in nonsyndromic autism spectrum disor-der), or many neurological disorders (e.g. abnormal muscle tone). In sum, the 2010 criteria require that, in addition to a history of regression, individuals with atypical RTT must have at least two of the four main criteria and five of 11 supportive criteria (Table 1.1).

Atypical RTT is a heterogeneous entity. Although some specific clinical presentations or variants have long been recognized (see below), many patients are better defined as simply having a milder or more severe atypical RTT presentation. A recent study used scores on the Clinical Severity Scale, a commonly applied instrument of RTT clinical severity (Cuddapah et al. 2014), to divide individuals with atypical RTT into better function and poorer function categories (Neul et al. 2014). In addition to the developmental and neuro-logical phenotype differences, the better function group had a close association to *MECP2* mutations (92% vs 80.5% in the poorer function group), although lower than in those with typical RTT (97.8% in the same study). These genotype–phenotype profiles are in line with the characteristics of the variants described below (see also Fig. 1.1).

Three atypical/variant forms of RTT have been delineated: the preserved speech vari-ant, the early seizure variant, and the congenital variant (Fig. 1.1). The preserved speech (Zappella) variant (Zappella 1992; Renieri et al. 2009) would correspond to the better func-tion category, with milder clinical features as well as *MECP2* mutations in the majority of individuals. The other two variants have a more severe clinical profile; therefore, the congenital (Rolando) and early seizure (Hanefeld) variants would be considered poorer function forms of atypical RTT (Hanefeld 1985; Rolando 1985). In both, *MECP2* muta-tions have only rarely been identified. Indeed, the early seizure variant is closely linked to mutations in the *CDKL5* gene (Artuso et al. 2010). A relatively larger number of individuals with *CDKL5* mutations have been identified in genetic screens for epileptic (early onset)

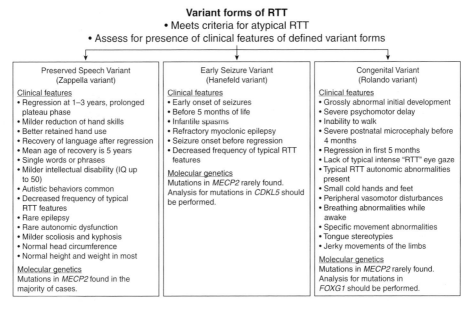

Fig. 1.1. Flow diagram of specific atypical (variant) forms of RTT. Reproduced from Neul et al. Rett syndrome: revised diagnostic criteria and nomenclature. *Ann Neurol* 68: 944–950 © 2010 with permission from John Wiley and Sons Ltd.

encephalopathy (Gursoy and Ercal 2016; von Deimling et al. 2017). Although the delineation of the phenotype associated with *CDKL5* mutations is work in progress, there is substantial evidence for a distinctive neurodevelopmental disorder (Fehr et al. 2013). Characterization of the congenital variant, linked to *FOXG1* mutations (Mencarelli et al. 2010), is still incomplete (Ma et al. 2016). However, as for *CDKL5* mutations, data suggest that a clinical entity defined by mutations in *FOXG1* and not phenotype deserves consideration.

EARLY DIAGNOSIS

Because *MECP2* testing is included in the diagnostic work up of individuals with global developmental delay (Moeschler et al. 2014) or autism spectrum disorder (Schaefer et al. 2013), mutations are now identified in some individuals prior to any clear evidence of regression. Consequently, we recommend the diagnosis of 'possible' RTT should be given to individuals under 3 years old who have not lost any skills but present with clinical features suggestive of RTT. These individuals should be reassessed every 6–12 months for evidence of developmental regression. If regression manifests, the diagnosis should then be changed to definite RTT, either typical or atypical. However, if the child does not show any evidence of regression by 5 years, the diagnosis of RTT should be questioned since loss of skills is unusual after this age (Neul et al. 2010, 2014).

Genotype–phenotype correlations and Rett syndrome diagnosis

There is a strong but imperfect correlation between *MECP2* mutations and phenotype. While most individuals with pathogenic mutations in *MECP2* present with RTT, others do not have the clinical features of the disorder. The phenotypical spectrum of *MECP2* mutations includes, at one end, asymptomatic female carriers found in familial RTT, who have extreme skewing of their X chromosome inactivation that allows a typical development (Wan et al. 1999; Lombardi et al. 2015). At the opposite extreme are boys with *MECP2* mutations known to cause typical RTT in girls, but presenting with severe early postnatal encephalopathy, early death, and absence of the distinctive clinical features of RTT (Wan et al. 1999; Kankirawatana et al. 2006). There are also multiple reports of rare individuals with *MECP2* mutations who present with other neurodevelopmental or neuropsychiatric disorders, including autism spectrum disorder (Carney et al. 2003; Li et al. 2005; Campos et al. 2011), Angelman syndrome-like presentation (Watson et al. 2001), attention-deficit–hyperactivity disorder (Adegbola et al. 2009), nonspecific intellectual disability (Grozeva et al. 2015; Bianciardi et al. 2016), bipolar disorder (Klauck et al. 2002), and schizophrenia (Cohen et al. 2002). Although most of these individuals have developmental abnormalities, they lack features that characterize RTT, including the defining one, a history of regression. These clinical phenotypes emphasize that mutations in *MECP2* are not synonymous with RTT and that a mutation in *MECP2* is not sufficient to make the diagnosis of RTT. In 2010, we proposed that all individuals with clinical disorders and MECP2 mutations be called MECP2-related disorders, which includes RTT and other neurological conditions associated with *MECP2* mutations (Neul et al. 2010).

As mentioned in the preceding section, typical RTT has the strongest association with *MECP2* mutations, followed by the milder forms of atypical RTT, with the lowest proportion of *MECP2* positive individuals in the severe presentation of atypical RTT. Since the publication of the current diagnostic guidelines (Neul et al. 2010), efforts at applying newer genetic methods such as whole exome sequencing (i.e. coding regions) to identify the bases of mutation negative cases have narrowed the *MECP2*-RTT gap. These studies have also tested the limits of the RTT's phenotypical profile by investigating the relationship between RTT-related features, beyond the diagnosis of RTT, and mutations in *MECP2* and other genes. They have confirmed the preferential association between typical RTT and *MECP2* mutations (Olson et al. 2015; Sajan et al. 2017). However, these studies have also found in individuals with typical RTT mutations in genes involved in chromatin regulation, neuronal homeostasis, and synaptic activity (Lucariello et al. 2016; Sajan et al. 2017). These investigations have also reported the association of atypical RTT with mutations in genes implicated in chromatin regulation, glutamatergic and GABAergic function, or synaptic ion channels (Lucariello et al. 2016; Sajan et al. 2017), some of them previously reported in other neurodevelopmental disorders (e.g. *TCF4*, linked to Pitt-Hopkins syndrome). As expected, mutations in genes linked to epileptic encephalopathy tend to be found in individuals with early onset seizure variant (Sajan et al. 2017). Interestingly, Olson and colleagues (2015) reported that females showing some RTT features but not meeting all criteria for atypical RTT could have abnormalities in the same genes found to have sequence abnormalities in RTT (i.e. *IQSEC2, SCN8A, FOXG1*). All these studies have shown that sequencing techniques fail to identify mutations in a small proportion of individuals with typical or atypical RTT. Higher resolution analyses of copy number variations and sequencing of noncoding regions have rarely been applied to RTT.

Thus, in the future, the proportion of mutation negative RTT cases will be most likely to decrease further.

The aforementioned studies highlight the close but not absolute association between *MECP2* mutations with typical RTT and the greater variety of genetic abnormalities in atypical RTT, particularly in the more severe cases, which appear to extend to individuals with borderline features of RTT. Despite this complex picture, genotype–phenotype correlations are relatively consistent for individuals with RTT and *MECP2* mutations. Distinctive profiles of severity can be identified for each common *MECP2* mutation (Bebbington et al. 2008; Neul et al. 2008), which are more evident when examining longitudinal trajectories (Cuddapah et al. 2014). The 2010 publication on diagnostic criteria also includes a section on nomenclature, focused on *MECP2* mutations (Neul et al. 2010).

More detailed information about diagnostic issues and clinical presentation, with emphasis on genetics, can be found in Chapter 3 on the Clinical Genetics of RTT and Chapter 4 on Genetic Sources of Variation in RTT.

Rett syndrome spectrum vs *MECP2* spectrum

The continuous progress in the delineation of the features of RTT, and their relationship with specific genetic abnormalities, has raised the question about the existence of more than one disorder under the RTT umbrella. Typical RTT with *MECP2* mutation would constitute the 'core' disorder of this spectrum (i.e. some propose the term RTT disorder for these individuals; Kerr et al. 2001b), which would also include atypical RTT presentations linked to other genes, and even individuals with most but not all diagnostic features of RTT (e.g. one main criterion plus six supportive criteria). An easily identifiable common manifestation of the RTT spectrum would be hand stereotypies. An advantage of this approach would be the interpretation of genetic findings, already reported in RTT and in individuals who do not meet RTT criteria (Olson et al. 2015). On the other hand, the value of a RTT spectrum is already questioned for most individuals with *CDKL5* or *FOXG1* mutations who do not present with RTT-like features. In these instances, a diagnosis based on genotype similar to that of fragile X syndrome (Hagerman et al. 2009) seems more sensible. The development of targeted therapies based on the primary genetic defect, as the case of *MECP2* deficit mutations (Kaufmann et al. 2016), further supports the rationale for separating some groups of atypical RTT from the spectrum.

The identification of *MECP2* duplications, with a relatively distinctive clinical presentation quite different from RTT (Van Esch 2012) and a pathophysiology linked to increased MeCP2 function, has led to the proposal of a *MECP2* spectrum of disorders (Lombardi et al. 2015). As for the RTT spectrum, there are advantages and shortcomings of this classification. While a *MECP2* disorders category would help to understand the effect of gene dosage upon neural function, and the consequent development of MeCP2-focused treatments, other practical diagnostic and management applications are less clear.

In future years, the greater ability to identify *MECP2* pathogenic mutations prior to the development of overt neurodevelopmental abnormalities will test the current diagnostic criteria of RTT. In addition, sensitive sequencing techniques are revealing an increased number of variants of unknown significance and even multiple genetic abnormalities, which require careful interpretation in the clinical context. This is particularly difficult in individuals with atypical RTT since many of their manifestations are relatively non-specific. Although in the distant future, newborn screening for *MECP2* mutations will be the ultimate challenge for the concept of RTT.

Conclusion

The continuous expansion of our knowledge on RTT, *MECP2*, and related disorders has already required several revisions of diagnostic criteria. Fifty years after its original description, and 15 years after the association of *MECP2* mutations with RTT, the diagnosis of RTT remains clinical and challenges to the delineation and classification of RTT variants have arisen. The 2010 diagnostic criteria are the first with some level of validation in RTT; however, their eventual obsolescence is already anticipated by the emergence of new entities (e.g. CDKL5 disorder) and the increasing complexity of the genetics of RTT. It is important to remember the multiple implications of a diagnosis, including clinical practice, epidemiology, and research. However, the ultimate goals of a diagnosis are management and prognosis. Any future revision of RTT diagnostic criteria needs to take these factors into consideration. A similar mechanism to the one used in the generation of the 2010 criteria, through RettSearch or another authoritative group, followed by an assessment of the guidelines in an appropriate clinical sample will certainly be necessary. The constitution of a permanent entity updating RTT-related criteria and nomenclature may even be needed. Diagnostic confusion cannot only have negative impact upon research endeavors, but also on clinical management decisions and patient identity.

REFERENCES

Adegbola AA, Gonzales ML, Chess A, LaSalle JM, Cox GF (2009) A novel hypomorphic MECP2 point mutation is associated with a neuropsychiatric phenotype. *Hum Genet* 124(6): 615–623.

Amir RE, Van den Veyver IB, Wan M, Tran CQ, Francke U, Zoghbi HY (1999) Rett syndrome is caused by mutations in X-linked MECP2, encoding methyl-CpG-binding protein 2. *Nat Genet* 23(2): 185–188.

Anderson A, Wong K, Jacoby P, Downs J, Leonard H (2014) Twenty years of surveillance in Rett syndrome: What does this tell us? *Orphanet J Rare Dis* 9: 87.

Artuso R, Mencarelli MA, Polli R et al. (2010) Early-onset seizure variant of Rett syndrome: Definition of the clinical diagnostic criteria. *Brain Dev* 32(1): 17–24.

Baikie G, Ravikumara M, Downs J et al. (2014) Gastrointestinal dysmotility in Rett syndrome. *J Pediatr Gastroenterol Nutr* 58(2): 237–244.

Barnes KV, Coughlin FR, O'Leary HM et al. (2015) Anxiety-like behavior in Rett syndrome: Characteristics and assessment by anxiety scales. *J Neurodev Disord* 7(1): 30.

Bebbington A, Anderson A, Ravine D et al. (2008) Investigating genotype-phenotype relationships in Rett syndrome using an international data set. *Neurology* 70(11): 868–875.

Bianciardi L, Fichera M, Failla P et al. (2016) MECP2 missense mutations outside the canonical MBD and TRD domains in males with intellectual disability. *J Hum Genet* 61(2): 95–101.

Blue ME, Boskey AL, Doty SB, Fedarko NS, Hossain MA, Shapiro JR (2015) Osteoblast function and bone histomorphometry in a murine model of Rett syndrome. *Bone* 76: 23–30.

Campos M Jr, Pestana CP, dos Santos AV et al. (2011) A MECP2 missense mutation within the MBD domain in a Brazilian male with autistic disorder. *Brain Dev* 33(10): 807–809.

Carney RM, Wolpert CM, Ravan SA et al. (2003) Identification of MeCP2 mutations in a series of females with autistic disorder. *Pediatr Neurol* 28(3): 205–211.

Carter P, Downs J, Bebbington A, Williams S, Jacoby P, Kaufmann WE, Leonard H (2010) Stereotypical hand movements in 144 subjects with Rett syndrome from the population-based Australian database. *Mov Disord* 25(3): 282–288.

Christen HJ, Hanefeld F (1995) Male Rett variant. *Neuropediatrics* 26(2): 81–82.

Cianfaglione R, Clarke A, Kerr M et al. (2015) A national survey of Rett syndrome: Behavioural characteristics. *J Neurodev Disord* 7(1): 11.

Cohen D, Lazar G, Couvert P et al. (2002) MECP2 mutation in a boy with language disorder and schizophrenia. *Am J Psychiatry* 159(1): 148–149.

Cuddapah VA, Pillai RB, Shekar KV et al. (2014) Methyl-CpG-binding protein 2 (MECP2) mutation type is associated with disease severity in Rett syndrome. *J Med Genet* 51(3): 152–158.

Einspieler C, Kerr AM, Prechtl HF (2005) Is the early development of girls with Rett disorder really normal? *Pediatr Res* 57(5 Pt 1): 696–700.

Fehr S, Wilson M, Downs J et al. (2013) The CDKL5 disorder is an independent clinical entity associated with early-onset encephalopathy. *Eur J Hum Genet* 21(3): 266–273.

Foley KR, Downs J, Bebbington A et al. (2011) Change in gross motor abilities of girls and women with Rett syndrome over a 3- to 4-year period. *J Child Neurol* 26(10): 1237–1245.

Grozeva D, Carss K, Spasic-Boskovic O et al. (2015) Targeted next-generation sequencing analysis of 1,000 individuals with intellectual disability. *Hum Mutat* 36(12): 1197–1204.

Gursoy S, Ercal D (2016) Diagnostic approach to genetic causes of early-onset epileptic encephalopathy. *J Child Neurol* 31(4): 523–532.

Hagberg B, Aicardi J, Dias K, Ramos O (1983) A progressive syndrome of autism, dementia, ataxia, and loss of purposeful hand use in girls: Rett's syndrome: report of 35 cases. *Ann Neurol* 14(4): 471–479.

Hagberg B, Goutieres F, Hanefeld F, Rett A, Wilson J (1985) Rett syndrome: Criteria for inclusion and exclusion. *Brain Dev* 7(3): 372–373.

Hagberg BA, Skjeldal OH (1994) Rett variants: A suggested model for inclusion criteria. *Pediatr Neurol* 11: 5–11.

Hagberg B, Hanefeld F, Percy A, Skjeldal O (2002) An update on clinically applicable diagnostic criteria in Rett syndrome. Comments to Rett Syndrome Clinical Criteria Consensus Panel Satellite to European Paediatric Neurology Society Meeting, Baden Baden, Germany, 11 September 2001. *Eur J Paediatr Neurol* 6(5): 293–297.

Hagerman RJ, Berry-Kravis E, Kaufmann WE et al. (2009) Advances in the treatment of fragile X syndrome. *Pediatrics* 123(1): 378–390.

Hanefeld F (1985) The clinical pattern of the Rett syndrome. *Brain Dev* 7(3): 320–325.

Jefferson A, Leonard H, Siafarikas A et al. (2016) Clinical guidelines for management of bone health in Rett syndrome based on expert consensus and available evidence. *PLoS One* 11(2): e0146824.

Kankirawatana P, Leonard H, Ellaway C et al. (2006) Early progressive encephalopathy in boys and MECP2 mutations. *Neurology* 67(1): 164–166.

Kaufmann WE, Johnston MV, Blue ME (2005) MeCP2 expression and function during brain development: Implications for Rett syndrome's pathogenesis and clinical evolution. *Brain Dev* 27(Suppl 1): S77–S87.

Kaufmann WE, Tierney E, Rohde CA et al. (2012) Social impairments in Rett syndrome: Characteristics and relationship with clinical severity. *J Intellect Disabil Res* 56(3): 233–247.

Kaufmann WE, Stallworth JL, Everman DB, Skinner SA (2016) Neurobiologically-based treatments in Rett syndrome: Opportunities and challenges. *Expert Opin Orphan Drugs* 4(10): 1043–1055.

Kerr AM, Nomura Y, Armstrong D et al. (2001a) Guidelines for reporting clinical features in cases with MECP2 mutations. *Brain Dev* 23(4): 208–211.

Kerr AM, Belichenko P, Woodcock T, Woodcock M (2001b) Mind and brain in Rett disorder. *Brain Dev* 23(Suppl 1): S44–S49.

Klauck SM, Lindsay S, Beyer KS, Splitt M, Burn J, Poustka A (2002) A mutation hot spot for nonspecific X-linked mental retardation in the MECP2 gene causes the PPM-X syndrome. *Am J Hum Genet* 70(4): 1034–1037.

Leonard H, Cobb S, Downs J (2017) Clinical and biological progress over 50 years in Rett syndrome. *Nat Rev Neurol* 13(1): 37–51.

Li H, Yamagata T, Mori M, Yasuhara A, Momoi MY (2005) Mutation analysis of methyl-CpG binding protein family genes in autistic patients. *Brain Dev* 27(5): 321–325.

Lombardi LM, Baker SA, Zoghbi HY (2015) MECP2 disorders: From the clinic to mice and back. *J Clin Invest* 125(8): 2914–2923.

Lucariello M, Vidal E, Vidal S et al. (2016) Whole exome sequencing of Rett syndrome-like patients reveals the mutational diversity of the clinical phenotype. *Hum Genet* 135(12): 1343–1354.

Ma M, Adams HR, Seltzer LE, Dobyns WB, Paciorkowski AR (2016) Phenotype differentiation of FOXG1 and MECP2 disorders: A new method for characterization of developmental encephalopathies. *J Pediatr* 178: 233–240.

Marschik PB, Kaufmann WE, Sigafoos J et al. (2013) Changing the perspective on early development of Rett syndrome. *Res Dev Disabil* 34(4): 1236–1239.

McCauley MD, Wang T, Mike E et al. (2011) Pathogenesis of lethal cardiac arrhythmias in Mecp2 mutant mice: Implication for therapy in Rett syndrome. *Sci Transl Med* 3(113): 113–125.

Mencarelli MA, Spanhol-Rosseto A, Artuso R et al. (2010) Novel FOXG1 mutations associated with the congenital variant of Rett syndrome. *J Med Genet* 47(1): 49–53.

Moeschler JB, Shevell M, Committee on Genetics (2014) Comprehensive evaluation of the child with intellectual disability or global developmental delays. *Pediatrics* 134(3): e903–e918.

Motil KJ, Caeg E, Barrish JO et al. (2012) Gastrointestinal and nutritional problems occur frequently throughout life in girls and women with Rett syndrome. *J Pediatr Gastroenterol Nutr* 55(3): 292–298.

Mount RH, Charman T, Hastings RP, Reilly S, Cass H (2002a) The Rett Syndrome Behaviour Questionnaire (RSBQ): Refining the behavioural phenotype of Rett syndrome. *J Child Psychol Psychiatry* 43(8): 1099–1110.

Mount RH, Hastings RP, Reilly S, Cass H, Charman T (2002b) Behaviour problems in adult women with Rett syndrome. *J Intellect Disabil Res* 46(Pt 8): 619–624.

Mount RH, Charman T, Hastings RP, Reilly S, Cass H (2003) Features of autism in Rett syndrome and severe mental retardation. *J Autism Dev Disord* 33(4): 435–442.

Neul JL, Fang P, Barrish J et al. (2008) Specific mutations in methyl-CpG-binding protein 2 confer different severity in Rett syndrome. *Neurology* 70(16): 1313–1321.

Neul JL, Kaufmann WE, Glaze DG et al. (2010) Rett syndrome: Revised diagnostic criteria and nomenclature. *Ann Neurol* 68(6): 944–950.

Neul JL, Lane JB, Lee HS et al. (2014) Developmental delay in Rett syndrome: Data from the natural history study. *J Neurodev Disord* 6(1): 20.

Nissenkorn A, Levy-Drummer RS, Bondi O et al. (2015) Epilepsy in Rett syndrome – Lessons from the Rett networked database. *Epilepsia* 56(4): 569–576.

Nomura Y, Segawa M, Hasegawa M (1984) Rett syndrome – Clinical studies and pathophysiological consideration. *Brain Dev* 6(5): 475–486.

Olson HE, Tambunan D, LaCoursiere C et al. (2015) Mutations in epilepsy and intellectual disability genes in patients with features of Rett syndrome. *Am J Med Genet A* 167A(9): 2017–2025.

Percy AK (2016) Progress in Rett syndrome: From discovery to clinical trials. *Wien Med Wochenschr* 166(11–12): 325–332.

Percy AK, Neul JL, Glaze DG et al. (2010) Rett syndrome diagnostic criteria: Lessons from the Natural History Study. *Ann Neurol* 68(6): 951–955.

Renieri A, Mari F, Mencarelli MA et al. (2009) Diagnostic criteria for the Zappella variant of Rett syndrome (the preserved speech variant). *Brain Dev* 31(3): 208–216.

Rett A (1966) On an unusual brain atrophy syndrome in hyperammonemia in childhood. *Wien Med Wochenschr* 116(37): 723–726.

Rolando S (1985) Rett syndrome: Report of eight cases. *Brain Dev* 7(3): 290–296.

Ross PD, Guy J, Selfridge J et al. (2016) Exclusive expression of MeCP2 in the nervous system distinguishes between brain and peripheral Rett syndrome-like phenotypes. *Hum Mol Genet* 25(20): 4389–4404.

Sajan SA, Jhangiani SN, Muzny DM et al. (2017) Enrichment of mutations in chromatin regulators in people with Rett syndrome lacking mutations in MECP2. *Genet Med* 19(1): 13–19.

Schaefer GB, Mendelsohn NJ, Professional Practice and Guidelines Committee (2013) Clinical genetics evaluation in identifying the etiology of autism spectrum disorders: 2013 guideline revisions. *Genet Med* 15(5): 399–407.

Suter B, Treadwell-Deering D, Zoghbi HY, Glaze DG, Neul JL (2014) Brief report: MECP2 mutations in people without Rett syndrome. *J Autism Dev Disord* 44(3): 703–711.

Tarquinio DC, Motil KJ, Hou W et al. (2012) Growth failure and outcome in Rett syndrome: Specific growth references. *Neurology* 79(16): 1653–1661.

Tarquinio DC, Hou W, Berg A et al. (2017) Longitudinal course of epilepsy in Rett syndrome and related disorders. *Brain* 140(Pt 2): 306–318.

The Rett Syndrome Diagnostic Criteria Work Group (1988) Diagnostic criteria for Rett syndrome. *Ann Neurol* 23(4): 425–428.

Van Esch H (2012) MECP2 duplication syndrome. *Mol Syndromol* 2(3–5): 128–136.

von Deimling M, Helbig I, Marsh ED (2017) Epileptic encephalopathies-clinical syndromes and pathophysiological concepts. *Curr Neurol Neurosci Rep* 17(2): 10.

Wan M, Lee SS, Zhang X et al. (1999) Rett syndrome and beyond: Recurrent spontaneous and familial MECP2 mutations at CpG hotspots. *Am J Hum Gene,* 65(6): 1520–1529.

Watson P, Black G, Ramsden S et al. (2001) Angelman syndrome phenotype associated with mutations in MECP2, a gene encoding a methyl CpG binding protein. *J Med Genet* 38(4): 224–228.

Zappella M (1992) The Rett girls with preserved speech. *Brain Dev* 14(2): 98–101.

2

THE NATURAL HISTORY OF RETT SYNDROME: BUILDING ON RECENT EXPERIENCE

Alan K Percy and Daniel G Glaze

Introduction

The first widely-read publication by Hagberg et al. (1983) on Rett syndrome (RTT) (Rett, 1966a, b) spawned a remarkable surge in our understanding of this unique neurodevelopmental disorder, from both the clinical and laboratory perspectives. Critical elements from the clinical perspective were the development of consensus criteria as detailed in Chapter 1 and a firm conceptualization of the disease profile. The hallmark features of RTT are profound cognitive impairment, poor communication skills, stereotypic hand movements, motor impairments, and pervasive growth failure beginning between 6 and 18 months of age. These follow a period of *apparently* typical development during which initial fine motor skills and spoken communication are acquired. During the regression period, fine motor skills, effective eye contact, and communication are lost and inconsolable crying or irritability may occur. The limited eye contact and poor socialization or interaction, often lead to consideration of autism. Typically, the autistic features are transient, lasting from weeks to many months, and certainly by school age, intense eye gaze and interaction with others return, yet spoken communication does not. As such, a rather typical temporal profile characterizes RTT, namely: (1) apparently typical early development; (2) arrest of developmental progress at 6–18 months; (3) followed by frank regression of social contact, language, and finger skills; (4) subsequent improvement in social contact and eye gaze by age 5; and (5) thereafter demonstrating effective social interaction throughout life with gradual slowing of motor functions into adulthood (Box 2.1).

BOX 2.1 Temporal profile for Rett syndrome

- Apparently normal early development: 6–18 months
- Arrest of developmental progress
- Regression, including poor social contact and finger skills
- Stabilization: better social contact and eye gaze by age five in most
- Thereafter demonstrating effective social interaction throughout life with gradual slowing of motor functions into adulthood

---

Hagberg and Witt-Engerström (1986) introduced a four-stage model to provide a conceptual framework for understanding the sequential pattern of clinical features in RTT. Briefly, these were characterized as follows: Stage I arrest of development; Stage II regression; Stage III pseudo-stationary or plateau without further regression; and Stage IV motor deterioration with loss of ambulation. During the early period of studying RTT, this staging system was extremely helpful; however, as diagnostic acumen advanced successively during the next 15–20 years leading to increasingly sophisticated therapeutic interventions and with the identification of *MECP2* mutations as the principal etiology, application of the complete staging system began to create some confusion, especially among caregivers. Stages I and II overlap directly with the second and third items in the temporal profile described above. Although Stage III does reflect the improvement in interaction, it was also limited to those individuals who were ambulatory, while excluding those who were similarly more interactive socially, but were not ambulatory. This posed a dilemma for clinicians in correctly assigning a proper stage. As intensive physical and occupational therapies were increasingly implemented and attention given to management of progressive scoliosis and other neuromuscular problems including rigidity and dystonia, the neuromotor deformities for Stage IV became less clear-cut. Witt-Engerström (1992) provided a modified substaging, Stage III/IV, in an attempt to resolve the dilemma between those who would be in Stage III in terms of social interaction, but in Stage IV by virtue of being nonambulatory. Over time, this substaging proved not to be completely satisfactory. As such, the temporal profile, by incorporating the principal features of the staging system while resolving the main issues of the latter phases of the staging system, has become a preferred descriptor.

With the increasing appearance of clinical trials for potential disease-modifying or potentially fundamental therapies aimed at reversing RTT, the age at diagnosis has been a key point of study. During the course of the US Natural History Study (NCT00299312), the average age at diagnosis has fallen from 4 years to 2.7 (Tarquinio et al. 2015a). This is regarded as very positive, but inasmuch as the diagnosis is made mainly by subspecialists, that is, child neurologists, developmental pediatricians, and geneticists; current efforts are being made to promote the warning signs of a neurodevelopmental disorder to pediatricians and general physicians. These include the abnormal deceleration of the rate of head growth, signs of delayed or plateaued development, and appreciation of the parents' concerns that the infant is 'too good' during the early months. This may further reduce the age at diagnosis.

Developmental features: pre- and post-regression

Clinical features of RTT are not evident in the first few months of life. Generally, the period of early infancy is regarded as typical. On closer inspection of this period one can detect suggestions of deviations from what is typical; however, for most families, these alterations of typical development are not noteworthy except in hindsight. Still, careful assessment has been conducted based on early videos suggesting clear changes in typical development (Einspieler et al. 2005a, b). For most parents, this is a period during which little attention is devoted to this aspect. Indeed, from the Natural History study (Neul et al. 2014) currently in progress in the United States, for 765 individuals with classic RTT, early gross motor (rolling from back to front or front to back, sitting when placed) and cognitive (social smile, quieting to voice, and cooing and babbling) skills occur in most at the expected time periods. For later developing skills including gross motor (coming to a sit, walking with support or independently, and negotiating stairs), all fine motor and cognitive (single words, phrases, inhibiting to 'No', or follow commands with or without a gesture) delays are evident. Therefore, skills emerging beyond the 6-month period are delayed or absent in this cohort (Table 2.1). The period from 6 to 18 months marks the beginning of stagnation and frank regression in all spheres with a substantial loss in all skills, whether gross or fine motor, or cognitive. While some children regain these skills after the period of regression, this number is generally quite small.

For most individuals with atypical RTT, development is significantly delayed overall and in some instances very significantly so, for example, for early gross and fine motor skills, and cognitive features.

The issue of autism is prominent with respect to RTT (Percy 2011). In general, children with RTT have features consistent with autism only during the period of regression. It is during this time that some do not like being held and become visually and aurally inattentive. This period is transient in most cases, as is seen in Table 2.2. Of the 765 individuals in the Natural History Study, 714 liked being held and roughly one-half stopped being visually (409) and aurally (343) attentive. The majority of individuals maintained their desire to be held and regained their ability to be visually and aurally attentive and only a relatively small number lost these again. As such, for the great majority, features consistent with autism spectrum disorder are not persistent in RTT. Indeed, after the regression period individuals with RTT are defined for the most part by their intense eye-contact, their direct interaction with others, and their ability to communicate using picture boards or interactive computers, quite distinct from most individuals with autism.

Main clinical features

GROWTH FAILURE

Growth is a major issue for most children with RTT. This was recognized at the outset by Andreas Rett in his early writings, namely describing abnormal postnatal deceleration in the rate of head growth and later by Schultz et al. (1993, 2009) in separate publications dealing with height, weight, and head circumference and hand and foot growth. Most recently, through the Natural History Study and the International Rett Syndrome Foundation, a much larger study (Tarquinio et al. 2012) has validated and extended these findings. From 793 female participants, more than 9100 observations were observed, combining cross-sectional and longitudinal data. The mean growth for classic RTT fell below the normative population for weight (6 months), height (17 months), and head circumference (1.5 months). Normal pubertal increases in weight and height were absent. Body mass index curves, however, did not differ from the normative population. Furthermore, classic and atypical RTT cohorts showed similar growth patterns in all parameters. Of interest, mutation type did not appear to have any impact on growth, whereas early gross and fine motor development was associated with much better growth. Language abilities, on the contrary, were not correlated with growth. Although not part of this study, the Natural History Study has similar data showing that hands and feet tend to be significantly smaller, feet more so than hands.

16

TABLE 2.1
Comparison of development in children with Rett syndrome and typically developing children

Parameter	Rett syndrome (n=765) age, n (%)	Typically developing children, age
Rolling	5.5 months 726 (95)	5 months
Sit alone	10.5 months 619 (81)	7 months
Crawl	11.8 months 527 (69)	10 months
Walk alone	20.7 months 439 (57)	18 months
Climb steps	29.1 months 189 (25)	24 months
Reach for objects	7.0 months 733 (96)	4 months
Finger feed	10.8 months 697 (91)	6–7 months
Pincer grasp	11.5 months 557 (73)	10–12 months
Social smile	3.4 months 752 (98)	2–3 months
Coo	3.5 months 697 (91)	3–4 months
Babble	8.2 months 711 (93)	6 months
Single words	12.2 months 590 (77)	12 months
Phrases	21.5 months 172 (23)	18 months
Fix and follow	7.1 months 693 (91)	3–4 months
Quiet to voice	5.2 months 636 (83)	3–5 months
Follow command with gesture	23.3 months 412 (54%)	12 months
Follow command without gesture	27.2 months 341 (45)	15 months

Data obtained from the Natural History Study (Neul et al. 2014); total classic, 772.

TABLE 2.2
Features of autism in classic and variant Rett syndrome

Classic Rett syndrome n=765			Variant Rett syndrome n=140		
Liked being held n (%)	Lost visual attention n (%)	Lost aural attention n (%)	Liked being held n (%)	Lost visual attention n (%)	Lost aural attention n (%)
714 (93) Acquired	409 (53) Lost	343 (46) Lost	126 (90) Acquired	42 (30) Lost	38 (27) Lost
139 (18) Lost	309 (40) Regained	246 (32) Regained	15 (11) Lost	27 (19) Regained	21 (15) Regained
100 (13) Regained	40 (5.2) Lost again	26 (3.4) Lost again	8 (5.7) Regained	5 (3.6) Lost again	3 (2.1) Lost again
675 (88) Retained	625 (82) Retained	642 (84) Retained	119 (85) Retained	120 (86) Retained	120 (86) Retained

Data obtained from the Natural History Study (Neul et al. 2014).

The period of childhood is often marked by difficult feeding or persistent primary aspiration associated with feeding, as well as, poor somatic growth. For these issues, gastrostomy feeding is strongly recommended (Motil et al. 2009). This is a relatively straightforward procedure that should be coupled with fundoplication, particularly if gastroesophageal reflux is problematic. Parents of children who have had this procedure are uniform in their acceptance of the decision. One potential concern is that once puberty has been completed, it is very important to watch for more rapid weight gain, as caloric needs become less. In addition to somatic growth failure and feeding dysfunction, during childhood and adulthood, osteopenia (and bone fractures), and insufficient vitamin D levels are prevalent problems that require attention.

HAND-STEREOTYPIES

Stereotypic hand movements are pathognomonic of RTT. They appear around the time of regression, especially being associated with decline in fine motor skills. Each girl has her own repertoire of movements that may vary over time, are absent during sleep, and are often increased during periods associated with stress or anxiety. Interestingly, they also tend to decline or be absent during periods of intercurrent illness or other episodes affecting general health and well-being; a feature commented upon frequently by Andreas Rett. They may consist of hand-clapping, tapping, or hand-wringing most commonly, but can also consist of hand clasping, squeezing, or hand-mouthing (unilateral or bilateral), or feature the hands being separated with asymmetric movements including patting of clothes or others, playing or pulling her hair, and finger rubbing with unusual crossing of the fingers. The mouth and feet may also be involved to a lesser extent, but can be increased by suppressing the movements in the hands. Hand stereotypies tend to decrease with age after puberty and may become virtually non-existent in adulthood.

Awake-breathing dysrhythmia in the form of breath-holding, hyperventilation, or both occurs during wakefulness and is noted quite commonly, although not uniformly, in RTT (Glaze et al. 1987). From the Natural History Study (unpublished data), periodic breathing occurred in 77% of 653 girls with classic RTT and 61% of 112 girls with atypical RTT. It tends to appear after the regression period increasing in frequency between 5 and 15 years, and then begins to taper off with notably fewer women demonstrating significant breathing issues. As with hand stereotypies, periodic breathing is often increased by stress or anxiety-provoking issues yet goes away during sleep. Noisy breathing during sleep (snoring) is a common complaint during childhood. In such children, sleep studies are recommended to rule in obstructive issues such as enlarged tonsils or adenoid, if these are not evident on general examination. Occasionally, the sleep study will reveal evidence of central apnea. The experience of some clinicians indicates that continuous positive pressure may be helpful in relieving obstructive sleep apnea that persists despite tonsillectomy and adenoidectomy, as well as the central sleep apnea and the awake-breathing dysrhythmia, especially when it is frequent and associated with cyanosis.

SLEEP DYSFUNCTION

Sleep dysfunction is a major problem in RTT involving 70% of affected individuals. Twenty years ago, Glaze et al. (1987) described abnormal sleep patterns in individuals with RTT, including abnormal sleep stages and reduced stage rapid eye movement (REM) sleep. Common sleep problems in RTT include insomnia characterized by difficulties initiating and maintaining sleep, and prolonged night-time awakenings, as well as circadian sleep disorders characterized by irregular sleep/wake patterns. Other sleep disorders such as sleep disordered breathing, nocturnal events such as seizures and parasomnias, may also be experienced by individuals with RTT. Other medical problems including gastroesophageal reflux diseases (GERD) and constipation may contribute to disruption of sleep. Therapeutic options include maintaining a strict sleep/wake schedule, sleep hygiene including the use of light therapy, management of comorbid sleep disorders and medical problems, and pharmacotherapy, including melatonin. No approved medications exist for insomnia experienced by children; however, drugs such as trazodone and clonidine may be helpful.

EPILEPSY

Epilepsy in RTT syndrome has been reported in 50–80% of individuals, but prior reports often reflected small sample size, parent-completed questionnaires, and failure to consider the specific *MECP2* mutation. Using the Rare Disease Clinical Research Consortium (RDCRC) National Health Service (NHS) study database, epilepsy was evaluated based on classic or variant RTT, *MECP2* mutation, clinical severity, and presence, frequency, and treatment of seizures (Glaze et al. 2010). In 2008, 360 (60%) parents or caregivers reported seizures including 315 (60%) with classic and 45 (61%) with atypical RTT; however, physician assessment of these individuals indicated that 48% had seizures. Individuals who were regarded as having seizures were noted to have greater overall clinical severity with substantially increased difficulties with ambulation, hand use, and communication. Specific *MECP2* mutations were most frequently associated with seizures, p.Thr158Met (74%) and p.Arg106Trp (78%), whereas others mutations were associated less commonly, but still represented a significant percentage of these individuals, p.Arg255X and p.Arg306Cys (both 49%).

Seizures were noted infrequently before age 2 years and tended not to occur after age 20 years. Seizures begin to appear after age 2 years, but reach their peak, as with periodic breathing, during the period from age 5 to 10 years and then increase less through the next 5 years. At any given time, approximately 30–40% of children with RTT will have clinical seizures, while by age 16, 86% will have had seizures at some period from age 2.

Beginning around age 2, the EEG becomes decidedly abnormal with slowing background rhythms and multifocal epileptiform spike or spike-wave activity (Glaze 2005); however, this does not translate to clinical epilepsy in general. As such, clinical events resembling seizures must be compared by simultaneous video-EEG recording to verify whether these are actually epileptic in nature or are associated with some other event such as periodic breathing or other non-epileptiform event. No evidence exists that these are modified in any way by standard antiepileptic medication(s) and utilization of them is regarded as an unnecessary risk exposure.

Numerous different medications have been utilized for documented seizures, but the greatest experience in the United States has been with carbamazepine and lamotrigine (Glaze et al. 2010). Slightly more than one-half were managed on no medication (20%) or a single antiepileptic drug (37%), whereas 8% required three medications. A smaller number, about 12–13%, had either received a vagal nerve stimulator or had been on the ketogenic diet, in addition to being on antiepileptic medication. In some children, topiramate or levetiracetam was an effective agent, but a number of children who had untoward side effects were also noted.

SCOLIOSIS

Scoliosis is present in most individuals (85%) with RTT by age 16 (Percy et al. 2010); however, the mean age of individuals with scoliosis was 15 years and those without was 6 years. Surgical correction of scoliosis was required in 13% of cases. Most parents reported a remarkably better quality of life for those following surgery (Kerr et al. 2003). From analyses of multiple risk factors, overall clinical severity score, later acquisition, loss of or absent walking, and constipation were associated with scoliosis. Two of the most common *MECP2* mutations, p.Arg294X and p.Arg306Cys, had reduced risk for scoliosis.

More recent information indicates a striking relationship between the occurrence of scoliosis and ambulation skills. In stepwise fashion, increasing difficulties with ambulation is noted between no scoliosis, scoliosis without surgery, and scoliosis with surgery.

GASTROINTESTINAL DYSFUNCTION

The greatest change in natural history has been recognized over the past 10–15 years with respect to the frequency of gastrointestinal dysfunction and difficulties in multiple other features of RTT (Motil et al. 1999). It is clear that gastrointestinal dysfunction may provide an explanation for many other evident abnormalities including growth and nutrition, periodic breathing, sleeping, self-abusive behaviors, and even the so-called absent spells. Issues with GI dysfunction may run the gamut of the alimentary canal including chewing and swallowing, esophageal, gastric, and intestinal function, as well as gallbladder function. As such, gastrointestinal dysfunction is a major source of concern for many of the clinical issues of RTT and should be ruled out before moving on to consider other possibilities.

SEXUAL MATURATION

Sexual maturation in terms of age at menarche in RTT occurs nearly at the same time as in typically developing females (12.5 years), namely, about 13.0 years (Killian et al. 2014). This is one aspect that parents should not associate with much greater concern. Nevertheless, 25–28% reach puberty prematurely, 4–5% are delayed, and nearly 20% have delayed onset of menarche. Furthermore, the median time from onset of puberty to onset of menarche is 3.9 years versus 3.0 years in typically developing females. Regardless of the timing, this does place women with RTT at risk for unwanted exploitation. Systems should be in place to prevent unwanted contact. Typical menstrual management strategies can be employed that are determined by parental wishes and the individual needs of the person with RTT. Because of concerns about bone health and excessive weight gain, we recommend avoiding the use of medroxyprogesterone acetate. Regular care by an adolescent medicine physician or a gynecologist should be considered.

QUALITY OF LIFE

The clinical features and genetics of RTT have been well studied, but examination of quality of life (QOL) is limited. From the Natural History Study (Lane et al. 2011), the impact of clinical severity on QOL among female children and adolescents with classic RTT was examined over 2 years in more than 200 participants from 5 to 18 years of age (Lane et al. 2011). After adjusting for their *MECP2* mutation type and age at enrollment, the association between clinical status and QOL was evaluated. Poor physical QOL was significantly associated with worse motor function and earlier age at onset of RTT stereotypies, but better psychosocial QOL. On the reverse side, poorer psychosocial QOL was associated with better motor function, or stated differently, psychosocial QOL assessment for children and adolescents with RTT is inversely related to their level of motor function.

Understanding the caregiver QOL for RTT is also critical. Utilizing the Optum SF-36v2 Health Survey in the NHS, physical QOL was found to be superior to mental QOL, as seen in other disorders (Killian et al. 2016). However, increased disease severity in the girls or women with RTT led to poorer physical and better mental QOL while problems related to feeding led to decline in both scores. In addition, if the caregivers' personal time was limited or if there was conflict at home, the physical QOL was adversely affected.

In the NHS, more than 97% or individuals with RTT, either classic or atypical, live at home. For classic RTT, 17 (2.2%) live in a group home and three (0.4%) in an institution; for atypical, three (2.1%) live in an institution.

The North American Database, created through the International Rett Syndrome Foundation, was assessed to evaluate longevity in a large cohort (1928 individuals with RTT) from the USA and Canada (Kirby et al. 2010). With birth-date data extending well into the mid-20th century, most respondents had survived into middle age, the 50% mean survival being just beyond 50 years. Mortality was greater for individuals with typical than those with atypical RTT. These data indicate that significant longevity is possible for individuals with RTT and supports the need for careful planning for long-term care of these women.

A recent analysis of survival (Tarquinio et al. 2015b) provided a quite different perspective from that of Kerr et al. (1997). With the improvement in diagnosis, health maintenance, nutrition, and physical, occupational, and communication therapies, not only has survival improved, but also the cause of death is rarely related to extreme frailty associated with malnutrition. For both classic and atypical RTT, survival was greater than 70% at age 45. Still, the leading cause of death remains a cardiorespiratory event, reminding us that we need to be ever mindful of these issues.

Conclusion

RTT is a complex disorder, with a wide range of neurobehavioral and systemic abnormalities. However, even more challenging than its frequently severe symptomatology is its dynamic nature. Therefore, a careful characterization of the natural history of the disorder is critical. This has been pursued since the early characterizations of RTT because of the seminal observations of Andreas Rett and Bengt Hagberg and the early proponents of international collaboration, as noted by Kathy Hunter and Alison Kerr. Nonetheless, it has only been in the past two decades, in part since the identification of mutations in the gene, *MECP2*, and the elaboration of clearly defined consensus criteria that large-scale studies have demonstrated the temporal aspects and relationships between clinical manifestations. In the future, we will learn more about the challenges of adulthood with RTT and probably also about subtle developmental abnormalities before obvious symptoms emerge, filling, in this way, gaps of knowledge. Advancements in our understanding of the evolution of RTT will also come from applying new technologies for data collection, such as devices for measuring autonomic or motor function, and improved data analysis. Ultimately, greater knowledge about the natural history of RTT will inform clinical practice and the development of novel treatments for this unique disorder.

REFERENCES

Einspieler C, Kerr AM, Prechtl HF (2005a) Is the early development of girls with Rett disorder really normal? *Pediatr Res* 57(5 Pt 1): 696–700.

Einspieler C, Kerr AM, Prechtl HF (2005b) Abnormal general movements in girls with Rett disorder: The first four months of life. *Brain Dev* 27(Suppl 1): S8–S13.

Glaze DG (2005) Neurophysiology of Rett syndrome. *J Child Neurol* 20(9): 740–746.

Glaze DG, Frost JD Jr, Zoghbi HY, Percy AK (1987) Rett's syndrome: Characterization of respiratory patterns and sleep. *Ann Neurol* 21(4): 377–382.

Glaze DG, Frost JD Jr, Zoghbi HY, Percy AK (2010) Epilepsy and the natural history of Rett syndrome. *Neurology* 74(11): 909–912.

Hagberg B, Witt-Engerström I (1986) Rett syndrome: A suggested staging system for describing impairment profile with increasing age towards adolescence. *Am J Med Genet* 24(Suppl 1): 47–59.

Hagberg B, Aicardi J, Dias K, Ramos O (1983) A progressive syndrome of autism, dementia, ataxia, and loss of purposeful hand use in girls: Rett's syndrome: Report of 35 cases. *Ann Neurol* 14(4): 471–479.

Kerr AM, Armstrong DD, Prescott RJ, Doyle D, Kearney DL (1997) Rett syndrome: Analysis of deaths in the British survey. *Eur Child Adolesc Psychiatry* 6(Suppl 1): 71–74.

Kerr AM, Webb P, Prescott RJ, Milne Y (2003) Results of surgery for scoliosis in Rett syndrome. *J Child Neurol* 18(10): 703–708.

Killian JT, Lane JB, Cutter GR et al. (2014) Pubertal development in Rett syndrome deviates from typical females. *Pediatr Neurol* 51(6): 769–775.

Killian JT Jr, Lane JB, Lee H-S et al. (2016) Caretaker quality of life in Rett syndrome: Disorder features and psychological predictors. *Pediatr Neurol* 58: 67–74.

Kirby RS, Lane JB, Childers J (2010) Longevity in Rett syndrome: Analysis of the North American Database. *J Pediatr* 156(1): 135–138 e1.

Lane JB, Lee H-S, Smith LW et al. (2011) Clinical severity and quality of life in children and adolescents with Rett syndrome. *Neurology* 77(20): 1812–1818.

Motil KJ, Schultz KJ, Browning K, Trautwein L, Glaze DG (1999) Oropharyngeal dysfunction and gastroesophageal dysmotility are present in girls and women with Rett syndrome. *J Pediatr Gastroenterol Nutr* 29: 31–37.

Motil KJ, Morrissey M, Caeg E, Barrishs JO, Glaze DG (2009) Gastrostomy placement improves height and weight gain in girls with Rett syndrome. *J Pediatr Gastroenterol Nutr* 49(2): 237–242.

Neul JL, Jane B, Lee H-S et al. (2014) Developmental delay in Rett syndrome: data from the natural history study. *J Neurodev Disord* 6(1): 1–20.

Percy A (2011) Rett syndrome: Exploring the autism link. *Arch Neurol* 68(8): 985–989.

Percy AK, Lee H-S, Neul JL et al. (2010) Profiling scoliosis in Rett syndrome. *Pediatr Res* 67(4): 435–439.

Rett A (1966a) Uber ein eigenartiges hirnatrophisches Syndrom bei Hyperammonamie im Kindesalter. *Wiener Medizinische Wochenschrift* 116: 723–726.

Rett A (1966b) *Uber ein cerebral-atrophisches Syndrom bei Hyperammonaemie.* Wien: Bruder Hollinek.

Schultz RJ, Glaze DG, Motil KJ et al. (1993) The pattern of growth failure in Rett syndrome. *Am J Dis Child* 147: 633–637.

Schultz R, Glaze D, Motil K, Hebert D, Percy AK (1998) Hand and foot growth failure in Rett syndrome. *J Child Neurol* 13: 71–74.

Tarquinio DC, How W, Neul JL et al. (2015a) Age of diagnosis in Rett syndrome: Patterns of recognition among diagnosticians and risk factors for late diagnosis. *Pediatr Neurol* 52(6): 585-91 e2.

Tarquinio DC, Hou W, Neul JL et al. (2015b) The changing face of survival in Rett syndrome and MECP2-related disorders. *Pediatr Neurol* 53(5): 402–411.

Witt Engerström I (1992) Age-related occurrence of signs and symptoms in the Rett syndrome. *Brain Dev* 14:(Suppl): S11–S20.

3
THE CLINICAL GENETICS OF RETT SYNDROME

Hayley Archer, John Christodoulou and Angus Clarke

Introduction

Pediatricians are usually the clinicians who first encounter a child with suspected Rett syndrome (RTT) on their journey to a diagnosis. Once they reach the clinical geneticist, many of the primary investigations have already been carried out and the family will have often already been given the diagnosis by the pediatrician or the pediatric neurologist. The family will attend the genetics clinic for further information about the clinical aspects of RTT, its pattern of inheritance, and the recurrence risks. The context may be very different if the patient being assessed is an adult with profound impairments who has not had a diagnostic evaluation for 2 or 3 decades. It will be important to understand what has triggered the reassessment and to learn what investigations have been performed. This section of the chapter discusses the clinical and investigative approach to a child with suspected RTT. The differential diagnosis is discussed later in this chapter.

The child with suspected RTT is usually, although not always, female. Enquiry into the early history aims to identify prenatal factors that may have caused brain injury. Was the mother unwell in some way during the pregnancy? Was there exposure to teratogens, such as drugs or infections? Was placental function adequate? Has there been any postnatal evidence of perinatal problems on ultrasonic, X-ray, or magnetic imaging? The possibility of perinatal hypoxia or infection should be considered. Preterm birth is unusual in RTT, as is intrauterine growth retardation, but neither excludes the diagnosis. In the neonatal period, infection, seizures, or metabolic disturbances may have caused developmental issues.

The primary presentation of RTT is often of a child who was making 'adequate' progress but in whom delay then became apparent, followed by concerns that she might have lost skills. The regression may have been first recognized around the time of an immunization (e.g. the MMR triple immunization against measles, mumps, and rubella). This co-occurrence is usually irrelevant and potentially confusing, unless there is clear evidence of encephalitis. Some parents report regression occurring with infection. This will usually be another distracting coincidence, although there may be rare instances when infection has played a role in the regression. In RTT, it is unusual for seizures to occur immediately prior to the onset of regression and this should trigger a different diagnostic pathway relating to the epileptic encephalopathies of infancy.

In RTT, the regression is usually gradual and always finite. RTT shows some overlap with the features of the autism spectrum disorder (ASD), but the *Diagnostic and Statistical Manual of Mental Disorders*, 5th edition (DSM-5; APA 2013) no longer includes RTT as one of the ASDs. As in RTT, regression is temporary in the ASDs, but the clinical picture does not usually include loss of manual dexterity and locomotor skills. Hand stereotypy and loss of social interaction are part of the autistic picture, but in RTT the loss of social interaction is usually temporary. Persistence of autistic features is more common in those with the preserved speech variant (Neul 2012). These mildly affected children with RTT may have an early label of atypical autism; the diagnosis is often only considered in later years when scoliosis develops. Hand stereotypy and breathing irregularity may be subtler, only manifesting when the person is anxious (as when entering the clinic room).

Ongoing regression implies a neurodegenerative process that requires further investigation. Metabolic disorders, including storage disorders, need to be considered and excluded by investigation. Mitochondrial abnormalities may be found in some but, unless a clear diagnosis emerges, this could still represent part of the RTT spectrum (Clarke et al. 1990). MRI brain imaging may provide clues to the underlying pathogenesis in some neurodegenerative disorders. An MRI of the brain in RTT is usually normal, though the brain will most often be small and occasionally interpreted as 'cerebral atrophy' on the basis of a single scan.

Adults with undiagnosed intellectual disability may also present to the genetics clinic. The early history is often lost if parents are no longer able to attend appointments. In older individuals in addition to the other differential diagnoses, the effects of antipsychotic drugs may also need to be considered. The clinical picture may be of a lady with hand stereotypies, who walks with support, and may have occasional words. She may demonstrate other signs of RTT, such as scoliosis, epilepsy, and breathing irregularity. The diagnosis is much more difficult in an older person but, when made, is often helpful as the carers are then better able to understand the particular needs and interests of their client.

History of the genetics of Rett syndrome

COMPETING MODELS OF INHERITANCE

Once the RTT clinical entity had been recognized as the evolving temporal pattern of a single diagnostic entity (Rett 1966 [in German]; Rett 1977 [in English]; Hagberg et al. 1983), thoughts turned to its causation. The condition was known to be rare and to affect girls almost exclusively. It was thought likely to be genetic in origin rather than an acquired condition because of the sex asymmetry and because no association with infection or other potential trigger had been noted. Other disorders restricted to females were known and it was suggested that pattern of inheritance most resembled the X-linked dominant, male-lethal (XDML) pattern of inheritance found in incontinentia pigmenti. The one difference would be that in RTT, the girls were too severely impaired to reproduce, so that every case would represent a new mutation.

This model would account for many of the clinical observations, including the sometimes striking differences in severity between affected females in the same family. Such differences would be expected, even when two individuals had precisely the same mutation, as a result of the anticipated differences in pattern of X chromosome inactivation

(XCI) between females. This would be especially evident in monozygous twins, where the phenotypic differences could be especially striking.

An alternative explanation for the almost complete female preponderance was proposed by Thomas (1996). The same observations could be explained if the gene were on the X chromosome and if all (or almost all) mutations occurred at spermatogenesis: (almost) all cases would then be females. This has turned out to be the case.

Before turning to the research that led to the identification of *MECP2* as the RTT gene, we will briefly detour through some of the other avenues that turned out afterward to have been distractions. This area is examined in more detail elsewhere (Clarke et al. 2001). One observation that tantalized some Swedish scholars emerged from genealogical work on the families of females with RTT in Sweden; this showed that many females in Sweden could trace their ancestry back to just a few localities (Akesson et al. 1996). Models that could account for this were proposed but were complex and implausibly inelegant. Another suggestion that appeared unlikely, but remained a formal possibility until 1999, was that of metabolic interference for a locus on the X chromosome. This would affect only heterozygous females (and, similarly, males with a 47,XXY constitutive karyotype). Such mechanisms are very rare but an example, craniofrontonasal dysplasia, has recently been elucidated (Twigg et al. 2013). A model that would account for the features of RTT would be especially complex, involving interactions between the X chromosome and autosomal loci (Buhler et al. 1990).

Finally, before turning to the molecular genetics, mention should be made of aspects of the RTT phenotype that have received less attention recently; whether they will turn out to have been distractions is still not entirely clear. In particular, a range of metabolic anomalies, some indicating mitochondrial dysfunction such as impairment of ornithine carbamoyltransferase or elevated lactic acid (Haas et al. 1986; Clarke et al. 1990, 2001), as well as structural and morphological mitochondrial abnormalities (Jellinger et al. 1990; Eeg-Olofsson et al. 1989; Ruch et al. 1989; Wakai et al. 1990; Dotti et al. 1993; Cornford et al. 1994), and reduced enzyme activity measured in muscle biopsies and skin fibroblasts from patients (Eeg-Olofsson et al. 1989; Armstrong 1992; Dotti et al. 1993; Ruch et al. 1999) have been reported in a proportion of affected girls. However, most of this work was published before the usual genetic basis of RTT had been clarified and it has not recently been re-examined.

DISCOVERY OF THE CAUSATIVE GENE

Two routes to the discovery of 'the gene' appeared available: cytogenetic anomalies, especially translocations where the X chromosome breakpoint might indicate the RTT locus and families with multiple cases. Several X chromosome translocations were identified in females with RTT-like phenotypes, but these did not lead to the RTT locus. Indeed, as these cases would be expected to be affected as severely as if they were males, they 'should' have died *in utero* if the XDML model of RTT had been accurate. The few familial cases were investigated intensively by several teams, seeking to identify those sections of the maternal X chromosome shared by two affected sisters (or half-sisters). Most families studied had only two affected individuals (full sisters, sometimes twins) (e.g. Curtis et al. 1993), and these efforts depended upon assumptions that often turned out (in hindsight) to have been false. The most helpful study proved to be of an extensive Brazilian family with obligate female carriers and a male with a neonatal onset encephalopathy, so that phase was known in the linkage analysis (Schanen et al. 1998). This led the Baylor group to focus their gene sequencing efforts on plausible candidate loci at Xq28, leading to the recognition that mutations in the *MECP2* locus are the usual cause of classic RTT (Amir et al. 1999).

The fact that males carrying a mutation that would usually cause RTT in a female, but instead are affected by a more severe encephalopathy rather than RTT, is not surprising, given what is known of X chromosome biology. It does, however, point to some interesting consequences. Males with a classic RTT phenotype and a pathogenic *MECP2* mutation are usually either mosaic for a somatic mutation or have Klinefelter syndrome (47,XXY); in either case, their cells are functionally mosaic with some being MeCP2-competent and the others MeCP2-incompetent. This suggests that the RTT phenotype emerges from a brain that is mosaic for expression of the MeCP2 protein.

As expected, there is a relationship between the *MECP2* gene mutation and the severity of the phenotype (e.g. Cheadle et al. 2000; Cuddapah et al. 2014; Neul et al. 2014). This relationship is statistically robust, but is complicated by differences in pattern of XCI. It is difficult to study this directly and the studies that have done so indicate a need for caution in attempting to predict the clinical severity of an affected girl from the pattern of XCI in her peripheral blood leukocytes (Gibson et al. 2005; Archer et al. 2007). This topic is pursued further in Chapter 4 of this volume.

Differential diagnosis of Rett syndrome

RTT is a disorder of profound learning difficulty with a typical clinical history. One of the important features of classic RTT is a limited period of regression, which includes loss of social contact, verbal communication, manual dexterity, and locomotor skills. A striking feature is the development of hand stereotypies and another is the autonomic dysfunction that presents during or after regression, with episodes of hyperventilation and breath-holding. Individuals with RTT have small cold peripheries and, in severe cases, chilblains. There are clinical criteria that define classic RTT (Neul et al. 2010). The greatest diagnostic challenges arise with those who do not fulfill the RTT diagnostic criteria, but whose phenotype is reminiscent of RTT; those with a less obvious period of regression, who have not regressed in all the required areas, or those with an early and severe presentation. Another area of diagnostic difficulty lies with the RTT-like boys who present with intellectual disability, stereotypies, and breathing irregularity. The key features and genes associated with the disorders most often considered in the differential diagnosis of RTT are shown in Table 3.1. Note that many of these are associated with hyperventilation.

RETT SYNDROME AND ITS VARIANTS

Classic RTT is usually caused by mutations in the *MECP2* gene; only 5% do not have an identifiable alteration (Neul et al. 2010, 2014). Alterations in the *FOXG1* gene are often identified in the 'congenital variant' of RTT, but this term may be thought of as a misnomer because there is no regression and so patients do not fulfill the criteria even for atypical RTT

TABLE 3.1
Differential diagnoses of RTT; most are associated with breathing irregularity

Category	Syndrome	Genetic or metabolic investigation	Key clinical features	Sex prevalence
RTT and RTT-like	RTT	*MECP2*	See diagnostic criteria	Predominantly female
	CDKL5 (EIEE2)	*CDKL5*	Early severe epilepsy before 12 months of age	Predominantly female
	'Congenital' RTT	*FOXG1* (may be found on array CGH)	Markedly abnormal development before 6 months of age Movement disorder	Male and female
Angelman and Angelman-like	Angelman syndrome	Methylation *UBE3A*	Love of water No regression Difficult epilepsy	Male and female
	Pitt-Hopkins syndrome	*TCF4*	Distinctive face No regression	Male and female
	MEF2C	*MEF2C* (most found on array CGH)	Distinctive face	Male and female
	Christiansen syndrome	*SLC9A6*	Angelman-like males	Mostly males
	Pitt-Hopkins-like syndrome 2	*NRXN1*	Pitt-Hopkins-like May have early seizures	Male and female
	Pitt-Hopkins-like	*CNTNAP2*	Pitt-Hopkins-like ID seizures	Male and female
Joubert and Joubert-related spectrum disorders	Joubert syndrome	Numerous genes	Early (neonatal onset) panting Molar tooth sign on MRI brain scan Renal cysts and other physical anomalies	Male and female
Metabolic	Lysosomal storage disorders	Lysosomal enzymes	Ongoing regression and a variety of physical signs	Male and female
	Mucopolysaccharidoses: an important subgroup of the lysosomal storage disorders	Screening by urinary glycosamino-glycans	Ongoing regression Typical physical signs	Male and female
	Glut 1 deficiency syndrome 1	*SLC2A1*	Early seizures Low CSF glucose and lactate	Male and female
Chromosomal/ other genetic/ syndromal cause	Numerous deletion and some duplication syndromes	Array CGH or exomic sequencing	Likely to have additional features, e.g. dysmorphology, organ anomalies	Male and female

CGH, comparative genomic hybridization; CSF, cerebrospinal fluid; ID, intellectual disability; MRI, magnetic resonance imaging.

28

(Florian et al. 2012). Only a single case has been reported as meeting the criteria for classic RTT (Philippe et al. 2010). All have a movement disorder that may include chorea, athetosis, hyperkinesis, stereotypies, and/or dystonia (Papandreou et al. 2016).

Mutations in the *CDKL5* gene were thought to cause the early seizure (Hanefeld) variant but, as more cases have been ascertained, it has been recognized that this is a clinically distinct disorder (Fehr et al. 2013). The differential diagnosis of the early seizure variant includes many of the infantile epileptic encephalopathies (Mastrangelo et al. 2012). Those with *MEF2C* alterations, usually found on array comparative genomic hybridization (CGH), also present with early seizures but have less hand stereotypy and tend not to regress. The key difference is that they have a distinctive facial phenotype with hypotonic facies, broad forehead, tented upper lip, large ears with fleshy ear lobes, widely spaced teeth, and mildly upslanting palpebral fissures (Zweier and Rauch 2012).

ANGELMAN AND ANGELMAN-LIKE CONDITIONS

Aside from the RTT variants, the most frequently encountered differential diagnoses of classic RTT are Angelman syndrome and its close phenotypic relations. Angelman syndrome is well recognized amongst pediatricians for the distinctive facial appearance, cheerful disposition, broad-based unsteady gait, hand flapping, and typical EEG changes (Clayton-Smith and Laan 2003). Christiansen syndrome is an X-linked Angelman-like condition, which predominantly affects males. Apart from the Angelman-like features, an X-linked family history of intellectual disability, ophthalmoplegia (found in some), rapid activity on EEG, and persistent issues with weight gain may be helpful clues (Gifflian et al. 2008). Making a diagnosis of Christiansen syndrome is important, as the recurrence risk for a further affected boy is usually 25%, whereas the recurrence risk for the other Angelman-like conditions is usually low but is 50% in a small number of Angelman syndrome families. Pitt-Hopkins syndrome causes a characteristic dysmorphic appearance with features such as a notably wide mouth, distinctive facial profile, and facial coarsening with age (Zweier et al. 2008). Other clues to the diagnosis are lack of regression, long slim fingers, long slim feet, and myopia. Seizures and hyperventilation, when they arise, usually occur after 5 years of age.

OTHER CONDITIONS

Other conditions to consider in a child with suspected RTT include the Joubert spectrum disorders, which often present with episodic panting in early life that resolves with time (Kamdar et al. 2011). There are various other physical abnormalities that are not usually associated with RTT, such as retinal dystrophy, and renal and hepatic abnormalities. The 'molar tooth' sign on MRI brain imaging is extremely helpful in diagnosing Joubert syndrome, though it is not pathognomonic of this group of conditions. Most of the Joubert related spectrum disorders are autosomal recessive with a recurrence risk of 25% for a further affected child.

A range of metabolic and neurodegenerative disorders are most commonly considered in the differential diagnosis during the period of regression, when the full features of classic RTT may not yet have manifested.

Congenital anomalies, dysmorphic facial features, and brain malformations are very rarely reported in RTT and usually indicate an alternative diagnosis.

NEW GENETIC TECHNOLOGIES AND RETT SYNDROME

Other syndromal diagnoses may be identified by array CGH studies, where a chromosomal deletion or duplication syndrome may be identified. Next generation sequencing for RTT-like disorders, with the simultaneous analysis of a panel of loci associated with RTT or RTT-like phenotypes, may enable professionals to target their investigations in the most appropriate way. The simultaneous analysis of many genes will identify the correct molecular diagnosis for many children. Whole exome sequencing, which involves sequencing the coding regions of all known protein-coding genes, is beginning to supersede array CGH. While this has the potential to identify some smaller deletions and duplications, mosaicism, and sequence alterations, numerous challenges remain before the interpretation of sequence variants can be managed at high volumes. Furthermore, although there have been exciting advances in the capability of genetic technology, testing will not currently identify the underlying molecular genetic basis of the phenotype for everyone. For some, the diagnosis will remain clinical. For managing these cases, a good understanding of the differential diagnosis will be important.

Molecular genetic basis of Rett syndrome

MECP2 AND CLASSIC RETT SYNDROME

Classic RTT is usually caused by a mutation in the *MECP2* gene. Mutations are much less frequently identified in those with atypical RTT, with the exception of the preserved speech variant and other milder atypical presentations, where a mutation is often identified. There are eight common point mutations in *MECP2* that arise at CpG hotspots. In addition, C-terminal deletions and exonic deletions are frequently found. Together, these 10 mutation types account for up to 85% of pathogenic alterations in *MECP2* (Neul et al. 2010, 2014).

PATHOGENESIS OF RETT SYNDROME VARIANTS

MECP2 mutations are very rarely found in the more severe RTT variants – the early seizure (Hanefeld) and congenital variants. Mutations in the *CDKL5* gene have been found in many thought to have the Hanefeld variant (Bahi-Buisson et al. 2012). The phenotype associated with *CDKL5* mutations is more commonly of a severe clinically distinct early onset epileptic encephalopathy or West syndrome, rather than the Hanefeld variant of RTT (Weaving et al. 2004; Fehr et al. 2013). *FOXG1* mutations were initially found on array CGH and subsequent sequence alterations found in some with the congenital variant of RTT (Ariani et al. 2008). In addition, there have been a number of recent reports of individuals with the so-called FOXG1 disorder phenotype who had large deletions in the 14q13 region, but not encompassing *FOXG1*, suggesting that there may be important sequences in the deleted region which are long range regulators of *FOXG1* expression (Ellaway et al. 2013).

THE PROBLEM OF VARIANTS OF UNKNOWN SIGNIFICANCE

Molecular genetic investigation will often yield a clear result; however, genetic alterations of uncertain pathogenicity may be found, that is, variants of unknown significance (VOUS).

These are difficult to classify for several reasons. Most often, the variant has not been identified in a person with RTT before. A careful investigative approach aimed at categorizing the variant may fail to provide a clear answer regarding its significance. Molecular approaches include parental studies to identify whether the mutation has arisen de novo, whether there has been a change of charge on the corresponding amino acid, an *in silico* approach to elucidate pathogenicity, and base conservation across species and prediction of the effect of the alteration on RNA transcripts and protein structure. Further in vitro studies of RNA and functional work mostly occur in a research setting and so are not routinely available. VOUS are increasingly being identified as genetic technology progresses to whole exome and genomic approaches to genetic investigation.

Genetic modifiers of the clinical picture associated with *MECP2* mutations

The clinical variability associated with each mutation in *MECP2* is vast and can only partially be explained by our current knowledge of other genetic modifiers. Our current knowledge is limited to the effects of XCI and of variation in the *BDNF* gene. There have been no studies to date to evaluate the molecular basis of clinical variability associated with mutations in either the *CDKL5* or *FOXG1* genes.

X-CHROMOSOME INACTIVATION

X-chromosome inactivation (XCI) is the process by which one of the X-chromosomes is randomly selected for switching off during blastogenesis. In RTT, and in X-linked dominant conditions, when skewing of XCI occurs, it is usually preferentially towards expression of the normal allele (Archer et al. 2007). The degree to which XCI is skewed, particularly in the brain, will have an effect on the clinical picture. The clinical utility of XCI studies is limited because X-chromosome studies on lymphocytes may not accurately reflect the XCI pattern in the brain, or indeed regional variation within the brain (Gibson et al. 2005; Watson et al. 2005). Attempts have been made to evaluate phenotypes in large groups of patients with the same *MECP2* gene alteration (Cuddapah et al. 2014). Genotype–phenotype correlations, taking into account XCI, can only be made when large numbers of patients are included and should also include a robust method for determining the direction as well as the extent of skewing (Archer et al. 2007). The pattern of XCI in peripheral blood leukocytes only accounts for approximately 20% of the variance in clinical severity, perhaps reflecting the limited correlation between the XCI patterns in leukocytes and in various regions of the brain, leaving open the impact of other complex genetic influences on the clinical severity in RTT (Archer et al. 2007).

EFFECT OF THE BDNF POLYMORPHISM

Variation in the *BDNF* gene at codon 66 is referred to as the common *BDNF* polymorphism. Genotype–phenotype studies and RTT population studies have demonstrated that those with the val/met alleles rather than val/val or met/met are more likely to have severe disease (Ben-Zeev et al. 2009). Those with the p.Arg168X mutation and val/met are more likely to have epilepsy. In another study, the val/val polymorphism was associated with earlier seizures (Nectoux et al. 2008).

Effects of variations within the *MECP2* untranslated region and introns are not widely described and have rarely been demonstrated as causing RTT (Saxena et al. 2006). Key regulatory elements are contained within the untranslated regions of genes. There is evidence that deletions on chromosome 14, close to the *FOXG1* gene, but not including it, give rise to the clinical picture of FOXG1 disorder (Ellaway et al. 2013). In two cases, a reduction in the level of FOXG1 was demonstrated, implying that the deletion caused misregulation of FOXG1 expression. Effects of more remote changes on *MECP2* expression are not well understood.

Genetic counseling in the context of Rett syndrome

FRAMING THE PROBLEMS

Genetic counseling is the process through which families are enabled to find out more about a (likely) genetic condition in the family and through which they are supported in adjusting to the diagnosis and making decisions about it. The first element of genetic counseling is listening with the professionals listening to the concerns and questions of the client, patient, or family; these concerns may be spoken or unspoken, but both must be heard. Then the professionals gather information about the affected person in the family – the patient – and the family as a whole. This will involve asking questions about the patient and the rest of the family and will often involve examining the patient and arranging investigations. Then – perhaps after a long interval if it is necessary to wait for test results – the professionals do their best to answer the family's questions.

The parents' questions about serious problems with their child's development will often include the wish for an explanation as to why their child has such problems – the nature of the condition and its genetic basis – and may also relate to the making of practical life decisions, and better when based upon accurate information. Questions may relate to the child's future – the likely course of the condition or of the child's life and any scope for treating or ameliorating the condition. Many families also have questions about reproductive options. Accurate information about the risk of recurrence for such a condition in the family and the applicability of different approaches to rational treatment will often require a thorough knowledge of the molecular pathology in each affected individual.

Genetic diagnosis and counseling also gives access to the relevant family support groups and to additional sources of information. Through genetic counseling, the clinical geneticist and genetic counselor help families to understand their situation and their choices, as well as support them in adjusting to their new situation and making their decisions.

Families come to the genetics clinic with different questions. This is often dependent upon where they are in the diagnostic process and which phase of life they are in. The initial question is usually centered on establishing the diagnosis. If there is a diagnosis, information about the condition and what they should expect as their child becomes older is sought. Parents are frequently concerned about prognosis and whether this can be predicted through genetic testing. They usually want to know if their child will survive to adulthood. Initially, there is a concern about premature loss of a child. Later, this may change into concern about planning for the future as the parents age. Parents may wonder where the mutation arose.

For couples of childbearing age, there may be questions about the possibility of recurrence in a future pregnancy and the options available to them. If they have a new partner, the question may be raised again. As their healthy children grow up, the parents and their other children may be concerned about the chances of affected children arising in the next generation, for the nieces or nephews of the affected individual. The genetics clinic provides a space within which these difficult questions about RTT and related disorders can be explored by families at their own pace.

DECISIONS ABOUT TESTING

For children with an intellectual disability, the family's initial question is often about the diagnosis. What has caused the problem? What is it called? Those parents who have realized that their child's developmental progress is seriously impaired may be actively looking for an answer and, indeed, relieved to find one. Other parents may not be ready for a diagnostic label for many reasons, perhaps because they are still coming to terms with the idea that their child's progress may be slower than that of their peers. Perhaps they would prefer to cope with their child's problems as they arise. Parents are often – very appropriately – frightened of what the diagnosis and its implications for the future might be. The way in which the diagnosis is given will live on with the parents and may affect their ability to accept it. For many parents, the diagnosis of RTT or an RTT-related disorder will cause enormous distress, however earnestly they want a name for the condition. The diagnosis, particularly in a very young child, takes away the hope of a 'normal' future. The information about the condition, particularly of other problems that may develop, can cause additional distress. Parents may also be aware, through the internet, of the increased mortality rate in RTT and feel as though they are sitting on a time bomb. Careful explanation about the condition and the problems that may arise can alleviate some of the fears. Sometimes a number of sessions are required, though this may not always be feasible within service constraints. Time usually heals the acute distress, although it will leave a long-lasting sadness that may recur intermittently in a more intense form, triggered by a variety of circumstances over the years. When a diagnosis is made in an older patient, whose parents have long ago recognized the gravity of the condition, the parents may feel relief that there is finally an explanation for their child's problems; at this stage other parents may be indifferent to the diagnosis as it tells them nothing they have not already discovered for themselves with the passage of time.

When the question of diagnosis is raised in an adult with an intellectual disability, the advantages and disadvantages of making a diagnosis for that individual must be carefully considered. If there is a conceivable benefit to the individual, then genetic testing may be appropriate. Sometimes it is possible to make a clinical diagnosis; however, many adults are in care and it may be difficult or impossible to find out key information about their early history. This makes a purely clinical diagnosis of RTT much more difficult. If it would cause distress to the affected person to go through a diagnostic assessment, especially if that entailed venepuncture or sedation for imaging studies, then it may be difficult to justify. Each case will require a careful assessment of the best interests of the affected individual, although this can incorporate a recognition of their place within a wider family network for whom the value of a confirmed diagnosis in the patient may be greater than it would be to the patient themselves. To what extent investigations may be justified by the possibility of rational treatments yet to be developed is another consideration, but could be exploited by investigative enthusiasts at the expense of raising too many false hopes.

If a child attends the clinic with a clinical diagnosis of RTT, the questions are often different. If a mutation is identified in a gene, the parents often enquire as to what the mutation means for their child's general and developmental prognosis. They may also have heard of XCI studies or the *BDNF* polymorphism and wonder about their value in giving a prognosis. It is not possible to provide accurate information about prognosis based on a particular mutation, even if XCI and *BDNF* polymorphism status is known. This question is discussed in Chapter 4, on genotype–phenotype relationships. The best clue to a child's long term outcome at any age is likely to be their current clinical severity and their developmental progress so far. Parents may also wonder what the mutation means for healthy siblings and close relatives.

If a child does not have an alteration in the *MECP2* gene but has a clinical diagnosis of RTT, parents often feel uncertainty. Is the diagnosis correct? Why was a mutation not found? What are we going to do about having more children? Can we risk this happening again? If the child has classic RTT, the lack of a mutation is most likely due to the limitations of the technology for genetic testing. The technology does not detect all disease-causing mutations and does not explore the non-coding regions of *MECP2*. Even those with atypical RTT, according to the new diagnostic criteria, are still most likely to have RTT, even if a mutation is not found. However, for some there may be an alternative underlying genetic basis.

For those with a suspected RTT-like disorder but without clear evidence of regression, a question mark remains over the diagnosis. It is not possible to provide accurate information to families when the diagnosis is not known and they can find this disconcerting. The hope, that new technologies may extend our understanding of RTT-like phenotypes, can provide encouragement to families. At present, this is a growing area of research, but caution is needed if we are to avoid unfairly raising expectations.

Perhaps even more confusing than the complete failure to find a mutation in the *MECP2* gene is the identification of a variant of unknown significance, a VOUS. This often leads to genetic testing of a number of healthy relatives to see whether the alteration has arisen as a de novo event, or whether it is present in perfectly healthy family members (especially hemizygous males). Further testing often does not provide the answer. This leaves uncertainty over the genetic basis of the child's condition and even over the diagnosis itself.

For those parents whose child has an alteration in one of the other genes associated with a RTT-like clinical picture, they often ask whether their child has RTT, what they should expect the future to hold for their child, and whether there are other parents who have similarly affected children. The finding of an alteration in a different gene can mean changing the name of their child's diagnosis, sometimes after many years. This can be difficult for families to adjust to. However, others feel relief, as their child's problems may never really have fitted in with those of others given a definite and confirmed diagnosis of RTT.

There is a worldwide effort to search for rational therapies and treatments for people with RTT (see Chapter 14 on therapies). If identified, these may also be of benefit to those with RTT-related disorders. Whilst at present it may be difficult to justify working toward a diagnosis in some individuals, if effective therapies are found then an early diagnosis would become increasingly important, as early treatment may affect the long term outcome.

REPRODUCTIVE ISSUES

Once a child has a diagnosis, parents may ask questions about the implications for future children. They often wait until the diagnosis in their child becomes clear before considering extending their family. Reproductive decision-making is a very personal process that requires a sensitive and specialist approach. The genetic counselor carefully facilitates the couple's exploration of their views on prenatal testing in the face of the stated (usually rather low) level of genetic risk. Discussions can address how the couple might make decisions about embarking upon a pregnancy, about prenatal diagnosis and, just possibly, the question of the selective termination of an affected pregnancy. Some of the topics addressed and questions raised may be personally challenging and difficult for one or both members of the couple; the tightrope of remaining sensitive and empathic, whilst dealing with sensitive and challenging information, may need to be walked.

Reproductive decision-making is preferably discussed in advance of a pregnancy. This allows time for the couple to consider their options in an unpressured situation. For the moment, prenatal testing usually remains an invasive procedure that carries a risk of miscarriage. Couples will need carefully to weigh up the risks and benefits of a prenatal test alongside their predicted risk of having a further affected child. For some, the chance of having a child with a chromosome problem such as Down syndrome is more likely than the chance of having a child with RTT or related disorder. The risk of recurrence of RTT may be considered alongside the risk of a completely different problem arising. This perspective can help people make difficult decisions.

If a couple decide that they would like prenatal testing, they need to inform their genetic service at an early stage in the pregnancy. Parents may feel more confident in extending their family once they are aware of the available prenatal testing options.

RECURRENCE RISKS IN RETT SYNDROME AND RELATED DISORDERS

Recurrences of RTT in the same family are uncommon but not rare. The recurrence risk for RTT caused by *MECP2* mutations is less than 1% if there is no identifiable mutation in the maternal lymphocytes. This risk equates to the germline mosaicism risk, that is, the chance that there is a mutation in a proportion of either the mother's oocytes or the father's spermatogonia.

Assessing from which parent the mutation arose (parent of origin) is not routine clinical practice, although this does affect the recurrence risks. More than 90% of mutations in the *MECP2* gene are of paternal origin and arise during the process of spermatogenesis (Trappe et al. 2001; Zhu et al. 2010; Zhang et al. 2012). There is only one reported case of paternal germline mosaicism where RTT recurred in a second child (Evans et al. 2006). Parental origin has not always been determined, even when there has been a familial recurrence, so if the mutation is of paternal origin, the recurrence risk is likely to be low although a precise risk cannot be given. There is less than a 10% chance of the mutation being of maternal origin, although the mother is unlikely to be a carrier. If a healthy mother has a *MECP2* mutation in her white blood cells, she would be considered a 'carrier' of an *MECP2* mutation if she was unaffected by the condition herself. Her healthy status is usually a consequence of skewing of XCI favoring the normal *MECP2* allele. When a mother does carry the mutation (constitutionally, not in mosaic form), the risk of recurrence is 50% for both male and female offspring; an affected daughter would have RTT and an affected son a more severe, usually lethal, neonatal-onset encephalopathy. If the mother is not a constitutional carrier of the *MECP2* mutation, there is a gonadal mosaicism risk of about 1%, that is, where there is a mutation harbored in a proportion of her oocytes.

Recurrences of *CDKL5* mutations, another X-linked 'dominant' condition, also appear to be rare. There are over one hundred reported cases in the medical literature and more than this in RettBASE (http://mecp2.chw.edu.au). So far, there has been only one reported case of maternal germline mosaicism and no cases of healthy carrier mothers (Weaving et al. 2004). There are no studies on the parent of origin of the mutations. Whilst there are no scientific papers on recurrence risk, the evidence so far suggests that the recurrence risk is low.

FOXG1 mutations cause a severe autosomal dominant RTT-like condition. The recurrence risk for this condition is yet to be determined, but is likely to be confined to germline mosaicism; so far, there have been few reported familial cases (McMahon et al. 2015).

GENETIC TESTING OF THE WIDER FAMILY

Healthy relatives of affected individuals with RTT or related disorders may seek genetic counseling to discuss their risk of being a carrier and of having an affected child themselves. This is clearly different to offering a genetic test for a sibling or relative with severe learning difficulties where there is a question about the diagnosis.

Genetic testing for carrier status would not usually be offered until a healthy child has reached their country's age of majority, or the age of consent for sexual intercourse and/ or marriage where that is younger. However, genetic counseling is appropriate at any age, even long before the age of majority, to allow the child to ask their own questions about the condition in their family and how it may affect them. The family will usually have discussed the situation with the child in an age-appropriate way as he or she has been growing up alongside their affected sibling, so that the child will then have lived through powerful and sometimes difficult experiences that may enable them to discuss the issues with real insight and maturity at a young age.

Unless the mother of an affected and a healthy daughter is known to be a carrier for one of the X-linked dominant conditions, the chances of the healthy daughter being a carrier are very low. The reason is that a number of rare events would have to occur, not simply a single rare event. First, the mother would need to be a gonadal mosaic for the X-linked condition. She would then have to pass the alteration to the unaffected daughter, who would require skewed X-chromosome inactivation in order to be unaffected. The chance of this sequence of two rare events occurring is very low. However, a daughter may choose to have a genetic test, effectively for reassurance, although the discussion around testing should always help to prepare the individual for the unlikely event of a positive (unfavorable) or an incidental, unanticipated result. The chance of healthy siblings having an alteration in one of the autosomal dominant genes is extremely low, although a test could be offered for reassurance.

However, if the mother of an affected girl carries a mutation in *MECP2* or *CDKL5*, the risk of her healthy daughter being a carrier is low, but not zero. The chance of the mother's healthy sister being a carrier is very low, although she may be concerned and seek testing. Genetic counseling should allow the consultand to explore her feelings about possibly being a carrier, and what that might mean to her now and in the future. Possible female carriers should be given the opportunity to consider how they might feel if they knew they were a carrier rather than simply at risk, and how they might feel if they received a different result to one of their sisters.

PRENATAL TESTING FOR RETT SYNDROME AND RELATED DISORDERS

Although the recurrence risks for the conditions discussed in this chapter are generally low, many families will consider prenatal genetic testing. This may provide the confidence to proceed with another pregnancy.

There are various options available to families. The first is that they may elect to have no testing at all and wait to see whether the infant develops problems. Alternatively, they may choose to have a test during pregnancy, either of a chorionic villus sample or of amniotic fluid. These are invasive tests and there is a risk of miscarriage for both, which, though small, is dependent upon the operator. There is also a chance that the sample may not be suitable for analysis. By using these invasive prenatal techniques, the presence or absence of the known genetic alteration can be confirmed.

There may also be a useful role for non-invasive prenatal testing through the examination of the cell-free DNA in the mother's blood for the specific mutation found in the family. This could be used to look for a recurrence of RTT to a couple, although we are not aware of this having yet happened.

Some couples may elect to have a genetic test that will enable them to avoid a potential termination of pregnancy. Pre-implantation genetic diagnosis (PGD) is an in vitro fertilization technique that permits the selection of embryos that do not harbor the family's known genetic mutation. Only embryos without the family's mutation would be implanted. This technology is available in many countries, through public or private health services. Some PGD centers will only offer their services to couples with a high recurrence risk. The couples considered to be at high risk of a recurrence would be carrier mothers of X-linked conditions such as *MECP2* and *CDKL5*, or those with chromosomal rearrangements that create an increased risk of recurrence of *FOXG1*. There may also be maternal age restrictions for treatment. Different centers have different pregnancy success rates and this should be considered in selecting a PGD center. The process of PGD is often stressful as well as expensive and lengthy – it can be 'draining' in many ways.

Conclusion

The clinical genetic approach allows careful evaluation of the individual and their family regarding the suspected diagnosis of RTT. This will allow the clinician to address the concerns expressed by the family and to supply additional information and advice that they may find helpful, concerning the natural history of the condition and the practical and emotional adjustments they may be able to make in living with the condition. Furthermore, a correct diagnostic label will become increasingly important as new rational therapies are developed for RTT and related disorders.

Affected adults, as well as children, should be able to access genetics services or specialized neurology clinics, not only to enhance the understanding of their carers, but also to facilitate access to the best current management and to the anticipated new treatments as they develop in the future.

Although there have been, and will be further, exciting advances in genetic technology and the molecular evaluation of disease, there will be some cases where it does not prove possible to identify the underlying genetic basis: the clinical geneticist will keep these cases under review, aiming to determine the cause of the patient's disease phenotype as knowledge advances. For those where a molecular cause is eventually found, its precise nature will be highly relevant in determining which therapy or treatment is most appropriate. It is likely that disease mechanisms of fundamental biological importance remain to be determined through the pursuit of understanding the basis of disease in particular individuals. Equally, efforts to understand those aspects of the disease phenotype that have so far resisted investigation, such as the intriguing metabolic aspects of RTT, are likely to repay the efforts of biomedical scientists with both new insights and improved patient outcomes.

REFERENCES

Akesson HO, Hagberg B, Wahlstrom J (1996) RTT, classical and atypical: Genealogical support for common origin. *J Med Genet* 33: 764–766.

Amir RE, van den Veyver IB, Wan M, Tran CQ, Francke U, Zoghbi HY (1999) RTT is caused by mutations in X-linked MECP2, encoding methyl-CpG-binding protein. *Nat Genet* 23: 185–188.

APA (2013) Diagnostic and Statistical Manual of Mental Disorders, 5th edition, DSM-5. Washington, DC: American Psychiatric Association.

Ariani F, Hayek G, Rondinella D et al. (2008) FOXG1 is responsible for the congenital variant of Rett syndrome. *Am J Hum Genet* 83: 89–93.

Archer HL, Evans JE, Leonard H et al. (2007) Correlation between clinical severity in patients with RTT with a p.R168X or p.T158M MECP2 mutation, and the direction and degree of skewing of X chromosome inactivation. *J Med Genet* 44: 148–152.

Armstrong DD (1992) The neuropathology of Rett syndrome. *Brain Dev* 15: 103–106.

Bahi-Buisson N, Villeneuve N, Caietta E et al. (2012) Recurrent mutations in the CDKL5 gene: Genotype:phenotype relationships. *Am J Med Genet* 158A: 1612–1619.

Ben-Zeev B, Bebbington A, Ho G et al. (2009) The common BDNF polymorphism mat be a modifier of disease severity in RTT. *Neurol* 72: 1242–1247.

Buhler EM, Malik HJ, Alkan M (1990) Another model for the inheritance of RTT. *Am J Med Genet* 36: 126–131.

Cheadle JP, Gill H, Fleming N et al. (2000) Long-read sequence analysis of the MECP2 gene in RTT patients: Correlation of disease severity with mutation type and location. *Hum Molec Genet* 9: 1119–1129.

Clarke A, Gardner-Medwin D, Richardson J et al. (1990) Abnormalities of carbohydrate metabolism and of OCT gene function in the RTT. *Brain Dev* 12: 119–124.

Clarke AJ, Schanen C, Anvret M (2001) Towards the genetic basis of RTT. In: Kerr A and Witt-Engerstrom I, editors. *Rett Disorder and the Developing Brain*. Oxford: Oxford University Press, 27–56.

Clayton-Smith J, Laan L. (2003) Angelman syndrome: A review of the clinical and genetic aspects. *J Med Genet* 40: 87–95.

Cornford ME, Phillipat M, Jacobs B, Scheibel AB, Vinters HV (1994) Neuropathology of Rett syndrome: Case report with neuronal and mitochondrial abnormalities in the brain. *Neuroped* 26: 63–66.

Cuddapah VA, Pillai RB, Shekar KV et al. (2014) Methyl-CpG-binding protein 2 (MECP2) mutation type is associated with disease severity in Rett syndrome. *J Med Genet* 51: 152–158.

Curtis ARJ, Headland S, Lindsay S et al. (1993) S: X chromosome linkage studies in familial Rett syndrome. *Hum Genet* 90: 551–555.

Dotti MT, Manneschi L, Malandrini A, De Stefano N, Caznerale F, Frederico A (1993) Mitochondrial dysfunction in Rett syndrome: An ultrastructural and biochemical study. *Brain Dev* 15: 103–106.

Eeg-Olofsson O, al-Zuhair AG, Teebi AS, al-Essa MM (1989) Rett syndrome: Genetic clues based on mitochondrial changes in muscle. *Am J Med Genet* 32: 142–144.

Ellaway C, Ho G, Knapman A et al. (2013) 14q12 microdeletions excluding FOXG1 give rise to the congenital variant Rett syndrome-like phenotype. *Eur J Hum Genet* 21: 522–527.

Evans JC, Archer HL, Whatley SD, Clarke AJ (2006) Germline mosaicism for a MECP2 mutation in a man with two Rett daughters. *Clin Genet* 70: 366–368.

Fehr S, Wilson M, Downs J et al. (2013) The CDKL5 disorder is an independent clinical entity associated with early onset encephalopathy. *Eur J Hum Genet* 21: 266–273.

Florian C, Bahi-Buisson N, Bienvenu T (2012) FOXG1 related disorders: From clinical description to molecular genetics. *Mol Syndromol* 2: 153–163.

Gibson JH, Williamson SL, Arbuckle N, Christodoulou J (2005) X chromosome inactivation patterns in brain in Rett syndrome: Implications for the disease phenotype. *Brain & Development* 27: 266–270.

Gifflian GD, Selmer KK, Roxrud I et al. (2008) SLC9A6 mutations cause X-linked mental retardation, microcephaly and ataxia, a phenotype mimicking Angelman syndrome. *Am J Hum Genet* 93: 1003–1010.

Haas RH, Rice MA, Trauner DA, Merritt TA (1986) Therapeutic effects of a ketogenic diet in RTT. *Am J Med Genet* 24: 225–246.

Hagberg B, Aicardi J, Dias K, Ramos O (1983) A progressive syndrome of autism, dementia, ataxia and loss of purposeful hand use in girls: Rett's syndrome: Report of 35 cases. *Ann Neurol* 14: 471–479.

Jellinger K, Grisold W, Armstrong D, Rett A (1990) Peripheral nerve involvement in the Rett syndrome. *Brain Dev* 12: 93–96.

Kamdar BB, Nandkumar P, Krishnan V, Gamaldo CE, Collop NA (2011) Self-reported sleep and breathing disturbances in Joubert syndrome. *Pediatr Neurol* 45: 395–399.

Mastrangelo M, Leuzzi V (2012) Genes of early onset encephalopathies: From genotype to phenotype. *Paed Neurol* 46: 24–31.

McMahon KQ, Papandreou A, Ma M et al. (2015) Familial recurrences of FOXG1-related disorder: Evidence for mosaicism. *Am J Med Genet Part A* 167A: 3096–3102.

Neul JL, Kaufmann WE, Glaze DG et al. for the Rett Search Consortium (2010) Rett syndrome: Revised diagnostic criteria and nomenclature. *Ann Neurol* 68: 951–955.

Neul J (2012) The relationship of RTT and *MECP2* disorders to autism. *Dialogues Clin Neurosci* 14: 253–262.

Neul JL, Fang P, Barrish J et al. (2008) Specific mutations in methyl-CpG binding protein 2 confer different severity in Rett syndrome. *Neurology* 70: 1313–1321.

Neul J, Lane JB, Lee H-S et al. (2014) Developmental delay in Rett syndrome, data from the natural history study. *J Neurodev Dis* 6: 20.

Nectoux J, Bahi-Buisson N, Guellec I et al. (2008) The p.Val66Met polymorphism in the BDNF gene protects against early seizures in RTT. *Neurol* 70: 2145–2151.

Papandreou A, Schneider RB, Augustine EF et al. (2016) Delineation of movement disorders associated with FOXG1 mutations. *Neurol* 86: 1794–1800.

Philippe C, Amsallem D, Francannet C et al. (2010) Phenotypic variability associated with FOXG1 mutations in females. *J Med Genet* 47: 59–65.

Rett A (1966) Uber ein eigenartiges hirnatrophisches syndrom bei Hyperammonamie im Kindesalter. *Wein Med Wochenschr* 116: 723–738.

Rett A (1977) Cerebral atrophy associated with hyperammonaemia. Chapter 16. In: PJ Vinken and GW Bruynin association with HL Klawans HL, editors. *Metabolic and Deficiency Diseases of the Nervous System III*, Vol. 26, *Handbook of Clinical Neurology*. Amsterdam: Elsevier/North Holland Biomedical Press.

Ruch A, Kurcczynski TW, Velasco ME (1989) Mitochondrial alterations in Rett syndrome. *Paed Neurol* 5: 320–323.

Saxena A, de Lagarde D, Leonard H et al. (2006) Lost in translation: Translational interference from a recurrent mutation in exon 1 of MECP2. *J Med Genet* 43: 470–477.

Schanen NC, Francke U (1998) A severely affected male born into a RTT kindred supports X-linked inheritance and allows extension of the exclusion map. *Am J Hum Genet* 63: 267–269.

Thomas GH (1996) High male:female ratio of germ-line mutations: An alternative explanation for postulated gestational lethality in males in X-linked dominant disorders. *Am J Hum Genet* 58: 1364–1368.

Trappe R, Laccone F, Cobilanschi J et al. (2001) MECP2 mutations in sporadic cases are almost exclusively of paternal origin. *Am J Hum Genet* 68: 1093–1101.

Twigg SR, Babbs C, van den Elzen ME et al. (2013) Cellular interference in craniofrontonasal syndrome: Males mosaic for mutations in the X-linked EFNB1 gene are more severely affected than true hemizygotes. *Hum Mol Genet* 22: 1654–1662.

Wakai S, Kameda K, Ishikawa Y et al. (1990) Rett syndrome: Findings suggesting axonopathy and mitochondrial abnormalities. *Paed Neurol* 6: 339–343.

Watson CM, Pelka GJ, Radeziewic T et al. (2005) Reduced proportion of Purkinje cells expressing paternally derived mutant Mecp2308 allele in female mouse cerebellum is not due to a primary skewed pattern of X-chromosome inactivation. *Hum Mol Genet* 14: 1851–1861.

Weaving LS, Christodoulou J, Williamson SL et al. (2004) Mutations of CDKL5 cause a severe neurodevelopmental disorder with infantile spasms and mental retardation. *Am J Hum Genet* 75: 1079–1093.

Zhang J, Bao X, Cao G et al. (2012) What does the nature of the MECP2 mutation tell us about parental origin and recurrence risk in Rett syndrome? *Clin Genet* 82: 526–533.

Zhu X, Li M, Pan H, Bao X, Zhang J, Wu X (2010) Analysis of the parental origin of de novo MECP2 mutations and X chromosome inactivation in 24 sporadic patients with Rett syndrome in China. *J Child Neurol* 25: 842–848.

Zweier M, Rauch A (2012) The MEF2C related and 5q14.3q15microdeletion syndrome. *Mol Syndromol* 2: 137–152.

Zweier C, Sticht H, Bijlsma EK et al. (2008) Further delineation of Pitt–Hopkins syndrome: Phenotypic and genotypic description of 16 novel patients. *J Med Genet* 45: 738–744.

4

GENETIC SOURCES OF VARIATION IN RETT SYNDROME

Sonia Bjorum Brower, Helen Leonard, Francesca Mari, Alessandra Renieri and Jeffrey L Neul

Introduction

Among people who display all the typical features of Rett syndrome (RTT) (Neul et al. 2010), loss of previously acquired language and hand skills, distinctive repetitive stereotypies, and gait abnormalities, the majority have mutations in the X-linked gene Methyl-CpG-binding protein 2 (MECP2) (Amir et al. 1999; Neul et al. 2008).

There are a variety of sources of clinical variation in RTT. Known causes of this variation include different specific mutations found within MECP2, skewing of X chromosome inactivation (XCI), and genetic modifiers. In this chapter we seek to outline and describe the known genetic sources of clinical variation in RTT and speculate on possible additional genetic causes of variation.

Classification of genotype–phenotype

The major contribution to variation in clinical severity lies in the different *MECP2* mutations. The relationship between the specific *MECP2* mutations (the genotype) and clinical severity (the phenotype) in RTT has now been studied for over a decade. Early studies (Huppke et al. 2000) comparing phenotypes between missense and truncating (nonsense and frameshift) mutations initially failed to show any robust differences. A substantial improvement was made when the truncating mutation group was divided into early versus late truncating mutations, defined with respect to the proposed nuclear localization sequence (NLS). It was found that mutations which lead to complete or partial truncation of coding regions at or before the NLS, thus disrupting the NLS, tend to have a more severe phenotype (De Bona et al. 2000; Huppke et al. 2002; Colvin et al. 2004).

More recently, two large scale studies were performed to further examine the genotype–phenotype relationship of specific mutations (Bebbington et al. 2008; Neul et al. 2008). In comparison to previous studies, the categorization of mutations has now extended into more specific classifications based on mutation type; one for each of the eight most common point mutations, one for larger DNA deletions/rearrangements, and one for C-terminal truncations.

There are eight point mutations that account for approximately 70% of mutations found in typical RTT (Bebbington et al. 2008; Neul et al. 2008). These mutations are comprised of both nonsense (p.Arg168X, p.Arg255X, p.Arg270X, and p.Arg294X) and missense (p.Arg106Trp, p.Arg133Cys, p.Thr158Met, and p.Arg306Cys) mutations, all of which are the result of C–T transitions at mutational 'hot-spots'. Another 7–12% of the mutations are small insertions/deletions in the carboxyl-terminal domain (CTD), leading to frameshift mutations and late truncation of MeCP2 protein (De Bona et al. 2000; Bebbington et al. 2008; Neul et al. 2008). Finally, large DNA deletions that remove the bulk of the coding sequence account for about 7% of identified mutations (Neul et al. 2008).

When the genotypes were categorized according to the above classifications, phenotypical differences were found in each study (summarized below) (Bebbington et al. 2008; Neul et al. 2008). In terms of both overall severity and individual clinical features, statistically significant differences could only be found at the extremes, that is, between the most severe and the least severe phenotypes. Nevertheless, some of the mutations were clearly associated with increased overall severity; specifically, the point mutations p.Arg168X, p.Arg255X, p.Arg270X, and large DNA arrangements/deletions (Bebbington et al. 2008; Neul et al. 2008) showed increased overall severity, which could be attributed to problems in specific clinical areas. As a group, people with these mutations had a greater reduction in ambulation, hand use, and language skill, as well as an earlier onset of hand stereotypies (Bebbington et al. 2008; Neul et al. 2008). Furthermore, regression tended to occur earlier in people with these mutations (Bebbington et al. 2008). Recent work has found that some of these mutations (p.Arg168X, p.Arg255X, and p.Arg270X) are associated with a greater susceptibility to develop scoliosis compared with a less severe mutation, p.Arg294X (Percy et al. 2010). Despite an increase in overall severity in people with these mutations, some clinical features may be less severe in these cases. For example, people with the p.Arg255X mutation have a lower occurrence of seizures (Glaze et al. 2010) than those people with other mutations. Thus, assessment of overall severity may not be the only measure of disease burden and the use of mutation type to judge the severity should be discouraged in the clinical practice.

At the other end of the clinical spectrum, the point mutations p.Arg133Cys, p.Arg294X, p.Arg306Cys, and CTD truncations have been found to be associated with the less severe phenotypes. As a group, they also have lower clinical severity scores and are more likely to maintain more ambulation, hand use, and language skills (Bebbington et al. 2008; Neul et al. 2008). Individuals with the p.Arg294X and p.Arg306C mutations were also found to have a lower occurrence of seizures (Jian et al. 2007; Glaze et al. 2010) and are also at a reduced risk of developing scoliosis (Percy et al. 2010).

The point mutation p.Thr158Met has been associated with an intermediate phenotype, depending on the clinical scale used to determine overall severity and the individual clinical features examined. When evaluated with one particular severity scale, the Percy scale, people with the p.Thr158Met mutations were found to have an intermediate phenotype (Neul et al. 2008). In contrast, when the Kerr scale was used, people with this mutation were found to have a more severe phenotype (Bebbington et al. 2008). The difference may be due to the different nature of the clinical severity scales as the Kerr scale has an age-dependence, whereas the Percy scale is weighted more towards early developmental features. When individual clinical features were examined, the percentage of people who were able to walk, had language skills, and hand use was intermediate compared to the other mutations (Neul et al. 2008). The risk of seizure only increased for p.Thr158Met when compared to the other mutations (Glaze et al. 2010).

The largest genotype–phenotype study in RTT was published in 2014 (Cuddapah et al. 2014). In general, the findings were consistent with previous studies described above. For example, the point mutations p.Arg168X, p.Arg255X, p.Arg270X, and large DNA arrangements/deletions were more severe. Notably, the larger sample size allowed the determination that in addition to these severe mutation groups, p.Arg106Trp, p.Arg255X, p.Arg270X, splice sites, and smaller insertions and deletions were more severely affected. In general, less severe mutation groups were diagnosed later than more severe mutation groups. Clinical severity increased over age in all groups; however, the increase was more dramatic in the less severely affected groups. This study systematically explored the genotype–phenotype relationship in atypical forms of RTT, revealing that mutations that were less severe in typical RTT had even lower severity in atypical RTT, while mutations that were more severe in typical RTT had greater severity in atypical RTT.

X chromosome inactivation as a source of variation in Rett syndrome

One of the first recognized sources of clinical variation in RTT is skewing of XCI. Although the majority of cases of RTT are caused by de novo mutations in *MECP2*, in a small number of cases, the mother also has the mutation but is unaffected (Zappella et al. 2001). One explanation for these asymptomatic carriers is skewing of XCI (Zappella et al. 2001). In most women, including most girls and women with typical RTT, the X-chromosomes are randomly inactivated, resulting in about 50% of the cells expressing genes from the paternal chromosome and 50% expressing genes from the maternal chromosome. Thus, in most people with RTT, approximately half the cells express the wild-type *MECP2* allele and half express the mutant *MECP2* allele; however, asymptomatic carriers of *MECP2* mutation have skewed XCI with most cells in the body expressing the wild-type copy of *MECP2* (Wan et al. 1999). This finding led to the hypothesis that skewing of XCI within individuals with RTT might account for some of the clinical variation observed. To examine the extent that skewing modifies the phenotype of specific mutations, Archer et al. (2006) examined the degree and direction of skewing in patients with either the p.Thr158Met or the p.Arg168X mutation and the resulting phenotype. They found that there was a correlation between clinical severity and the amount of active mutant allele; that is, the more skewing there was in the direction towards the p.Thr158Met or p.Arg168X allele, the more severe the clinical presentation. When the two mutational groups were combined, the increase in clinical severity was again correlated to the amount of active mutant allele. Finally, they determined that 19% of variance in phenotypic outcome is due to the direction of XCI (Archer et al. 2006); however, there is concern that XCI status determined on blood is not representative of XCI status in the brain (Zoghbi et al. 1990). Nonetheless, recent studies have demonstrated a consistent relationship between peripheral blood and central nervous system (CNS) patterns of XCI (Shahbazian et al. 2002; Gibson et al. 2005), with the exceptional outlier that showed marked variation in XCI between brain regions (Gibson et al. 2005). Thus, although some of the observed variance in severity can be attributed to XCI, there must be additional factors that are responsible for the phenotypic variation observed.

OTHER POTENTIAL NONCODING GENETIC CHANGES CAUSING CLINICAL VARIATION

In addition to the type of mutations and the degree and direction of XCI, there may be other unknown modifiers yet to be identified responsible for the clinical variation observed in individuals with RTT. These may be either *trans* modifiers such as sequence changes or mutations in other loci that act as genetic modifiers or *cis* modifiers. Several findings within the 3' untranslated region (3'UTR) suggest that the noncoding regions of *MECP2* may be acting as *cis* modifiers in the severity of RTT. First, the 3'UTR of *MECP2* sequence is highly conserved suggesting that this region may have a role in *MECP2* regulation (Samaco et al. 2008). Additionally, the microRNA, miR132, was found to bind to the 3'UTR and regulate MeCP2 translation (Klein et al. 2007). Finally, there are multiple polyadenylation sites in the 3'UTR which result in the generation of four 3'UTR isoforms (Coy et al. 1999). Therefore, it is possible that mutations are present in the 3'UTR in people both with, and without, mutations in the *MECP2* coding region, and that these 3'UTR mutations alter the expression level of MeCP2. One prediction from this is that there may be mutations within the 3'UTR that in themselves cause disease, which might present as RTT or as another neurodevelopmental disorder. In fact, recent reports have identified nucleotide changes within the 3'UTR of people with autism (Shibayama et al. 2004; Coutinho et al. 2007). Additionally, such alterations could be envisioned to modify the expression of mutated versions of MeCP2, which could further modify the clinical severity in RTT. Moreover, as is the case with the 3'UTR, alterations in the 5'UTR sequence may also affect severity by altering the expression of *MECP2* transcripts; however, little is known about how the 5'UTR regulates *MECP2* expression and further work is needed to understand how this regulation works and its relationship to the variation in the clinical severity of RTT.

GENETIC MODIFIERS

Beyond the sources of variation already mentioned, a theoretical source of clinical variation in RTT is sequence changes or mutations in other loci that act as genetic modifies of the severity in RTT. One approach to try to identify these *trans* modifiers is by considering likely candidates. Brain derived neurotrophic factor (BDNF) has been identified as one of these potential candidates because genetic manipulation of *Bdnf* levels in a mouse model of RTT clearly modified the phenotype (Chang et al. 2006). Additionally, a number of studies have demonstrated that manipulating *Bdnf* levels pharmacologically can also modify the phenotype. In humans, a common polymorphism is found which changes a valine at position 66 to a methionine (p.Val66Met). This change in amino acid alters the cellular trafficking and packaging of the precursor form of BDNF, pro-BDNF, which ultimately leads to less BDNF released (Egan et al. 2003). Not surprisingly, this polymorphism has been found to modify the phenotypes of neurological diseases and neuropsychiatric disorders such as Alzheimer disease, schizophrenia, and depression (Hong et al. 2011 and references therein); however, the mechanism by which this polymorphism modifies the phenotype in these illnesses is unclear. Given the evidence from the mouse model and the apparent effect of p.Val66Met allele in other neurological disorders, the relationship between p.Val66Met polymorphism and RTT has now been explored in a clinical population. Using time-to-event analysis to investigate relationships with seizure onset a combined Israeli–Australian study (Ben Zeev et al. 2009) found, as would be predicted, that those with an *MECP2* mutation who were heterozygous for the p.Val66Met allele, had overall increased clinical severity and a slightly earlier seizure onset. This increase was greater in patients who had the p.Arg168X mutation; however, a French study (Nectoux et al. 2008), which categorized seizure onset by age group, rather than treating it as a continuous variable, and did not use time-to-event analysis to account for those who may not yet have developed seizures, reported contradictory results. Further, adequately powered collaborative studies are needed to provide more insight to the relationship between the different alleles of *BDNF* and the severity of RTT in terms of seizure onset and other clinical aspects. While the exact effect *BDNF* has on the severity of RTT is not yet clear, these results demonstrate that another gene can modify the severity of RTT.

The introduction of exome sequencing technologies opens the possibility to explore other potential sources of clinical variability. A pilot study of exome sequencing in two pairs of sisters with discordant phenotypes was performed (Grillo et al. 2013). As expected, exome analysis showed the presence of approximately 50 potentially harmful rare variants in each of the four individuals; however, among these, a few dozen might be responsible for the phenotype discordance. For example, a potentially damaging change in *CNTNAP2*, a gene mutated in neurodevelopmental disorders, was found in the severely affected sisters but not in their mildly affected sisters. Similarly, the more affected sisters had damaging mutations identified in genes involved in the catabolic pathway of squalene, which has been implicated in the mouse model of RTT as altering clinical severity (Buchovecky et al. 2013). Although this was a small-scale study, it suggests that use of advanced genetic technology will allow the discovery of genetic modifiers of RTT. The highly limited number of discordant sisters limits the utility of this specific approach; however, this methodology is likely to be useful when applied systematically to a large series of individuals at the two opposite ends of the phenotypic spectrum.

Atypical Rett syndrome

In addition to typical RTT, a number of RTT variants have been identified with the four most commonly reported forms being *forme fruste* variant (Hagberg and Rasmussen 1986), Zappella variant, early seizure variant, and congenital variant. The clinical severity of these atypical forms ranges from less severe (Zappella variant, *forme fruste* variant), to more severe than typical RTT (early seizure variant and congenital variant) (Hagberg 1993). Thus, together with typical RTT, the atypical forms create a considerable continuum of severity (Fig. 4.1).

Atypical Rett syndrome with *MECP2* mutations

Similar to typical RTT, two variants, the *forme fruste* variant and preserved speech variant (PSV), are caused by mutations in *MECP2*. For most individuals, the *MECP2* mutations

RTT severity

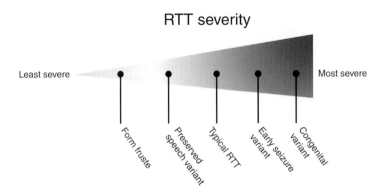

Fig. 4.1. A clinical severity continuum exists for RTT, spanning from least severe forms (*forme fruste* and preserved speech variant) to most severe forms (congenital variant and early seizure variant).

identified in these variants are those that are frequently associated with a milder typical RTT phenotype.

ZAPPELLA OR PRESERVED SPEECH VARIANT (ZAPPELLA/PSV)

Individuals with milder features of RTT, who are able to walk and have some speech, may be said to have the preserved speech variant of RTT. However, this form of RTT is characterized by other features, in addition to the preservation of some speech, as individuals with this are rather mildly affected in other ways, too. The term Zappella variant may be preferred as this Italian neuropsychiatrist described the overall pattern of this variant form of RTT (Zappella et al. 1998; Renieri et al. 2009). Clinically, they appear very different to the classic form and only experienced clinicians are likely to recognize those affected as having a form of RTT.

In this variant form of RTT, there is a recovery of some language after the regression period, ranging from single words to phrases (Renieri et al. 2009). Furthermore, although people with this variant will develop the hand stereotypies seen in typical RTT, they often have better retained hand use (Zappella et al. 1998; Zappella et al. 2001; Kerr et al. 2006; Renieri et al. 2009). A number of interesting features are found in individuals with Zappella/PSV that are not observed in typical RTT. First, it has been reported that the autistic traits first observed in the regression period continue beyond that period rather than being restricted to the regression period, as is the case in typical RTT (Zappella et al. 2003). Second, some individuals with this variant are overweight or obese, rather than suffering the much more usual growth failure (Renieri et al. 2009).

The main diagnostic handle is the persistent clinical course with four stages. At the beginning of the pseudostatinary stage (Stage 3) these people start to speak at perhaps 4 or even 5 years. Mutations found in patients with the Zappella/PSV are usually either missense mutations such as p.Arg133Cys, p.Thr158Met, p.Thr158Ala, p.Arg306Cys, or

CTD truncations (Zappella et al. 2001, 2003; Renieri et al. 2009). Occasionally, however, patients with this variant will be found to have mutations usually associated with the more severe phenotypes of typical RTT (Neul et al. 2008). This underlines the fact that other factors may influence their phenotype. The identification of other such genetic factors that influence clinical severity will be an important future direction of research.

Atypical Rett variants with mutations in other genes

The early seizure variant and congenital variant usually have a more severe phenotype than typical Rett or the other atypical Rett variants previously discussed. For both of these variants, *MECP2* mutations are less commonly found. Rather, mutations in other genes such as in *CDKL5* and *FOXG1* have at times been identified as the cause for these variants (Ariani et al. 2008; Artuso et al. 2010); however, the full spectrum of phenotypic problems associated with mutations in these genes is still being established.

Conclusion

Both typical and atypical RTT vary greatly in severity and the source of variation may be due to which locus is mutated, to which specific mutation occurs, to XCI, as well as to other genetic modifiers, most of which are yet to be identified. For typical RTT, the *forme fruste* variant and the preserved speech variant, mutations in the gene *MECP2* have been identified as the cause of RTT and the range in severity is due in part to the particular *MECP2* mutation present. For the early seizure variant and the congenital variant, mutations in *CDKL5* and *FOXG1* have been identified as the cause of these variant forms of RTT. To a limited extent, both the degree and direction of XCI affects clinical severity in individuals with *MECP2* or *CDKL5* mutations. Furthermore, polymorphisms of *BDNF* may account for some of the variation in severity observed in both RTT caused by a *MECP2* mutation and possibly also in the early seizure variant. Finally, sequence changes within the noncoding regions of *MECP2* may be a source of variation, as studies suggest that the 3'UTR may regulate MeCP2 translation and the expression of different *MECP2* isoforms.

Studies investigating the relationships between the different *MECP2* mutations and the resulting phenotypes can inform the potential clinical course a person with a particular *MECP2* mutation may take; however, the exact prediction of clinical severity for any individual is not possible unless all sources of variation are known. The pilot study on two pairs of sisters opens, for the first time, the possibility to shed light on other potential causes of variability, introducing the idea that the final phenotype of monogenic diseases may result from the combination of the mutation in the main gene together with some tens of functional variants in other genes, which may have been inherited or arisen de novo. Moreover, other potential sources of variation require additional investigation to understand their clinical implications. Understanding how each of these factors impact on RTT phenotypes will help further refine predictions of the potential clinical course of affected individuals with RTT, and help lead to personalized therapy for these people.

REFERENCES

Amir, RE, Van den Veyver IB, Wan M, Tran CQ, Francke U, Zoghbi HY (1999) Rett syndrome is caused by mutations in X-linked MECP2, encoding methyl-cpG-binding protein 2. *Nat Genet* 23(2): 185–188.

Archer H, Evans J, Leonard H et al. (2006) Correlation between clinical severity in patients with Rett syndrome with a p.R168X or p.T158M MECP2 mutation, and the direction and degree of skewing of X-chromosome inactivation. *J Med Genet* 44(2): 5.

Ariani, F, Hayek G, Rondinella D et al. (2008) FOXG1 is responsible for the congenital variant of Rett syndrome. *Am J Hum Genet* 83(1): 89–93.

Artuso R, Mencarelli MA, Polli R, Sartori S, Ariani F, Marozza A (2010) Early-onset seizure variant of Rett syndrome: Definition of the clinical diagnostic criteria. *Brain Dev* 32(1): 17–24.

Bebbington A, Anderson A, Ravine D et al. (2008) Investigating genotype-phenotype relationships in Rett syndrome using an international data set. *Neurology* 70(11): 8.

Ben Zeev B, Bebbington A, Ho G et al. (2009) The common BDNF polymorphism may be a modifier of disease severity in Rett syndrome. *Neurology* 72(14): 1242–1247.

Buchovecky C, Turley S, Brown HM et al. (2013) A suppressor screen in Mecp2 mutant mice implicates cholesterol metabolism in Rett syndrome. *Nat Genet* 45(9): 1013–1020.

Chang Q, Khare G, Dani V et al. (2006) The disease progression of Mecp2 mutant mice is affected by the level of BDNF expression. *Neuron* 49(3): 341–348.

Colvin L, Leonard H, de Klerk N et al. (2004) Refining the phenotype of common mutations in Rett syndrome. *J Med Genet* 41(1): 25–30.

Coutinho AM, Oliveira G, Katz C et al. (2007) MECP2 coding sequence and 3'UTR variation in 172 unrelated autistic patients. *Am J Med Genet B Neuropsychiatr Genet* 144B(4): 475–483.

Coy JF, Sedlacek Z, Bachner D et al. (1999) A complex pattern of evolutionary conservation and alternative polyadenylation within the long 3"-untranslated region of the methyl-cpG-binding protein 2 gene (MeCP2) suggests a regulatory role in gene expression. *Hum Mol Genet* 8(7): 1253–1262.

Cuddapah V, Pillai R, Shekar KV et al. (2014) Methyl-cpG-binding protein 2 (MECP2) mutation type is associated with disease severity in Rett syndrome. *J Med Genet* 51(3): 152–158.

De Bona C, Zappella M, Hayek G et al. (2000) Preserved speech variant is allelic of classic Rett syndrome. *Eur J Hum Genet* 8(5): 325–330.

Egan MF, Kojima M, Callicott JH et al. (2003) The BDNF val66met polymorphism affects activity-dependent secretion of BDNF and human memory and hippocampal function. *Cell* 112(2): 257–269.

Gibson JH, Williamson SL, Arbuckle S et al. (2005) X chromosome inactivation patterns in brain in Rett syndrome: Implications for the disease phenotype. *Brain Dev* 27(4): 266–270.

Glaze DG, Percy AK, Skinner S et al. (2010) Epilepsy and the natural history of Rett syndrome. *Neurology* 74(11): 4.

Grillo E, Lo Rizzo C, Bianciardi L et al. (2013) Revealing the complexity of a monogenic disease: Rett syndrome exome sequencing. *PLoS One* 8(2): e56599.

Hagberg, BA (1993) *Rett Syndrome – Clinical and Biological Aspects*. London: Mac Keith Press.

Hagberg B, Rasmussen P (1986) "Forme fruste" of Rett syndrome – a case report. *Am J Med Genet* Suppl 1: 175–181.

Hong C, Lioum Y, Tsai SJ (2011) Effects of BDNF polymorphisms on brain function and behavior in health and disease. *Brain Res Bull* 86(5–6): 287–297.

Huppke P, Laccone F, Kramer N, et al. (2000) Rett syndrome: Analysis of MECP2 and clinical characterization of 31 patients. *Hum Mol Genet* 9(9): 1369–1375.

Huppke P, Held M, Hanefeld F, Engel W and Laccone F (2002) Influence of mutation type and location on phenotype in 123 patients with Rett syndrome. *Neuropediatrics* 33(2): 63–68.

Jian L, Nagarajan L, de Klerk N et al. (2007) Seizures in Rett syndrome: An overview from a one-year calendar study. *Eur J Paediatr Neurol* 11(5): 310–317.

Kerr AM, Archer HL, Evans JC et al. (2006) People with MECP2 mutation-positive Rett disorder who converse. *J Intellect Disabil Res* 50(Pt 5): 386–394.

Klein ME, Lioy DT, Ma L et al. (2007) Homeostatic regulation of MeCP2 expression by a CREB-induced microRNA. *Nat Neurosci* 10(12): 1513–1514.

Nectoux J, Bahi-Buisson N, Guellec I et al. (2008) The p.Val66Met polymorphism in the BDNF gene protects against early seizures in Rett syndrome. *Neurology* 70(22 Pt 2): 2145–2151.

Neul JL, Fang P, Barrish J et al. (2008) Specific mutations in methyl-CpG-binding protein 2 confer different severity in Rett syndrome. *Neurology* 70(16): 1313–1321.

Neul JL, Kaufmann WE, Glaze DG et al. (2010) Rett syndrome: Revised diagnostic criteria and nomenclature. *Ann Neurol* 68(6): 944–950.

Percy AK, Lee HS, Neul JL et al. (2010) Profiling scoliosis in Rett syndrome. *Pediatr Res* 67(4): 435–439.

Renieri A, Mari F, Mencarelli A et al. (2009) Diagnostic criteria for the Zappella variant of Rett syndrome (the preserved speech variant). *Brain Dev* 31(3): 208–216.

Samaco RC, Fryer JD, Ren J et al. (2008) A partial loss of function allele of methyl-CpG-binding protein 2 predicts a human neurodevelopmental syndrome. *Hum Mol Genet* 17(12): 1718–1727.

Shahbazian MD, Sun Y, Zoghbi HY. (2002) Balanced X chromosome inactivation patterns in the Rett syndrome brain. *Am J Med Genet* 111(2): 164–168.

Shibayama A, Cook Jr EH, Feng J et al. (2004) MECP2 structural and 3'-UTR variants in schizophrenia, autism and other psychiatric diseases: A possible association with autism. *Am J Med Genet B Neuropsychiatr Genet* 128B(1): 50–53.

Wan M, Lee SS, Zhang X et al. (1999) Rett syndrome and beyond: recurrent spontaneous and familial MECP2 mutations at CpG hotspots. *Am J Hum Genet* 65(6): 1520–1529.

Zappella M, Gillberg C, and Ehlers S et al. (1998) The preserved speech variant: A subgroup of the Rett complex: A clinical report of 30 cases. *J Autism Dev Disord* 28(6): 519–526.

Zappella M, Meloni I, Longo I et al. (2001) Preserved speech variants of the Rett syndrome: Molecular and clinical analysis. *Am J Med Genet* 104(1): 14–22.

Zappella M, Meloni I, Longo I et al. (2003) Study of MECP2 gene in Rett syndrome variants and autistic girls. *Am J Med Genet B Neuropsychiatr Genet* 119B(1): 102–107.

Zoghbi HY, Percy AK, Schultz RJ, Fill C (1990) Patterns of X chromosome inactivation in the Rett syndrome. *Brain Dev* 12(1): 131–135.

5
COGNITION, COMMUNICATION AND BEHAVIOR IN INDIVIDUALS WITH RETT SYNDROME

Gillian S Townend, Walter E Kaufmann, Peter B Marschik, Rosa Angela Fabio, Jeff Sigafoos and Leopold MG Curfs

Introduction

One of the main criteria for clinical diagnosis of Rett syndrome (RTT), as defined by Neul et al. (2010), is that of 'partial or complete loss of acquired spoken language' (p. 946). For many parents, the communication difficulties experienced by their child (at any age) are one of the greatest challenges – and one of the greatest frustrations – they face. Questions of how an individual understands and interacts with the world, how they can best be helped to express themselves, how they can be educated and enabled to participate in society in a meaningful way are of fundamental importance and are grounded in the phenomenologically overlapping areas of cognition, communication, and behavior.

In this chapter, we will review the research to date and the current levels of knowledge and thinking with regard to cognition, communication, and behavior in individuals with RTT, including early development, later skills and deficits, and strategies for intervention and management.

Cognition

Relatively few studies to date have formally investigated information processing and learning abilities of individuals with RTT. By and large, this has been due to a lack of appropriate testing mechanisms and the difficulty of applying common or standardized instruments for the measurement of cognitive abilities in individuals with RTT. Traditionally, studies fall into two categories. The first assesses cognition directly [e.g. the Bayley Scales of Infant Development (Bayley 2006)] through verbal responses or manipulation tasks that require good hand control to demonstrate the development of concepts such as object permanence and means-end (cause and effect) as precursors to intentionality. The second assesses adaptive behaviors through parental/caregiver interviews and checklists [e.g. the Vineland Adaptive Behavior Scales (Sparrow et al. 2005)]. Early literature, utilizing such assessments, has tended to place individuals with RTT at a developmental age of between 1 and 18 months. A review published by Demeter (2000) at the turn of the century provides a useful synthesis of studies up to that date, pointing out the shortcomings of classical developmental tests when applied to individuals with RTT. 'If we define intelligence as the capacity to process information, we see, for instance, that the Bayley mental scales, the Uzgiris and Hunt scales and other diagnostic instruments only assess this capacity for a part of the (RTT) girls' world, a part they have showed a selective difficulty to handle efficiently. Therefore, we have to look to the interests of these girls, and use them to get a more complete image of their information processing capacity' (Demeter 2000, p. 230).

Demeter offers an alternative approach to testing based upon a parental questionnaire that recognizes differences in the types of stimuli that are of most relevance to individuals with RTT, is sensitive to the idiosyncratic and subtle ways in which individuals demonstrate learning, and accommodates fluctuations in cognitive performance and communication across time and place. More than a decade later, a review by Byiers and Symons (2012) suggests that a gap in practice still exists between knowing what form of assessment is desirable and what is available. Their review of 27 studies assessing intellectual and adaptive functioning of individuals with RTT is the most comprehensive to date and includes studies based on published and unpublished protocols, as well as estimates according to clinical judgment. In particular, they consider the appropriateness of the assessment tools utilized in the reviewed studies and conclude that 'developmental estimates for individuals with RTT based on sensorimotor assessments should be viewed with skepticism' (Byiers and Symons 2012, p. 163) and 'results of traditional cognitive assessments with individuals with RTT should not be over-interpreted' (Byiers and Symons 2012, p. 164).

Given that dys-/apraxia, or 'partial or complete loss of purposeful hand skills' (Neul et al. 2010, p. 946), is another of the main clinical features of RTT, accompanied by stereotypical hand movements, it is unsurprising that traditional tests relying on object manipulation are now recognized as inappropriate and their results called into question. In 2006, Baptista and colleagues (Baptista et al. 2006) published a study that pointed to the potential benefits of using 'new' eye gaze technologies to assess cognitive development more accurately. They showed, in a rudimentary way, through measurements of visual fixation, that individuals with RTT were capable of intentional eye gaze. Since then there has been increasing exploration of eye gaze/eye tracking technology to measure a range of cognitive processes in individuals with RTT. These forms of assessment recognize the importance of the 'intense eye communication – eye pointing' (Neul et al. 2010, p. 946), which is reported in almost all individuals with RTT. Of particular note are studies by research teams at Montefiore Medical Center in New York (Djukic and McDermott 2012; Djukic et al. 2012, 2014; Rose et al. 2013, 2016), Mackenzie Presbyterian University in São Paulo (de Lima Velloso et al. 2009; Schwartzman et al. 2015), and Boston Children's Hospital (Clarkson et al. 2017). Results to date have been mixed. Those studies which focus on measures of non-verbal cognition and visual preference/visual fixation verify a preference for social stimuli among individuals with RTT and suggest that eye gaze in RTT is intentional, thereby concluding that eye tracking technology can be used to study elements of cognition in this disorder. When using eye tracking to test attention and recognition memory (for both faces and patterns), Rose and colleagues (Rose et al. 2013), however, found that the performance of individuals with RTT was significantly poorer than their typically developing peers. When using eye tracking to test concept recognition, Velloso and colleagues (de Lima Velloso et al. 2009) had also concluded that individuals with RTT were unable to demonstrate reliable recognition of concepts of color, shape, size, and position to verbal command. A recent psychometric validation of a modified version of the Mullen Scales of Early Learning (MSEL) for individuals with RTT, which includes an eye-tracking component, confirmed average lower performance across developmental domains (Clarkson et al. 2017). However, it also demonstrated that some individuals have age- or above age-adequate abilities in the receptive language and visual reception (non-verbal) domains. This goes further than previous studies of adaptive behavior (Vignoli et al. 2010; Kaufmann et al. 2012; Barnes et al. 2015) in showing that, within the context of the aforementioned limitations, developmental skills measured by the MSEL can provide an overall assessment of cognition in RTT.

A number of studies have explored factors, such as hand stereotypies, which may influence attention in individuals with RTT (Matson et al. 2008; Fabio et al. 2009, 2011), and suggest that if the stereotypic behaviors are prevented, for example by embracing the individual or by restraining their hand, their attention to stimuli may improve. Fabio and colleagues (2016), along with other researchers, have explored associations between a broader range of cognitive, sensory, and neurophysiological features. For example, Vignoli and colleagues (2010) combined the use of EEG, eye tracking, and behavioral measures to examine links between epilepsy and cognition, whilst Stauder et al. (2006) and, more recently, Peters et al. (2015) considered links between auditory responses and (cortical) information processing. The Vignoli study (Vignoli et al. 2010) showed that the later the onset of seizures the greater the ability to respond to verbal commands, but that as seizure frequencies increase the ability to respond decreases. They also demonstrated that as the EEG abnormalities become more pronounced, cognitive performance, as marked by the ability to recognize and respond to instructions, decreases. The Stauder study (Stauder et al. 2006) tested visual and auditory event-related potentials, the results of which suggested slower information processing and reduced brain activation in a cohort of individuals with RTT compared with a control group. In the Peters study (Peters et al. 2015) measurement of gamma-band oscillatory responses during a passive voice discrimination test showed a decreased response to a familiar voice in individuals with RTT compared with individuals with *MECP2* duplication. This is tentatively interpreted as being indicative of greater social impairment in individuals with RTT. As the numbers in the study are small, however, Peters and colleagues recommend further testing in this area. Furthermore, they suggest that because 'this paradigm did not require any motor abilities or hand use, it can be more suitable as a measure of cognitive processing assessing recognition and discrimination as well as processing of socially relevant stimuli as compared to conventional behavioral/psychological measurements' (Peters et al. 2015, p. 150).

Such conclusions, pointing to limitations in cognitive capacity, seem to be at odds with the anecdotal evidence of many parents who report that their child is far more cognitively able than can be demonstrated on assessment or is suggested by current research. This mismatch may be answered, at least in part, by the apraxia which limits the ability to respond easily on command, meaning that it is not simply a matter of changing the access method for assessment of skills, but also the manner and style of presentation. At the current time, therefore, it can be concluded that although eye gaze and eye tracking technologies appear to offer the most appropriate access to assessments of cognition, there is still some way to go in order to develop robust assessments that can accurately capture the skills and abilities of individuals with RTT and that can be validated and set to appropriate norms (Byiers and Symons 2013).

Communication

COMMUNICATION SKILLS

Individuals with RTT demonstrate severe limitations in their ability to communicate through conventional channels, such as hand signs/gestures and speech (Cass et al. 2003; Urbanowicz et al. 2016a) which, according to the core clinical criteria (Neul et al. 2010), is due to a regression or loss of previously acquired skills and subsequent impairment in acquiring new ones. This is supported by findings from parental interviews and question-naire administration using population-based and international samples (Lee et al. 2013; Urbanowicz et al. 2015), which reveal that the level of expressive language acquisition is in general low, but to some extent influenced by genotype. In one study involving 542 individuals with classic RTT and 96 with atypical RTT enrolled in the US-based Natu-ral History Study, 77% of those with classic RTT were reported to have acquired single words, but only 18% phrases. Of those with atypical RTT, 94% of individuals classified as 'atypical better' acquired single words and 54% phrases, whilst only 36% of those classified as 'atypical poorer' acquired single words and 6.7% phrases (Neul et al. 2014). Analysis of early communicative behaviors through the application of retrospective video-analysis and/ or parental interviews or questionnaires, which probe the pre-diagnosis period (Tams-Little and Holdgrafer 1996; Leonard and Bower 1998; Burford et al. 2003; Fehr et al. 2011; Marschik et al. 2012a, b, 2013, 2014; Bartl-Pokorny et al. 2013; Townend et al. 2015) has shed further light on early development. This has demonstrated that in many cases devel-opment in the first year of life is not as asymptomatic as previously thought and deviations from typical development can be identified prior to, as well as after, the onset of regression. For example, with a reduction in gestural and vocal repertoire, abnormal quality of (ingressive) vocalizations, failure to reach milestones such as canonical babbling and deficits in sociocommunicative behaviors (joint attention and reciprocity).

The lack of ability to communicate is recognized as being due, at least in part, to the influence of apraxia (an inability to control purposeful, voluntary movements) (Djukic and McDermott 2012), although the extent to which this, as opposed to deeper language and/ or cognitive impairments are to blame, is a subject for ongoing debate. A number of studies have sought to probe deeper into the communicative behaviors of individuals with RTT, to explore levels of underlying intentionality and the range of functions, as well as the means by which they are able to express themselves. Sigafoos et al. (2011) offer a systematic review of eight studies that were conducted prior to 2006, whilst later studies (Hetzroni and Rubin 2006; Didden et al. 2010; Bartolotta et al. 2011; Julien et al. 2015; Urbanowicz et al. 2016b) have either collected parental reports through questionnaires and structured interviews, or applied behavioral or observational checklists (such as the Inventory of Potential Commu-nicative Acts (IPCA), Sigafoos et al. 2000a) and/or experimental paradigms. In general, their findings suggest that the majority of individuals with RTT operate at pre-linguistic, pre-intentional levels of communication, with their behaviors interpreted by caregivers and communication partners as 'potential communicative acts' (Sigafoos et al. 2000b). Behaviors may include the use of stereotyped hand movements, facial expressions, body movements, undifferentiated vocalizations, and hyperventilation, with eye gaze reported as the most frequent form of expressive communication behavior across the studies. Some authors have suggested that the eye gaze may be limited to fixating on an object, indicating need or preference at a pre-intentional level and they question whether individuals with RTT can use truly referential eye gaze, demonstrating communicative intent by switching gaze between a desired object and a partner (Cass et al. 2003; Bartolotta et al. 2011). Hetzroni and Rubin (2006), however, have demonstrated that this behavior can be trained in individuals with RTT and, more recently, Urbanowicz and colleagues have shown that eye gaze can be used effectively by some individuals with RTT to make choices and requests (Urbanowicz et al. 2016a, 2017). The functions attributed to communication behaviors are commonly acknowledged as being to seek attention, to protest, to request, and/or to make choices. At the present time there is little published literature that demonstrates the use of higher level communication skills, although there is much anecdotal evidence shared between parents and professionals, for example through Facebook posts.

Several of the aforementioned studies also point to apparently low levels of receptive language, especially when standardized tests are employed. The limitations of such tests have already been discussed and, in studies where parents have been interviewed, they frequently express the view that their children know more than they are able to express or to demonstrate on assessment (Bartolotta et al. 2011; Urbanowicz et al. 2016b) leading once more to calls for the development of more objective (eye tracking-based) language assessments, which can be used to validate data gathered from parental reports. Alongside these studies, research profiling genotype–phenotype relationships also delineate more specific speech-language profiles according to both variant and *MECP2* mutation type (Uchino et al. 2001; Kerr et al. 2006; Bebbington et al. 2008; Urbanowicz et al. 2015). In particular, those who are diagnosed with 'milder' mutations such as p.Arg133Cys (often associated with the so-called preserved speech variant, PSV), present with a somewhat milder phenotype, being likely to develop more words pre-regression and retaining or regaining an ability to speak and using single words or simple sentences post-regression, as well as retaining or regaining more control over hand function and an ability to walk (Zappella et al. 2005; Renieri et al. 2009; Neul et al. 2014; Urbanowicz et al. 2015).

COMMUNICATION INTERVENTION AND MANAGEMENT

Intervention studies employing the use of augmentative and alternative communication (AAC) to improve the communication skills of individuals with RTT are increasingly being reported in the published literature. A systematic review conducted by Sigafoos and colleagues (2009) identified nine small studies (with a total of 31 participants) in which various forms of AAC had been introduced, including the use of gestures, picture symbol boards, and computers with speech output/speech generating devices (SGDs). The authors found broadly positive outcomes related to the use of AAC for individuals with RTT; however, they cautioned that the existing corpus of studies was relatively small-scale and few in number (*n*=9 studies with a total of 31 participants) and hampered by methodological limitations, such that the benefits of these studies could not be pronounced conclusive.

Since that time further studies have, in various ways, reported on the application of AAC to individuals with RTT. Surveys of speech-language pathologists (SLPs) and parents, for example those conducted by Wandin et al. (2015) in Sweden and Townend et al. (2016) in the Netherlands, have highlighted a range of AAC systems and strategies that are utilized by SLPs working with individuals with RTT. These include the use of pictures/objects of reference, communication charts and books, single- and multi-message SGDs, and communication apps. Many of these AAC systems are based on the use of picture symbols and may be accessed through direct touch or, increasingly, through eye gaze/eye tracking technology. AAC, in general, is reported by SLPs and parents to have a positive effect on the communication of individuals with RTT, especially at the levels of choice making and requesting, which are the most frequent goals for intervention, as reported by Wandin et al. (2015). At the level of experimental design studies, more recent publications have also supported this view. Studies by Byiers et al. (2014), Stasolla et al. (2014, 2015), and Simacek et al. (2016) have aimed to teach requesting and/or choosing behaviors through the use of a voice-output micro-switch or SGD, or through the manual exchange of picture symbols. As with the earlier studies reviewed by Sigafoos et al. (2011), the numbers across the four studies are small (a combined total of 11 participants), yet the results are promising, at least in relation to the development of requesting and choice-making behaviors.

Interest in eye gaze technology as a form of access, both in relation to assessment of cognitive and comprehension skills (as described above), and as a medium for intervention, has grown in the last several years. With increasing recognition of the influence of apraxia on the communication behaviors of individuals with RTT, eye gaze is acknowledged by many to be the most appropriate and reliable access method and intervention studies utilizing eye gaze/eye tracking technology are emerging. The above-mentioned modification of the Mullen Scales of Early Learning (MSEL) (Clarkson et al. 2017) includes two independent but complementary versions, the first consisting of adaptations on response timing and size and motivation-level of objects, the second completely eye tracking-based. Although promising, the latter measure highlights the limitation of this technology, since it is restricted to assessing receptive language and visual function. At the present time, differences in opinion and practice exist in relation to goals for intervention. There is a gap between the published studies (as reported above), where materials and options are limited to small numbers of choices, and interventions reported anecdotally where individuals with RTT are introduced to broad-based 'robust vocabularies' in the form of complex communication books or dynamic screen SGDs. In the latter scenario, the expectation is that individuals with RTT can achieve if given the right access to communication and through this can access education and participation in society. It is hoped that in the near future more studies will be published in this area so that a stronger body of evidence can be formed in relation to the use and benefits of AAC for individuals with RTT.

Additional areas for intervention, which are increasingly reported in relation to individuals with RTT, include developing reading and writing skills (Fabio et al. 2013) and providing training in partner communication strategies (Bartolotta and Remshifski 2013;

Wandin et al. 2015). The beneficial effects of music and music therapy on stimulating inter-action and communication between individuals with RTT and their caregivers have also long been acknowledged (Elefant 2009; Wigram and Elefant 2009; Bergstrom-Isacsson et al. 2014).

Behavior

Although the diagnostic criteria for RTT primarily focus on communicative and motor features, behavioral abnormalities are also prominent. As reported by a recent study by Cianfaglione et al. (2015), who examined a group of 91 adults and children with RTT utilizing the 'Rett Syndrome Behaviour Questionnaire' (RSBQ) (Mount et al. 2002) and compared them with a cohort of individuals with six other syndromes associated with intellectual disability, the range of behavioral abnormalities is wide. Cianfaglione et al. (2015) found that hand stereotypies, breathing irregularities, night-time unrest, anxiety or inappropriate fear, and low or changeable mood were commonly reported in the RTT group. Self-injury was lower but, where reported, it was found to be related to over-activity and impulsivity, two features associated with milder forms of RTT and recognized predictors of self-injury in other syndromes and autism spectrum disorders (Arron et al. 2011; Richards et al. 2012). Whilst there were some differences in the weighting of behaviors between this and previously conducted studies (Mount et al. 2002; Robertson et al. 2006), that may be accounted for by the fact that previous studies reported on predominant child samples whilst Cianfaglione's cohort included both adults and children. One particularly significant feature compared to the contrast group in this study was the type of hand stereotypy observed in individuals with RTT, notably that of hand wringing. Hand stereotypies such as hand flapping may be found in other forms of intellectual disability, yet hand wringing appears to be unique to RTT and, according to Robertson et al. (2006) is especially evident in individuals with an p.Arg255X or p.Arg270X mutation but less likely in those with a p.Arg294X mutation.

The early focus on autistic behavior, which was included in the seminal publication by Hagberg and colleagues (1983), is a result of the impairment in communication, social withdrawal, and severe stereotypies that are observed during the regressive phase of RTT. Most subsequent studies have emphasized the transient nature of these autistic features and their prominence in the context of a milder phenotype (i.e. better ambulation and hand use) (Young et al. 2008). A study by Kaufmann et al. (2012), however, found that although mild autistic behavior persisted beyond regression it was relatively independent of overall clin-ical severity. Kaufmann and colleagues suggest that differences in identification of autism may be due to methodological differences and argues for further research into the RTT phenotype utilizing 'more comprehensive cognitive and behavioral batteries, and examining their associations with physiological and/or neurological data (e.g. neuroimaging, electro-encephalogram)' (Kaufmann et al. 2012, p. 245). A similar argument is presented in another study by the same group. Barnes et al. (2015) describe the first attempt to systematically examine anxiety-like behaviors in individuals with RTT using standardized assessment tools. This is an important area for evaluation as anxiety is commonly reported (Halbach et al. 2013; Anderson et al. 2014; Cianfaglione et al. 2015), with fear/anxiety behaviors most frequently seen among individuals with p.Arg133Cys and p.Arg306Cys mutations (Robertson et al. 2006). Correct identification of such behaviors, and the mechanisms and functions underpinning them, in individuals who by virtue of their communication difficulties cannot easily draw attention to how they feel or how they perceive the world, carries implications for management and therapeutic intervention and must, therefore, be taken seriously.

TREATMENT OF BEHAVIOR

Behavioral intervention strategies have been used for the management of a variety of manifestations in RTT, including sleep dysfunction (Piazza et al. 1991), feeding skills (Piazza et al. 1993), and cognitive and communication skills (Byiers et al. 2014; Fabio et al. 2013, 2016). As for other areas covered by this chapter, these studies include small series of participants with a wide age range and different methodologies. Use of applied behavioral analysis has only been either theorized (Roane et al. 2001) or anecdotally reported (reviewed by Lotan 2007). When behavioral interventions or music therapy are not employed or are considered ineffective, psychopharmacology can be the treatment of choice for anxiety-like and disruptive behaviors. Again, virtually no publications are available in this area and the use of selective serotonin reuptake inhibitors (SSRIs) for anxiety is mentioned in a few reviews focused on novel drug interventions (Chapleau et al. 2013; Kaufmann et al. 2016). The recently reported mild improvements in social avoidance in an open label trial with insulin-like growth factor (IGF-1) are encouraging, but they should be taken with caution (Khwaja et al. 2014).

Conclusion

We have come a long way in our understanding of RTT in the 50 years since Andreas Rett [see Rett (2016) for a translation into English] first described the cluster of symptoms that later came to be known as RTT. Our knowledge and understanding of the phenotypic presentations and their underlying genetics has moved on considerably since the discovery of the *MECP2* gene in 1999 and we are now gaining new insights into the biological pathways influenced by *MECP2* (Ehrhart et al. 2016a, b). We have begun to separate out aspects of communication and behavior according to mutation, but we still have much further to go to fit together all the pieces of the jigsaw. Cognition, communication, and behavior are not simply a matter of genetics, but are the result of a complex interaction within and between each individual, the people around them, their environment, and the supportive strategies and tools that are offered to them. We recognize the influence of apraxia on the ability of individuals to respond to command, for example, and to execute actions under voluntary control, and we recognize the effect of other neurophysiological, sensory, and behavioral elements on communication and cognition. More specific tools need to be developed to evaluate the cognitive and communicative abilities, as well as abnormal behaviors, of individuals with RTT appropriately and accurately. Well-conducted assessments should underpin the formulation of appropriate goals that acknowledge the potential of the individual and offer appropriate support through the use of AAC, including but not limited to eye gaze and eye tracking technology. Furthermore, advances in the development of behavioral interventions and/or neurobiologically-based drug treatments offer potential avenues for future exploration.

REFERENCES

Anderson A, Wong K, Jacoby P, Downs J, Leonard H. (2014) Twenty years of surveillance in Rett syndrome: What does this tell us? *Orphanet J Rare Dis* 9: 87.

Arron K, Oliver C, Moss J, Berg K, Burbidge C (2011) The prevalence and phenomenology of self-injurious and aggressive behaviour in genetic syndromes. *J Intellect Dis Res* 55: 109–120.

Baptista PM, Mercadante MT, Macedo EC, Schwartzman JS (2006) Cognitive performance in Rett syndrome girls: A pilot study using eyetracking technology. *J Intellect Dis Res* 50(9): 662–666.

Barnes KV, Coughlin FR, O'Leary HM et al. (2015) 'Anxiety-like behavior in Rett syndrome: Characteristics and assessment by anxiety scales. *J Neurodev Disord* 7(1): 30.

Bartl-Pokorny KD, Marschik PB, Sigafoos J et al. (2013) Early socio-communicative forms and functions in typical Rett syndrome. *Res Dev Disabil* 34(10): 3133–3138.

Bartolotta TE Remshifski PA (2013) Coaching communication partners: A preliminary investigation of communication intervention during mealtime in Rett syndrome. *Commun Dis Quart* 34(3): 162–171.

Bartolotta TE, Zipp GP, Simpkins SD, Glazewski B (2011) Communication skills in girls with Rett syndrome. *Focus Autism Other Dev Disabil* 26(1): 15–24.

Bayley N (2006) *Bayley Scales of Infant and Toddler Development: Administration Manual.* San Antonio, TX: Harcourt Assessment.

Bebbington A, Anderson A, Ravine D et al. (2008) Investigating genotype-phenotype relationships in Rett syndrome using an international data set. *Neurol* 70: 868–875.

Bergstrom-Isacsson M, Lagerkvist B, Holck U, Gold C (2014) Neurophysiological responses to music and vibroacoustic stimuli in Rett syndrome. *Res Dev Disabil* 35(6): 1281–1291.

Burford B, Kerr AM, Macleod HA (2003) Nurse recognition of early deviation in development in home videos of infants with Rett disorder. *J Intellect Disabil Res* 47(Pt 8): 588–596.

Byiers B, Symons F (2012) Issues in estimating developmental level and cognitive function in Rett syndrome. In: Hodapp RM, editor. *International Review of Research in Developmental Disabilities*, San Diego, CA: Academic Press, Volume 43, 147–185.

Byiers B, Symons F (2013) The need for unbiased cognitive assessment in Rett syndrome: Is eye tracking the answer? *Dev Med Child Neurol* 55(4): 301–302.

Byiers BJ, Dimian A, Symons FJ (2014) Functional communication training in Rett syndrome: A preliminary study. *Am J Intellect Dev Disabil* 119(4): 340–350.

Cass H, Reilly S, Owen L et al. (2003) Findings from a multidisciplinary clinical case series of females with Rett syndrome. *Dev Med Child Neurol* 45: 325–337.

Chapleau CA, Lane J, Larimore J, Li W, Pozzo-Miller L, Percy AK (2013) Recent progress in Rett syndrome and MeCP2 dysfunction: Assessment of potential treatment options. *Future Neurol* 8(1): 21–28.

Cianfaglione R, Clarke A, Kerr M et al. (2015) A national survey of Rett syndrome: Behavioural characteristics. *J Neurodev Dis* 7(1): doi: 10.1186/s11689-015-9104-y.

Clarkson T, LeBlanc J, DeGregorio G et al. (2017) Adapting the Mullen Scales of Early Learning for a standardized measure of cognition in children with Rett syndrome. *Intellect Dev Dis*, Forthcoming.

de Lima Velloso R, de Araújo CA, Schwartzman JS (2009) Concepts of color, shape, size and position in ten children with Rett syndrome. *Arquivos de Neuro-Psiquiatria* 67(1): 50–54.

Demeter K (2000) Assessing the developmental level in Rett syndrome: An alternative approach? *Euro Child Adoles Psych* 9(3): 227.

Didden R, Korzilius H, Smeets E et al. (2010) Communication in individuals with Rett syndrome: An assessment of forms and functions. *Jo Dev Phys Dis* 22(2): 105–118.

Djukic A, McDermott MV (2012) Social preferences in Rett syndrome. *Pediatr Neurol* 46(4): 240–242.

Djukic A, Valicenti McDermott M, Mavrommatis K, Martins CL (2012) Rett syndrome: Basic features of visual processing-a pilot study of eye-tracking. *Pediatr Neurol* 47(1): 25–29.

Djukic A, Rose SA, Jankowski JJ, Feldman JF (2014) Rett syndrome: Recognition of facial expression and its relation to scanning patterns. *Pediatr Neurol* 51(5): 650–656.

Ehrhart F, Coort SLM, Cirillo E, Smeets E, Evelo CT, Curfs L (2016a) New insights in Rett syndrome using pathway analysis for transcriptomics data. *Wiener Medizinische Wochenschrift* 166(11–12): 346–352.

Ehrhart F, Coort SLM, Cirillo E, Smeets E, Evelo CT, Curfs LM (2016b) Rett syndrome – Biological pathways leading from MECP2 to disorder phenotypes. *Orphanet J Rare Dis* 11(1): 158.

Elefant C (2009) Music therapy for individuals with Rett syndrome. *Int J Dis Hum Dev* 8(4): 359–368.

Fabio RA, Antonietti A, Castelli I, Marchetti A (2009) Attention and communication in Rett syndrome. *Res Autism Spectrum Dis* 3(2): 329–335.

Fabio R, Giannatiempo S, Oliva P, Murdaca A (2011) The increase of attention in Rett syndrome: A pre-test/ post-test research design. *J Dev Phys Dis* 23(2): 99–111.

Fabio RA, Castelli I, Marchetti A, Antonietti A (2013) Training communication abilities in Rett Syndrome through reading and writing. *Front Psychol* 4: 911.

Fabio RA, Billeci L, Crifaci G, Troise E, Tortorella G, Pioggia G. (2016) Cognitive training modifies frequency EEG bands and neuropsychological measures in Rett syndrome. *Res Dev Disabil* 53–54: 73–85.

Fehr S, Bebbington A, Ellaway C, Rowe P, Leonard H, Downs J (2011) Altered attainment of developmental milestones influences the age of diagnosis of Rett syndrome. *J Child Neurol* 26(8): 980–987.

Hagberg B, Aicardi J, Dias K, Ramos O (1983) A progressive syndrome of autism, dementia, ataxia, and loss of purposeful hand use in girls: Rett's syndrome: Report of 35 cases. *Ann Neurol* 14(4): 471–479.

Halbach NS, Smeets EE, Steinbusch C, Maaskant MA, van Waardenburg D, Curfs LM (2013) Aging in Rett syndrome: A longitudinal study. *Clin Genet* 84(3): 223–229.

Hetzroni OE, Rubin C (2006) Identifying patterns of communicative behaviors in girls with Rett syndrome. *AAC: Augment Alt Commun* 22(1): 48–61.

Julien H, Parker-McGowan Q, Byiers B, Reichle J (2015) Adult interpretations of communicative behavior in learners with Rett syndrome. *J Dev Phys Dis* 27(2): 167–182.

Kaufmann WE, Tierney E, Rohde CA et al. (2012) Social impairments in Rett syndrome: Characteristics and relationship with clinical severity. *J Intellect Disabil Res* 56(3): 233–247.

Kaufmann WE, Stallworth JL, Everman DB, Skinner SA (2016) Neurobiologically-based treatments in Rett syndrome: Opportunities and challenges. *Expert Op Orphan Drugs* 4(10): 1043–1055.

Kerr AM, Archer HL, Evans JC, Gibbon F (2006) People with mutation positive Rett disorder who converse. *J Intellect Dis Res* 50: 386–394.

Khwaja OS, Ho E, Barnes KV et al. (2014) Safety, pharmacokinetics, and preliminary assessment of efficacy of mecasermin (recombinant human IGF-1) for the treatment of Rett syndrome. *Proc Natl Acad Sci USA* 111(12): 4596–4601.

Lee J, Leonard H, Piek J, Downs J (2013) Early development and regression in Rett syndrome. *Clin Genet* 84(6): 572–576.

Leonard H, Bower C (1998) Is the girl with Rett syndrome normal at birth? *Dev Med Child Neurol* 40(2): 115–121.

Lotan M (2007) Alternative therapeutic intervention for individuals with Rett syndrome. *Sci World J* 7: 698–714.

Marschik PB, Kaufmann WE, Einspieler C et al. (2012a). Profiling early socio-communicative development in five young girls with the preserved speech variant of Rett syndrome. *Res Dev Disabil* 33(6): 1749–1756.

Marschik PB, Pini G, Bartl-Pokorny KD et al. (2012b) Early speech-language development in females with Rett syndrome: Focusing on the preserved speech variant. *Dev Med Child Neurol* 54(5): 451–456.

Marschik PB, Kaufmann WE, Sigafoos J et al. (2013) Changing the perspective on early development of Rett syndrome. *Res Dev Disabil* 34(4): 1236–1239.

Marschik PB, Bartl-Pokorny KD, Tager-Flusberg H et al. (2014) Three different profiles: Early socio-communicative capacities in typical Rett syndrome, the preserved speech variant and normal development. *Dev Neurorehabil* 17(1): 34–38.

Matson JL, Dempsey T, Wilkins J (2008) Rett syndrome in adults with severe intellectual disability: Exploration of behavioral characteristics. *Eur Psychiatry* 23(6): 460–465.

Mount RH, Charman T, Hastings RP, Reilly S, Cass H (2002) The Rett Syndrome Behaviour Questionnaire (RSBQ): Refining the behavioural phenotype of Rett syndrome. *J Child Psychol Psychiatry* 43: 1099–1110.

Neul JL, Kaufmann WE, Glaze DG et al. (2010) Rett syndrome: Revised diagnostic criteria and nomenclature. *Ann Neurol* 68(6): 944–950.

Neul JL, Lane JB, Lee HS et al. (2014) Developmental delay in Rett syndrome: Data from the natural history study. *J Neurodev Disord* 6(1): 20.

Peters SU, Gordon RL, Key AP (2015) Induced gamma oscillations differentiate familiar and novel voices in children with MECP2 duplication and Rett syndromes. *J Child Neurol* 30(2): 145–152.

Piazza CC, Fisher W, Moser H (1991) Behavioral treatment of sleep dysfunction in patients with the Rett syndrome. *Brain Dev* 13(4): 232–237.

Piazza CC, Anderson C Fisher W (1993) Teaching self-feeding skills to patients with Rett syndrome. *Dev Med Child Neurol* 35(11): 991–996.

Renieri A, Mari F, Mencarelli MA et al. (2009) Diagnostic criteria for die Zappella variant of Rett syndrome (the preserved speech variant). *Brain Dev* 31: 208–216.

Rett A (2016) On a remarkable syndrome of cerebral atrophy associated with hyperammonaemia in childhood. *Wiener Med Wochenschrift* 166(11–12): 322–324.

Richards C, Oliver C, Nelson L, Moss J (2012) Self-injurious behaviour in individuals with autism spectrum disorder and intellectual disability. *J Intellect Dis Res* 56: 476–489.

Roane HS, Piazza CC, Sgro GM, Volkert VM, Anderson CM (2001) Analysis of aberrant behaviour associated with Rett syndrome. *Dis Rehab* 23(3–4): 139–148.

Robertson L, Hall SAE, Jacoby P, Ellaway C, Klerk ND, Leonard H (2006) The association between behavior and genotype in Rett syndrome using the Australian Rett Syndrome Database. *Am J Med Genet B: Neuropsych Genet* 141B(2): 177–183.

Rose SA, Djukic A, Jankowski JJ, Feldman JF, Fishman I, Valicenti-McDermott M (2013) Rett syndrome: An eye-tracking study of attention and recognition memory. *Dev Med Child Neurol* 55(4): 364–371.

Rose SA, Djukic A, Jankowski JJ, Feldman JF, Rimlerd M (2016) Aspects of attention in Rett syndrome. *Pediatr Neurol* 57: 22–28.

Schwartzman JS, Velloso Rde L, D'Antino ME, Santos S (2015) The eye-tracking of social stimuli in patients with Rett syndrome and autism spectrum disorders: A pilot study. *Arq Neuropsiquiatr* 73(5): 402–407.

Sigafoos J, Woodyatt G, Keen D et al. (2000a) Identifying potential communicative acts in children with developmental and physical disabilities. *Commun Dis Quart* 21(2): 77–86.

Sigafoos J, Woodyatt G, Tucker M, Roberts-Pennell D, Pittendreigh N (2000b) Assessment of potential communicative acts in three individuals with Rett syndrome. *J Dev Phys Dis* 12: 203–216.

Sigafoos J, Green VA, Schlosser R et al. (2009) Communication intervention in Rett syndrome: A systematic review. *Res Autism Spec Dis* 3(2): 304–318.

Sigafoos J, Kagohara D, van der Meer L et al. (2011) Communication assessment for individuals with Rett syndrome: A systematic review. *Res Autism Spec Dis* 5(2): 692–700.

Simacek J, Reichle J, McComas JJ (2016) Communication intervention to teach requesting through aided aac for two learners with Rett syndrome. *J Dev Phys Dis* 28(1): 59–81.

Sparrow SS, Cicchetti DV, Balla DA, Doll EA, Firm P A (2005) *Vineland-II: Vineland Adaptive Behavior Scales*. Minneapolis, MN: PearAssessments.

Stasolla F, De Pace C, Damiani R, Di Leone A, Albano V, Perilli V (2014) Comparing PECS and VOCA to promote communication opportunities and to reduce stereotyped behaviors by three girls with Rett syndrome. *Res Autism Spec Dis* 8(10): 1269–1278.

Stasolla F, Perilli V, Di Leone A et al. (2015) Technological aids to support choice strategies by three girls with Rett syndrome. *Res Dev Disabil* 36: 36–44.

Stauder JEA, Smeets EEJ, van Mil SGM, Curfs LGM (2006) The development of visual- and auditory processing in Rett syndrome: An ERP study. *Brain Dev* 28(8): 487–494.

Tams-Little S, Holdgrafer G (1996) Early communication development in children with Rett syndrome. *Brain Dev* 18(5): 376–378.

Townend GS, Bartl-Pokorny KD, Sigafoos J et al. (2015) Comparing social reciprocity in preserved speech variant and typical Rett syndrome during the early years of life. *Res Dev Disabil* 43–44: 80–86.

Townend GS, Marschik PB, Smeets E, van de Berg R, van den Berg M, Curfs LM (2016) Eye gaze technology as a form of augmentative and alternative communication for individuals with Rett syndrome: Experiences of families in The Netherlands. *J Dev Phys Disabil* 28: 101–112.

Uchino J, Suzuki M, Hoshino K, Monura Y, Segawa M (2001) Development of language in Rett syndrome. *Brain Dev* 23: S223(Suppl 1): S233–S235.

Urbanowicz A, Downs J, Girdler S, Ciccone N, Leonard H (2015) Aspects of speech-language abilities are influenced by MECP2 mutation type in girls with Rett syndrome. *Am J Med Genet A* 167A(2): 354–362.

Urbanowicz A, Downs J, Girdler S, Ciccone N, Leonard H (2016a) An exploration of the use of eye gaze and gestures in females with Rett syndrome. *J Speech Lang Hear Res* 59(6): 1373–1383.

Urbanowicz A, Leonard H, Girdler S, Ciccone N, Downs J (2016b) Parental perspectives on the communication abilities of their daughters with Rett syndrome. *Dev Neurorehabil* 19(1): 17–25.

Urbanowicz A, Ciccone N, Girdler S, Leonard H, Downs J (2017) Choice making in Rett syndrome: A descriptive study using video data. *Dis Rehabil*: doi: 10.1080/09638288.2016.1277392.

Vignoli A, Fabio RA, La Briola F et al. (2010) Correlations between neurophysiological, behavioral, and cognitive function in Rett syndrome. *Epilepsy Behav* 17(4): 489–496.

Wandin H, Lindberg P, Sonnander K (2015) Communication intervention in Rett syndrome: A survey of speech language pathologists in Swedish health services. *Disabil Rehabil* 37(15): 1324–1333.

Wigram T, Elefant C (2009) Therapeutic dialogues in music: Nurturing musicality of communication in children with autistic spectrum disorder and Rett syndrome. In: Malloch S, Trevarthen C editors. *Communicative Musicality: Exploring the Basis of Human Companionship*, 423–445. New York, NY: Oxford University Press.

Young DJ, Bebbington A, Anderson A et al. (2008) The diagnosis of autism in a female: Could it be Rett syndrome? *Eur J Pediatr* 167(6): 661–669.

Zappella M, Mari F, Renieri A (2005) Should a syndrome be called by its correct name? The example of the preserved speech variant of Rett syndrome. *Eur J Pediatr* 164(11): 710; author reply 711–712.

6
MOTOR ABNORMALITIES IN RETT SYNDROME

Jenny Downs and Teresa Temudo

Introduction

The early descriptions of Rett syndrome (RTT) by Andreas Rett (Rett 1966, 1977) and Bengt Hagberg (Hagberg 1983) highlighted altered movement skills which are now recognized as core features of the syndrome. For most individuals, there is initial developmental progress followed by regression at around 6–30 months. The classic signs of RTT then become apparent, including loss of hand and communication skills, the development of stereotypical hand movements, and impairment of gait (Neul et al. 2010). Therefore, RTT is essentially a movement disorder. These motor difficulties are further complicated by neurological signs of altered muscle tone and dyspraxia, and the effects of comorbidities including epilepsy, autonomic dysfunction, and orthopedic complications including scoliosis, hip dysplasia, and foot deformities.

Rett syndrome is characteristically associated with a mutation located within the Methyl-CpG Binding Protein 2 (*MECP2*) gene on the X chromosome (Amir et al. 1999), and while over 200 mutations have been described in the literature, most occur in one of eight hotspots (Amir and Zoghbi 2000). Large cross-sectional and population-based studies have shown relationships between the specific mutation and phenotype and those with mutations p.Arg168X, p.Arg255X, or p.Arg270X often manifest a relatively severe phenotypic expression, while those with mutations p.Arg294X or p.Arg133Cys are milder in comparison (Bebbington et al. 2008; Neul et al. 2008). It is not clear why different *MECP2* mutations can produce a particular phenotype, but one hypothesis is that some central nervous system areas are more susceptible than others to the degree of dysfunction of this protein. The different timing of disease onset among individuals with a *MECP2* mutation and the different neurological scenarios may be partially explained by the preferential function of MeCP2 in mature, rather than immature neurons (Shahbazian et al. 2002). It is possible that a less functional protein may affect more dramatically the brainstem and cerebellar structures, provoking, for instance, such a severe hypotonia that patients can never acquire an independent gait. Alternatively, a more functional (or less disruptive) protein may not affect severely the cerebellar structures, but absence of its full functionality may still be critical for other functions and, thus, provoke a milder phenotype. In the human brain, the number of MeCP2-expressing neurons increases dramatically throughout gestation and the percentage of neurons expressing MeCP2 in the cortex continues to increase to approximately 10 years of age (Shahbazian et al. 2002; Temudo et al. 2011). This may also contribute to explanation of the motor impairments of RTT and the later features of this disorder.

The disability is severe overall and those affected usually depend on carers for assistance with most daily living activities (Leonard et al. 2001). Consistent with the International Classification of Functioning, Disability and Health (ICF) (World Health Organization 2001), RTT affects body structure and function, activities of daily living, and abilities to participate in life opportunities. These aspects of function are affected by personal factors such as age and environmental factors such as therapy. This chapter will consider motor function from each of these perspectives.

Early development

The most recent diagnostic criteria require that early development is not grossly abnormal during the first 6 months of life, as indicated by the development of the very early skills of a social smile, head control, and swallowing (Neul et al. 2010). This criterion allows for considerable variability in early development; the more severe early presentations may never demonstrate normal early development, whereas other presentations acquire more functional skills prior to regression. The Australian population-based study investigating relationships between early presentation and the underlying genotype found that girls with a p.Arg270X mutation were less mobile at 10 months of age compared to those with the p.Arg306Cys mutation (Leonard et al. 2005).

Early infancy

Prior to regression, parents often notice subtle developmental deviations during infancy. In an early study using the Australian population database ($n=127$), parents reported unusual features during early infancy, often describing their child as 'placid' (15.7%) or 'floppy' (8.7%) (Leonard and Bower 1998). In retrospective studies observing home videos of infants who later developed RTT, health visitors and some midwives identified developmental deviations from birth, particularly in the areas of posture, movement, and social contact. However, these deviations were subtle and the health visitors felt that it was unlikely they would have noticed the developmental deviations or voiced concerns to parents at the time (Burford et al. 2003). Einspieler and colleagues applied standardized measures of early spontaneous movement to home videos of infants with RTT. They found that many of the infants displayed jerky uncoordinated movements with abnormal general and fidgety movements. Abnormal facial expressions, postural stiffness, and tremulous movements were also reported in some infants. These studies provide formative evidence that in some cases motor signs of RTT may manifest within the first few months of life (Einspieler et al. 2005a, b).

Beyond early infancy

The achievement of gross motor milestones by girls who subsequently develop RTT is of interest clinically, because both the developmental course and the manifestation of the specific features of RTT are watched carefully by families and clinicians as the diagnosis of RTT evolves. During typical development, learning to sit prior to 10 months and walking unassisted before 18 months is the norm internationally (WHO Multicentre Growth Reference Study Group 2006). Infants with RTT have been described as often experiencing delay reaching motor milestones such as rolling over, crawling, and sitting (Nomura and Segawa 2005). In 293 girls born since 1999 in the Australian Rett Syndrome Database or the International Rett Syndrome Phenotype Database, most girls learned to sit (91.5%) and less than half acquired the ability to walk unassisted (46.2%) prior to diagnosis (Fehr et al. 2011). For those who learned to sit, 79.9% sat before 10 months of age and of those who learned to walk, 45.5% walked prior to 18 months, indicating considerable motor delay in some. The acquisition of these milestones also varied by mutation type, with girls who had a p.Arg255X, p.Arg168X, p.Arg270X, or early-truncating mutations being less likely to achieve these early motor milestones. Conversely, learning to sit and walk was more frequent in those with a p.Arg133Cys, p.Arg306Cys, p.Arg294X, p.Arg106Trp, or C-terminal mutation (Fehr et al. 2011). These findings have been corroborated by recent analyses by the Natural History Study where early delay in the acquisition of fine motor tasks such as reaching for objects and grasping skills during early childhood was also reported (Neul et al. 2014). More general early developmental problems may, therefore, accompany the specific features of RTT.

Regression

Regression is a key feature of RTT and manifests as a combination of motor and behavioral features. Common features include loss of acquired purposeful hand and language skills, the development of stereotypic hand movements, a loss of interest in social contact, and inconsolable crying (Hagberg 2002; Lee et al. 2013). The age at onset of regression is variable ranging from 3 months to 4 years in 293 individuals born since 1999 in the Australian Rett Syndrome Database and the International Rett Syndrome Phenotype Database (Fehr et al. 2011). Presentation can be dramatic or very subtle. There are many characteristics of regression that are not yet clear, including the rate and duration of regression and relationships with genotype, and how other developmental skills such as those in the gross motor, social, or behavioral domains are affected and over what time frame (Lee et al. 2013).

Stereotypies

Stereotypies are involuntary, repetitive, and seemingly meaningless movements (Jankovic 2005). Abnormal hand movements such as stereotypies have been observed in infants who later developed RTT when they were as young as 3 months of age (Einspieler et al. 2005a, b) and at 19 months of age before the onset of other diagnostic criteria of RTT (Temudo et al. 2007a). In a Portuguese clinical study ($n=60$) the median (25th–75th centile) age at onset of stereotypies was reported as 20 (14.5–25.0) months (Temudo et al. 2008). Over time, stereotypies may be seen in any part of the body (Temudo et al. 2007b), although are more commonly seen in the hands. Different types of hand movements are seen including joined-hands stereotypies of wringing/clasping, clapping, mouthing, washing, and other more complex movements; and single-hand stereotypies of mouthing, clasping,

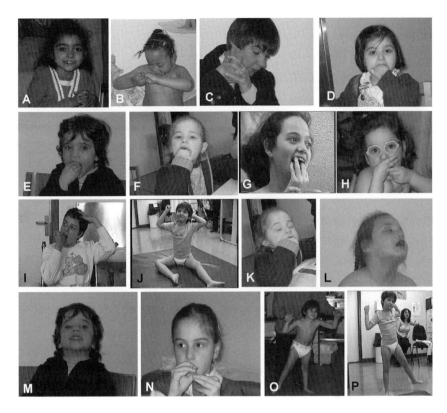

Fig. 6.1. Pictures of stereotypies of the hands including washing, mouthing, and hair pulling (A–J, N), retropulsion of the neck (K–M), and shifting of weight from one leg to the other forming part of an ataxic gait (O, P). Reproduced with permission from Wolters Kluwer Health: Neurology. Temudo et al. Stereotypies in Rett syndrome: Analysis of 83 patients with and without detected MECP2 mutations. 68: 1183–1187 © 2007.

tapping, 'sevillana', hair pulling, flapping, hand behind the neck, hair twirling, and other complex movements (Temudo et al. 2007b; Carter et al. 2010). The most common hand stereotypy seen is a midline wringing action; bruxism and trunk rocking are also commonly seen. Types of stereotypies are illustrated in Figure 6.1. In some cases, stereotypies may be so excessive that they become self-injurious; for example, there may be excessive rubbing of the hands, biting or chewing of the fingers and hands, and hand to head banging (Mount et al. 2001). Use of hand or elbow splints may be used to restrict hand stereotypies, and are recommended for specific time periods on a case by case basis, if reduction in self-injurious behaviors or better hand use can be demonstrated (Downs et al. 2014).

Predictors of stereotypies

Stereotypies in RTT become less prevalent with increasing age (Cass et al. 2003; Temudo et al. 2007b; Carter et al. 2010). In a video study undertaken on girls and women from the Australian population database ($n=144$), the median number of hand stereotypies per individual was two (range 0–6) and this number decreased with age. For example, over half (58.8%) of those younger than 8 years had three or more types of stereotypies, often including mouthing, compared with less than one-third (32.5%) of those older than 19 years. Diminishing variety of hand stereotypies is consistent with the overall picture of movement restriction in older women with RTT. Interestingly, those with independent gait have been observed to have more types of stereotypies compared to those who are unable to walk independently (Temudo et al. 2007b). Stereotypies such as hand-wringing have been observed in all categories of common mutation, although somewhat more frequently with certain mutations (C-terminal deletions, p.Thr158Met, and p.Arg294X) (Carter et al. 2010).

THE MECHANISM OF STEREOTYPIES

The physiological mechanism of stereotypies could, in part, be informed by neuroimaging studies in persons with physiological stereotypies and in those with RTT. In children with physiological stereotypies, a disproportionate reduction in volume of the frontal lobe white matter and decreased volume of the caudate nuclei were observed, suggesting that cortico-striatal-thalamo-cortical pathways may be involved (Kates et al. 2005). A relatively recent study in RTT showed selective gray matter reductions in the dorsal parietal lobe, possibly contributing to deficits in sequential movements and tactile information processing (Carter et al. 2008). Stereotypies developed before loss of hand skills in 56.6% of 83 girls with RTT, at around the same time in 30.1%, and beforehand skill loss in 13.2% (Temudo et al. 2007b). While stereotypies in RTT may relate to structural and functional abnormalities of the cortico-subcortical pathways, the precise neurobiological mechanisms related to their onset are not yet clear, nor are the functional relationships between the loss of hand function and the development of stereotypies.

Hand function

The loss of purposeful hand skills during the regression period is one of the most prominent features of RTT (Neul et al. 2010). Previously, measures of hand function in RTT have been relatively blunt and have rated hand function on a Likert scale in broad functional categories, including previous aspects of regression. More recently, a measure of hand function in RTT was developed with eight levels of function that are sequential in complexity and include skills of grasping, picking up, and holding of large and small objects (Downs et al. 2010). This eight-point scale allows greater characterization of hand function and focuses on current function, which may be amenable to change with therapeutic interventions.

HAND FUNCTION SKILLS

Total absence of hand function has been reported, although the ability to grasp has been described in 80% of girls and women, to hold an object in 70%, and self-feed in 25–43% (Cass et al. 2003; Larsson et al. 2005). Using videotaped footage of activities of daily living, our recent study assessed hand function using the above-mentioned eight-point scale on 144 girls and women with RTT (Downs et al. 2010). There was considerable variability in the hand function observed in this sample; approximately 47% (68/144) were unable to grasp or only able to hold a large object once placed in the hand and 12% (18/144) were able to grasp, pick up, and hold a large object. The remainder (40.3%, 58/144) could additionally grasp, pick up, and hold a small object, including 18 who were also able to transfer an object from hand to hand. Dyspraxia strongly influences hand function and it has been noted that the girl or woman with RTT often spends considerable time watching prior to grasping and picking up an object (Mount et al. 2002). Dystonic postures of the hands may be seen (FitzGerald et al. 1990; Temudo et al. 2008) and these also preclude hand function. Some girls cannot grasp objects, but can use switches for communication or other educative devices.

PREDICTORS OF HAND FUNCTION

A pattern of association between hand function and *MECP2* mutation type has been found, with girls and women with the p.Arg168X or p.Arg270X mutation generally having the poorest hand function whilst those with the p.Arg133Cys or p.Arg294X mutation generally have better hand function (Bebbington et al. 2008; Neul et al. 2008; Downs et al. 2010). Consistent with the thesis that functional skills in general deteriorate with age (Hagberg 2002), those who are older appear also to have the poorest hand function, although the magnitude of difference between age-groups is generally small (Downs et al. 2010). As also might be expected, milder symptoms of clinical severity, greater independence in activities of daily living, and better levels of mobility have been associated with better hand function, even after adjusting for genotype and age (Downs et al. 2010).

LONGITUDINAL COURSE OF HAND FUNCTION

Our Australian study has assessed changes in hand function in RTT over time in 72 girls and women whose family provided a video showing hand function at two time points 3–4 years apart (Downs et al. 2011). For those with some hand function at the time of the baseline video, approximately 60% retained their level of skill, a few gained skills, and the remainder lost skills. Those who had less mobility were more likely to lose skills; however, this time period of follow-up was short and more research is needed to identify the trajectory of hand function over longer periods.

Further evidence confirms general stability of hand function over time, reflected mainly in reports of self-feeding activities. A cross-sectional survey in Sweden (*n* = 121) found that many girls and women maintained self-feeding skills, and a small proportion of participants regained lost feeding abilities with training (3/46), or were taught how to self-feed when they had not previously been able to (2/38) (Larsson et al. 2005). A multiple baseline single case design study assessed a training program comprising prompting and reinforcement to promote self-feeding skills and gains were observed in five girls and women aged 3–23 years (Piazza et al. 1993). There appears to be phenotypic variability in the longitudinal course of hand function, which is likely to be related to genotype, but also influenced in some cases by motor activity including practice. Further studies are needed to define these treatment strategies more precisely.

Gross motor function

Many aspects of gross motor function are affected in RTT in association with altered muscle tone and dyspraxia, cognitive impairment, and comorbidities such as epilepsy and scoliosis. Clinical assessment is required to identify the presence of neurological signs, observation or parent-report have been used to assess functional skills, and accelerometers have been recently used to measure physical activity, namely walking as a reflection of participation in daily life. When defining gross motor function, the amount of assistance required for the performance of specific skills is typically observed. A 15-item Gross Motor Scale for Rett syndrome that assesses sitting, standing, walking, and transition skills was recently developed (Downs et al. 2008). This measure describes a broad range of gross motor skills and the calculation of sub-score values enables efficient statistical analysis with potential predictors such as age and genotype.

GROSS MOTOR SKILLS AND PHYSICAL ACTIVITY

Several large cross-sectional studies have reported gross motor function in samples of 87 (Cass et al. 2003), 125 (Larsson et al. 2005), and 99 (Downs et al. 2008) girls and women with RTT. The girls and women observed in the latter video study were broadly representative of the Australian population of girls and women with RTT, and the findings of the three studies are broadly consistent. Overall, most girls and women with RTT are able to sit (Downs et al. 2008), slightly less than half able to walk (Cass et al. 2003; Downs et al. 2008), or stand (Downs et al. 2008). For those who are able to walk, their gait may be characterized by rigidity, a lack of co-ordination in the upper extremities, and a wide base (Hagberg 2002); toe-walking and shuffling gait patterns have also been observed (Downs et al. 2008). Figure 6.1 (O, P) illustrates wide-based gait in RTT. A small proportion of individuals are able to transfer without assistance (Larsson and Engerstrom 2001; Larsson et al. 2005; Downs et al. 2008). The difficulties performing transitions are probably associated with the motor impairments of dyspraxia, altered muscle tone, and poor balance and co-ordination (Hagberg 2002). This limits spontaneity of movement and activity over the course of the day and represents a significant burden of care for families. If abilities to stand and walk are limited, many families and caregivers in developed (although not in resource-poor) countries will use specialized equipment, such as hoists, for transfers.

Physical activity involves the use of gross motor skills over the course of daily life. Understanding gross motor function, therefore, requires identification of gross motor skills to demonstrate what types of movements can be achieved and an understanding of participation in physical activity to identify how these movements are then utilized in daily life. For the general population, physical activity during childhood has many benefits, including positive effects on energy balance, bone mass, physical fitness, psychological well-being, and health benefits for later life (Biddle et al. 2004). The benefits for those with a disability are less well documented, but thus far include benefits for functional skills and fitness (Johnson 2009; Bartlo and Klein 2011). For RTT, it is believed that physical activity is important to prevent constipation and lower respiratory tract infections. Our recent study measured whole-day stepping activity using a StepWatch Activity Monitor™ (Modus Health LLC, Washington, DC) accelerometer in 12 girls and

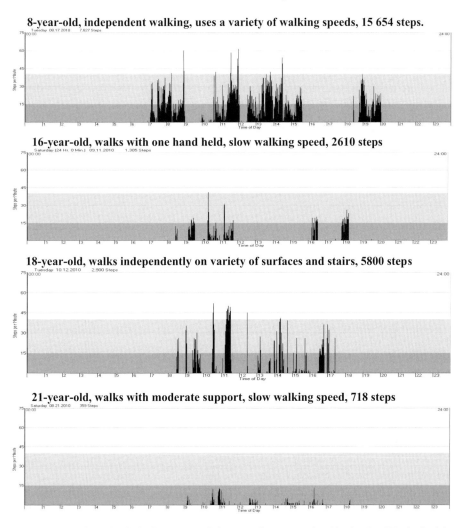

Fig. 6.2. Examples of whole-day step activity records measured with the StepWatch Activity Monitor™ (Modus Health LLC, Washington, DC) accelerometer in four individuals with RTT, illustrating variability of activity levels and the tendency for women to take less steps in a day even when able to walk.

women with RTT who were able to walk either independently or with assistance. The girls and women were sedentary for 64.8% (range 32.7–86.9%) of their awake hours, but recorded on average daily step count of 5652 ± 4185 steps (Downs et al. 2012). Figure 6.2 shows examples of physical activity over whole day periods in several girls and women with RTT. Each of these steps is important and represents an opportunity for participation in daily activities and exploration of the environment. Walking is also potentially protective against the severity of orthopedic complications such as scoliosis. Compared to those who are unable to walk, those able to walk either independently or with

69

assistance, experienced less marked progression of scoliosis after taking into account the effects of mutation group and age at scoliosis onset (Downs et al. 2016). Physical activity is a complex and multi-dimensional behavior that is affected by a composite of physical, psychosocial, and environmental characteristics (van Sluijs et al. 2007). For RTT, physical activity levels, in part, relate to complex daily needs and a very high level of dependency for daily activities (Leonard et al. 2001), but also to barriers in the provision of physical activity opportunities for persons with a severe disability. Girls and women with RTT are likely to benefit from a focus on optimal provision of physical activities in daily routines to support the maintenance of gross motor skills and the general benefits from a healthy lifestyle.

PREDICTORS OF GROSS MOTOR FUNCTION

Posture and motor control require interplay between musculoskeletal, neurological, and cognitive mechanisms in response to the requirements of the motor task and the contexts of the environment (Shumway-Cook and Woollacott 2007). Factors that could influence the level of gross motor skill and physical activity include genotype, neurological and musculoskeletal impairments, and age. Genotype influences the presentation of gross motor skills. Large cross-sectional studies have found that girls and women with mutation p.Arg270X or p.Arg168X present with a more severe phenotype in relation to motor abilities and are less likely to walk, whereas those with p.Arg133Cys, p.Arg294X, and C-terminal deletions are more likely to walk (Bebbington et al. 2008; Neul et al. 2008). Those with the p.Arg294X (Percy et al. 2010; Downs et al. 2016) or p.Arg306Cys (Percy et al. 2010) mutation are also less likely to develop scoliosis. For neuromuscular scoliosis, a larger curve can be associated with more difficulties sitting and walking (Berven and Bradford 2002). Other factors that influence the performance of motor skills in RTT include altered muscle tone, ataxia, and the poor initiation of movements consistent with dyspraxia. Over time, poorly controlled epilepsy and other orthopedic complications such as kyphosis, hip dysplasia, and foot deformities can also influence gross motor abilities. These impairments together form barriers to the development and maintenance of motor skills.

Age may influence the underlying neurological basis for movement and the performance of skills and activities. Muscle tone is typically low in younger girls, whereas increased muscle tone and rigidity are observed more commonly in those who are older (Cass et al. 2003). Following regression, motor skills may improve but over many years, the increased muscle tone and paucity of movement may contribute to loss of gross motor skills, including the ability to walk (Hagberg 2002). The findings of large cross-sectional studies are generally consistent with this view (Bebbington et al. 2008; Neul et al. 2008). A composite score describing 10 sitting, standing, walking, and transition skills was lower in older girls and women compared with those who were younger, whereas a composite score of five more complex skills such as walking on a slope or stepping over an obstacle did not vary with age (Downs et al. 2008). The greater stability of complex motor skills could represent a floor effect, but is also consistent with the finding that many older girls and women do maintain the ability to walk (Cass et al. 2003; Downs et al. 2008; Foley et al. 2011). Together, these findings illustrate variability in gross motor skills with age and highlight the need for the planning of movement opportunities for girls who maintain walking skills as they age.

The findings of cross-sectional studies can inform the course of RTT, but longitudinal studies are important to delineate more precisely how changes occur with time. Only one study has reported change in gross motor skills at different time points in the same individuals. Our Australian study (Foley et al. 2011) observed gross motor skills in 70 girls and women over a 3–4-year period, and found that skills were maintained or slightly improved in approximately 40% and slightly decreased in the remainder. Gains were more likely to have occurred in the general skills of sitting, standing, and walking, rather than more complex gross motor skills such as transition from the floor to standing. Approximately half of the individuals could walk at the initial observation and most maintained this ability over the 3-year period, with one girl learning to walk. This is important clinical information; on the one hand it was possible, but less usual, to acquire walking as a new skill but additionally, walking is a relatively stable feature of the phenotype over this time period. On the other hand, skills of sitting on the floor or a stool, transferring from sit to stand, or from the floor to standing, were more likely to decline.

There were no apparent relationships between age-group and change in the core skills of sitting, standing, and walking, although girls and women who were older showed less decline in complex skills if they were able to walk. The decline in complex gross motor skills in younger girls could have been associated with a longer than normal regression period, difficult-to-manage epilepsy during this period (Jian et al. 2007), or the development of early onset scoliosis (Downs et al. 2016). While possibly representing a survival effect, walking may have a protective influence on other motor skills that help in the negotiation of the various complexities within the environment. Life opportunities should be planned with the expectation of maintained mobility in women who retain the ability to walk (Foley et al. 2011). There is a need for further study of the longitudinal course of gross motor function in RTT in large but representative samples, to clarify the nature of gross motor trajectories and their relationships with genotype.

Physical therapy

Any neurological disorder is associated with the potential for loss of flexibility, weakness, and diminished abilities to carry out activities of daily living. Optimal performance of motor skills requires opportunities for practice of activities that are novel, challenging, and specific to motor performance needs (Gorman 2007). Apraxia is an additional feature of RTT, and strategies that decrease any anxieties associated with task demands and provide opportunities for repetition are recommended. This allows the girls and women to improve their abilities to progress from the planning to the performance of an activity (Downs et al. 2014). Therapy activities should aim to address each of these aspects within the context of a structured and enriched environment. *Mecp2* null mice housed in an enriched environment have demonstrated improved motor abilities, possibly associated with increased levels of BDNF and/or the reinforcement of neural synapses (Kondo et al. 2008;

Nag et al. 2009). With planning, an enriched environment can be achieved for every girl and woman with RTT.

Although a small body of literature, there is some research evidence that active therapy programs can contribute to improved functional abilities in RTT, although each of these studies were conducted with small samples and without a control group. For example, treadmill training improved aerobic fitness and gross motor function ($n=4$) (Lotan et al. 2004); walking and transfer skills improved with practice ($n=3$) (Larsson and Engerstrom 2001); an 8-week course of twice weekly hydrotherapy was associated with increased hand, feeding, and gross motor skills and interaction with the environment, and decreased hand stereotypies, hyperactivity, and anxiety ($n=1$) (Bumin et al. 2003); and intensive and structured supported feeding activities resulted in improved self-feeding skills ($n=5$) (Piazza et al. 1993). However, after a stable baseline period, three young girls who participated over 18 months in a conductive education program each gained gross motor skills (Lotan et al. 2012). While the evidence base is limited, girls and women with RTT have demonstrated responsiveness to activity programs and a proactive approach to the provision of opportunities for movement is recommended over their life span. Physical activity is associated with advantages for persons with a disability, such as reduction of the effects of deconditioning secondary to impairments, improvement of well-being, and family satisfaction (Johnson 2009; Bartlo and Klein 2011); these effects are likely in RTT, too. There are difficulties associated with assessing the effectiveness of therapies in rare disorders such as RTT, but creative multicenter studies using designs of all levels of evidence are needed to more clearly determine treatment effectiveness and to further develop therapeutic approaches.

Conclusion

The effects of RTT on movement are severe, but this chapter also speaks for the variability of clinical presentation, which is clearly associated with genotype and age. Our understanding of the movement disorders of RTT will be enhanced in future studies with larger, but representative samples, and the collection of detailed phenotypic data together with genetic information. There is a currently held view that using mobility and hand skills in opportunities for active participation in daily life helps to maintain and improve these motor skills. There may be additional benefits from participation in physical activity for general health and well-being, as well as meaningful involvement in social and community activities.

REFERENCES

Amir RE, Zoghbi HY (2000) Rett syndrome: Methyl-CpG-binding protein 2 mutations and phenotype-genotype correlations. *Am J Med Genet* 97: 147–152.

Amir RE, van den Veyver IB, Wan M, Tran CQ, Francke U, Zoghbi HY (1999) Rett syndrome is caused by mutations in X-linked MECP2, encoding methyl-CpG-binding protein 2. *Nature Genet* 23: 185–188.

Bartlo P, Klein P (2011) Physical activity benefits and needs in adults with intellectual disabilities: Systematic review of the literature. *Am J Intellect Dev Disabil* 116: 220–232.

Bebbington A, Anderson A, Ravine D et al. (2008) Investigating genotype-phenotype relationships in Rett syndrome using an international data set. *Neurology* 70: 868–875.

Berven S, Bradford DS (2002) Neuromuscular scoliosis: Causes of deformity and principles for evaluation and management. *Semin Neurol* 22: 167–178.

Biddle SJ, Gorely T, Stensel DJ (2004) Health-enhancing physical activity and sedentary behaviour in children and adolescents. *J Sports Sci* 22: 679–701.

Bumin G, Uyanik M, Yilmaz I, Kayihan H, Topçu M (2003) Hydrotherapy for Rett syndrome. *J Rehabil Med* 35: 44–45.

Burford B, Kerr AM, Macleod HA (2003) Nurse recognition of early deviation in development in home videos of infants with Rett disorder. *J Intellect Dis Res* 47: 588–596.

Carter JC, Lanham DC, Pham D, Bibat G, Naidu, S, Kaufmann WE (2008) Selective cerebral volume reduction in Rett syndrome: A multiple approach MRI study. *Am J Neuroradiol* 29: 436–441.

Carter P, Downs J, Bebbington A et al. (2010) Stereotypical hand movements in 144 subjects with Rett syndrome from the population-based Australian database. *Mov Dis* 25: 282–288.

Cass H, Reilly S, Owen L et al. (2003) Findings from a multidisciplinary clinical case series of females with Rett syndrome. *Dev Med Child Neurol* 45: 325–337.

Downs JA, Bebbington A, Jacoby P et al. (2008) Gross motor profile in Rett syndrome as determined by video analysis. *Neuropediatrics* 39: 205–210.

Downs JA, Bebbington A, Jacoby P et al. (2010) Level of purposeful hand function as a marker of clinical severity in Rett syndrome. *Dev Med Child Neurol* 52: 817–823.

Downs J, Bebbington A, Kaufmann W, Leonard H (2011) Longitudinal hand function in Rett syndrome. *J Child Neurol* 26: 334–340.

Downs J, Leonard H, Hill K (2012) Initial assessment of the StepWatch Activity Monitor (TM) to measure walking activity in Rett syndrome. *Dis Rehabil* 34: 1010–1015.

Downs J, Parkinson S, Ranelli S, Leonard H, Diener P, Lotan M (2014) Perspectives on hand function in girls and women with Rett syndrome. *Dev Neurorehabil* 17: 210–217.

Downs J, Torode I, Wong K et al. (2016) The natural history of scoliosis in females with Rett syndrome. *Spine* 41(10): 856–863.

Einspieler C, Kerr AM, Prechtl HF (2005a) Abnormal general movements in girls with Rett disorder: The first four months of life. *Brain Dev* 27(Suppl 1): S8–S13.

Einspieler C, Kerr AM, Prechtl HF (2005b) Is the early development of girls with Rett disorder really normal? *Pediatr Res* 57: 696–700.

Fehr S, Bebbington A, Ellaway C, Rowe P, Leonard H, Downs J (2011) Altered attainment of developmental milestones influences the age of diagnosis of Rett syndrome. *J Child Neurol* 26: 980–987.

Fitzgerald PM, Jankovic J, Percy AK (1990) Rett syndrome and associated movement disorders. *Mov Disord* 5: 195–202.

Foley KR, Downs J Bebbington A et al. (2011) Change in gross motor abilities of girls and women with Rett syndrome over a 3-to 4-year period. *J Child Neurol* 26: 1237–1245.

Gorman S (2007) Contemporary issues and theories of motor control, motor learning, and neuroplasticity: Assessment of movement and posture. In: Umphred D, editor. *Neurological Rehabilitation*, 5th ed. St Louis: Mosby Elsevier.

Hagberg B, Aicardi J, Dias K, Ramos O (1983) A progressive syndrome of autism, dementia, ataxia, and loss of purposeful hand use in girls: Rett's syndrome: report of 35 cases. *Ann Neurol* 14(4): 471–479.

Hagberg B (2002) Clinical manifestations and stages of Rett syndrome. *Ment Retard Dev Disabil Res Rev* 8: 61–65.

Jankovic J (2005) Stereotypies in autistic and other childhood disorders. In: Fernandez-Alvarez E, Arzimanoglou A, Tolosa E, editors. *Paediatric Movement Disorders: Progress in Understanding*. Montrouge: John Libbey Eurotext, 247–260.

Jian L, Nagarajan L, de Klerk N, Ravine D, Christodoulou J, Leonard H (2007) Seizures in Rett syndrome: An overview from a one-year calendar study. *Eur J Paediatr Neurol* 11: 310–317.

Johnson CC (2009) The benefits of physical activity for youth with developmental disabilities: A systematic review. *Am J Health Promot* 23: 157–167.

Kates W, Lanham D, Singer H (2005) Frontal white matter reductions in healthy males with complex stereotypies. *Pediatr Neurol* 32: 109–112.

Kondo M, Gray LJ, Pelka GJ, Christodoulou J, Tam PP, Hannan AJ (2008) Environmental enrichment ameliorates a motor coordination deficit in a mouse model of Rett syndrome – Mecp2 gene dosage effects and BDNF expression. *Eur J Neurosci* 27: 3342–3350.

Larsson G, Engerstrom IW (2001) Gross motor ability in Rett syndrome – the power of expectation, motivation and planning. *Brain Dev* 23(Suppl 1): S77–S81.

Larsson G, Lindstrom B, Engerstrom IW (2005) Rett syndrome from a family perspective: The Swedish Rett Center survey. *Brain Dev* 27(Suppl 1): S14–S19.

Lee J, Leonard H, Piek J, Downs J (2013) Early development and regression in Rett syndrome. *Clin Genet* 84: 572–576.

Leonard H, Bower C (1998) Is the girl with Rett syndrome normal at birth? *Dev Med Child Neurol* 40: 115–121.

Leonard H, Fyfe S, Leonard S, Msall M (2001) Functional status, medical impairments, and rehabilitation resources in 84 females with Rett syndrome: A snapshot across the world from the parental perspective. *Disabil Rehabil* 23: 107–117.

Leonard H, Moore H, Carey M et al. (2005) Genotype and early development in Rett syndrome: The value of international data. *Brain Dev* 27(Suppl 1): S59–S68.

Lotan M, Isakov E, Merrick J (2004) Improving functional skills and physical fitness in children with Rett syndrome. *J Intellect Disabil Res* 48: 730–735.

Lotan M, Schenker R, Wine J, Downs J (2012) The conductive environment enhances gross motor function of girls with Rett syndrome. A pilot study. *Dev Neurorehabil* 15: 19–25.

Mount RH, Hastings RP, Reilly S, Cass H, Charman T (2001) Behavioural and emotional features in Rett syndrome. *Disabil Rehabil* 23: 129–138.

Mount RH, Charman T, Hastings RP, Reilly S, Cass H (2002) The Rett Syndrome Behaviour Questionnaire (RSBQ): Refining the behavioural phenotype of Rett syndrome. *J Child Psychol Psych* 43: 1099–1110.

Nag N, Moriuchi J, Peitzman CGK, Ward B, Kolodny N, Berger-Sweeney J (2009) Environmental enrichment alters locomotor behaviour and ventricular volume in Mecp2 1lox mice. *Behav Brain Res* 196: 44–48.

Neul JL, Fang P, Barrish J et al. (2008) Specific mutations in methyl-CpG-binding protein 2 confer different severity in Rett syndrome. *Neurology* 70: 1313–1321.

Neul JL, Kaufmann WE, Glaze DG. et al. (2010) Rett syndrome: Revised diagnostic criteria and nomenclature. *Ann Neurol* 68: 944–950.

Neul JL, Lane JB, Lee HS et al. (2014) Developmental delay in Rett syndrome: Data from the natural history study. *J Neurodev Dis* 6: 20.

Nomura Y, Segawa M (2005) Natural history of Rett syndrome. *J Child Neurol* 20: 764–768.

Percy A, Lee H-S, Neul J et al. (2010) Profiling scoliosis in Rett syndrome. *Pediatr Res* 67: 435–439.

Piazza CC, Anderson C, Fisher W (1993) Teaching self-feeding skills to patients with Rett syndrome. *Dev Med Child Neurol* 35: 991–996.

Rett A (1966) On an unusual brain atrophy syndrome in hyperammonemia in childhood. *Wien Med Wochenschr* 116(37): 723–726.

Rett A (1977) Cerebral atrophy associated with hyperammonaemia. In: Vinken PJ, Bruyn GW, editors. *Handbook of Clinical Neurology,* Vol. 29, Amsterdam: North Holland, 305–329.

Shahbazian M, Antalffy B, Armstrong D, Zoghbi H (2002) Insight into Rett syndrome: MeCP2 levels display tissue- and cell-specific differences and correlate with neuronal maturation. *Hum Mol Genet* 11: 115–124.

Shumway-Cook A, Woollacott MH (2007) *Motor Control: Translating Research into Clinical Practice.* Philadelphia: Lippincott Williams & Wilkins.

Temudo T, Maciel P, Sequeiros J (2007a) Abnormal movements in Rett syndrome are present before the regression period: A case study. *Mov Disord* 22: 2284–2287.

Temudo T, Oliveira P, Santos M et al. (2007b) Stereotypies in Rett syndrome: Analysis of 83 patients with and without detected MECP2 mutations. *Neurology* 68: 1183–1187.

Temudo T, Ramos E, Dias K et al. (2008) Movement disorders in Rett syndrome: An analysis of 60 patients with detected MECP2 mutation and correlation with mutation type. *Mov Disord* 23: 1384–1390.

Temudo T, Santos M, Ramos E et al. (2011) Rett syndrome with and without detected MECP2 mutations: An attempt to redefine phenotypes. *Brain Dev* 33: 69–76.

van Sluijs EM, Griffin SJ, van Poppel MN (2007) A cross-sectional study of awareness of physical activity: Associations with personal, behavioral and psychosocial factors. *Int J Behav Nutr Phys Act* 4: 53.

WHO Multicentre Growth Reference Study Group (2006) WHO Motor Development Study: Windows of achievement for six gross motor development milestones. *Acta Paediatr* Suppl 450: 86–95.

World Health Organization (2001) *International Classification of Functioning, Disability and Health: ICF.* Geneva: World Health Organization.

7
ORTHOPEDIC ISSUES IN RETT SYNDROME

David P Roye Jr, Jenny Downs, Gordon Baikie and Brendan A Williams

Introduction

Neurological impairments and activity limitations in Rett syndrome (RTT) impose stress on the musculoskeletal system. This chapter reviews the prevalence, characteristics, and clinical management of orthopedic problems in RTT. Documentation of the epidemiology of scoliosis and fracture has been enhanced by interrogation of large databases, but the prevalence of other orthopedic disorders is estimated from smaller case series. In the absence of clinical trials that address outcomes specifically in individuals with RTT, management draws heavily on the clinical experience of experts and general principles that have been applied to children with other neurological disorders, including cerebral palsy.

The musculoskeletal system and Rett syndrome

RTT often presents with hypotonia and weakness, whereas hypertonia including dystonia and rigidity may develop in adulthood (Hagberg 2002). During early development, most girls learn to sit and approximately half learn to walk (Fehr et al. 2011). In those who can walk, gait lacks coordinated movement of the upper extremities, may be unsteady with a wide-base (Hagberg 2002), and toe-walking and shuffling gait patterns are also seen (Cass et al. 2003). The course of RTT has been conceptualized in four stages (Hagberg 2002), the last of which is the 'late motor deterioration phase'. Some individuals are able to maintain the ability to walk through adulthood (Foley et al. 2011), but others develop bradykinesia and increased muscle tone, and with increasing difficulty in maintaining an upright posture, the ability to walk is lost (Hagberg 2002).

Such neurological dysfunction may be associated with the development of deformity; for example, muscle weakness and disuse in combination with decreased blood supply reduces longitudinal bone growth (Salter 1999), and lack of regular stretching during functional activities reduces muscle growth (Graham and Selber 2003). Over time, the development of soft tissue contracture may cause joint deformity, bony torsion, and degenerative arthritis (Graham and Selber 2003). In RTT, dystonia in particular may be a factor in the development of scoliosis and foot deformities (FitzGerald et al. 1990; Temudo et al. 2008) and is also a likely risk factor for hip dysplasia.

Scoliosis and kyphosis

Scoliosis in RTT is currently believed to be neurogenic in origin, arising earlier in development, and with more rapid progression than idiopathic scoliosis (Lidstrom et al. 1994). Scoliosis can be C- or S-shaped, causing pain and deterioration of sitting and/or walking skills. Kyphosis is listed alongside scoliosis as one of the supportive criteria for the diagnosis of RTT (Neul et al. 2010), and similarly, may also lead to pain and difficulties in maintaining upright postures (Roussouly and Nnadi 2010). Little is known about the mechanism for the development of kyphosis in RTT, but over time, habitual postures associated with midline hand stereotypies and the limited focus of visual interest in the environment may contribute to its development (Kerr et al. 2003). During development, the spine grows in synchrony with the rib cage and lungs, and spinal deformity is associated with altered lung function consistent with a restrictive lung deficit (Sponseller et al. 2007). Therefore, spinal postures are closely related to later respiratory outcomes. As for other neurological disorders, the goal of management of spinal deformity is for the child to develop the largest and most symmetric thoracic shape.

EPIDEMIOLOGY AND RISK FACTORS

In 394 participants in the Australian Rett Syndrome Database, the median age at onset of scoliosis was 11 years with about 75% affected by the age of 15 years (Downs et al. 2016a). This study was population-based with a high rate of ascertainment, including those who are deceased, and provides a valuable estimate of incidence. A clinic survey of 554 girls and women aged between 1 and 57 years with a classic presentation, found scoliosis in 53% overall with higher prevalence in older age groups (Percy et al. 2010). Together, these findings demonstrate that scoliosis is a significant co-morbidity in RTT. Variability in phenotype is associated with genotype (Bebbington et al. 2008; Neul et al. 2008), and with regard to scoliosis, those with the p.Arg294X, p.Arg133Cys, or the p.Arg306Cys mutation appear less likely to develop scoliosis (Downs et al. 2016a; Percy et al. 2010). Never having learned to walk is associated with earlier development of scoliosis (Downs et al. 2016a; Percy et al. 2010), as seen in our case study described in Box 7.1.

The overall prevalence of kyphosis is not known, although several early clinical series, all undertaken over 20 years ago and therefore without genetic information, have described severe kyphosis in small proportions of their participants. For example, three of 36 (8.3%) participants had a structural hyperkyphosis (>55°) (Loder et al. 1989), eight of 258 (3.1%) had severe kyphosis (Bassett and Tolo 1990), and one participant of nine (10.1%) had both a thoracolumbar scoliosis and a 90° thoracic kyphosis (Guidera et al. 1991). Kyphosis has been described in younger girls and adolescents (Bassett and Tolo 1990), but appears more common when older (Bassett and Tolo 1990; Halbach et al. 2008). Some evidence of a genotype–phenotype relationship has also been found in a recent study, Seventy-nine participants with a C terminal deletion were compared with 832 cases with another pathogenic *MECP2* mutation recruited to either the International Rett Syndrome Phenotype Database or the Australian Rett Syndrome Database (Bebbington et al. 2010). The phenotype of the

BOX 7.1 Case study illustrating orthopedic issues of scoliosis, hip dysplasia, and fracture that are commonly seen in RTT

Early development to 3 years of age

- MA was born after a normal perinatal period and learned to sit at 5 months, stand at 18 months, and began cruising short distances shortly after. Hand stereotypies developed around 8 months and low muscle tone was noticed at approximately 16 months.
- She did not walk independently. Regression occurred just prior to the age of 2 years and she was diagnosed with RTT when 26 months old. She was found to have a large deletion of *MECP2*.
- Around the time of diagnosis, she rolled off a bed and sustained a right-sided distal tibial buckle fracture, which was treated with a cast for 6 weeks.
- Epilepsy developed at 3 years of age and has been managed with Topiramate 75 mg twice daily with reasonably good seizure control.

Development of spine and hip complications

- When starting school, MA was unable to stand or walk independently and had no purposeful hand function.
- Scoliosis developed when 5 years old with a right thoracic curve (T4–T11) of 14° and a left lumbar curve (T11–L4) of 16°. Six months later, the curves had progressed to 18° and 27°, respectively, and hip X-ray showed left hip subluxation.
- By 7 years, the lumbar curve progressed to 45° and left sided hip subluxation appeared to be worsening. She wore a Thoraco-Lumbar-Sacral-Orthosis and bilateral ankle-foot orthoses (AFOs) to maintain plantargrade feet when in her stander.

Surgical intervention for scoliosis

- At 8 years of age, her curve continued to progress but remained flexible. She was 50 inches (127 cm) tall and weighed 57 lbs (25.9 kg) (body mass index = 16). Otherwise, muscle tone of her lower limbs was variable with some cogwheel rigidity. She had good range of motion at upper and lower limb joints.
- Author DR advised surgical management and discussed options of growing instrumentation and definitive spinal fusion with parents. Discussion included the factors of current age, rapid progression of the curve, the likely small benefit from additional growth, and the difficulties of tolerating multiple surgical procedures. DR and parents agreed that spinal fusion was the preferred option.
- A posterior spinal instrumentation and fusion from T2 to the pelvis was performed. Somatosensory and motor–evoked potentials were robust and stable throughout the procedure and the estimated blood loss was 1000 cc. Postoperatively, MA was ventilated for 4 days and was discharged home on postoperative day 6. After returning home, MA was having difficulty with oral intake so received enteral feeding via a nasogastric tube for a short period at home.

Outcomes and monitoring following spinal fusion

- Three weeks postoperatively, MA had restarted usual oral feeds and had lost 5–7 lb in weight. At 6 weeks, she appeared pain free, was able to return to school, and her parents felt that her mobility was better than pre-operatively.
- At 6 months her parents described her sleeping through the night, sitting with a more upright posture, and generally being 'more alive and like herself'. X-rays showed excellent placement of instrumentation and good coronal alignment. After 1 year, there was good sitting balance and endurance, functional hip flexion, and activity levels. She has had no pulmonary issues since surgery.
- Annual follow-up will include antero-posterior X-ray for spine and hip surveillance.

C terminal deletion was generally milder and individuals were more likely to be able to walk, but they were also more likely to develop kyphosis.

ASSESSMENT

Recommendations regarding the surveillance and management of scoliosis in RTT were recently developed by consensus methods among an expert panel (Downs et al. 2009) and serve as the basis for many of the management principles outlined in this section. There was agreement that physical assessment of the spine should be conducted routinely following the diagnosis of RTT with orthopedic referral when there is clinical concern that a scoliosis has developed (Bassett and Tolo 1990; Downs et al. 2009), and that monitoring should continue at intervals of approximately 6 months until skeletal maturity (Downs et al. 2009). Traditional surveillance methods include initial antero-posterior and lateral X-ray films with antero-posterior films being sufficient at follow-up (Downs et al. 2009). MRI can evaluate for the presence of Arnold Chiari malformation, tether, or syrinx (Musson et al. 2010), which can occur rarely in association with scoliosis, although more commonly for scoliosis associated with myelodysplasia (Fribourg and Delgado 2004).

CONSERVATIVE MANAGEMENT

The management of scoliosis is largely guided by the magnitude of the Cobb angle and its progression. Management options can be grouped into two categories: conservative (bracing and physiotherapy) and surgical (growing and fusion strategies). The optimal treatment option is not always clear, and clinicians have to intervene according to the specific needs and functional status of their individual patient.

Limited evidence suggests that spinal bracing has little influence on the progression of scoliosis in neuromuscular scoliosis (Olafsson et al. 1999; Downs et al. 2009). Bracing is, however, sometimes used to delay the timing of surgery due to the risks associated with spinal fusion in a young child with early onset scoliosis. It may also assist in the maintenance of balanced sitting posture (Olafsson et al. 1999), although effectiveness probably decreases as scoliosis worsens (Kerr et al. 2003). In cases with an early onset scoliosis that is neuromuscular in origin, there is a lack of consensus among surgeons whether to observe or brace a curve of significant magnitude that has not yet reached the 'surgical' range (Corona et al. 2013). A functional benefit needs to be demonstrated, as bracing itself is not expected to prevent curve progression and may impair function.

Physiotherapy should focus on optimizing the strength of the back extensors, maintaining flexibility of the spine, and promoting participation in regular activities such as supported standing, walking, hydrotherapy, and hippotherapy (Downs et al. 2009). At this stage, no evidence that these strategies reduce the progression of scoliosis has been demonstrated, although in one case study, a regimen of over-corrected positioning that opposed the scoliosis in combination with physical activities for an 18 month period reduced the Cobb angle (Lotan et al. 2005). Physical activity is nevertheless associated with a broad spectrum of benefits related to gross motor function and contributes to quality of life. Appropriate support should also be provided to enable correct sitting and sleeping postures, including specific wheelchair supports.

SURGICAL MANAGEMENT

Surgical intervention of progressive scoliosis should be considered once the Cobb angle reaches 40–50° (Downs et al. 2009). Making a decision that surgery is the best option for their daughter is associated with a considerable physical and emotional burden for families (Marr et al. 2015), and management therefore needs to be comprehensive and family centered. A model of comprehensive care around the period of surgery is shown in Box 7.2. Spinal fusion carries risks related to the surgery itself and respiratory complications (Gabos et al. 2012), but long-term risks are not common and the consequences of not intervening include continued progression of the deformity, restrictive lung disease, worsening functional status and quality of life (Wazeka et al. 2004).

Spinal fusion approach

Posterior segmental instrumentation and fusion (PSIF) is the current mainstay of treatment for scoliosis in RTT (Downs et al. 2009). Modern segmental instrumentation materials, including pedicle screws, provide excellent control and stable curve correction and generally eliminate the development of crankshafting, a lordo-rotatory deformity resulting from continued anterior spinal growth in the setting of posterior tethering from spinal instrumentation. Therefore, there are currently few indications for anterior spinal surgery given improved control of the anterior spinal column and stable correction offered by modern posterior segmental instrumentation using pedicle screws.

Determination of levels to be fused

Longer rather than shorter fusion is recommended for individuals with RTT, because neurogenic scoliosis typically involves the entire spine. The general practice for nonambulatory individuals, or those with minimal remaining ambulatory potential, is to extend fusion levels to the pelvis to provide solid fixation for instrumentation and reduce the likelihood of future decompensation. However, pelvic fusion reduces lower lumbar motion and its outcomes in those who are ambulating are not clear. There was clinical equipoise on use of pelvic fixation for individuals with idiopathic or neuromuscular early onset scoliosis in a recent survey of expert pediatric spine surgeons (Corona et al. 2013; Vitale et al. 2011). In ambulating patients with RTT, the role of pelvic fusion is unresolved and clinicians currently determine use of pelvic fusion on a case by case basis.

Growing systems

Recently, instrumentation strategies including growing rods and Vertical Expandable Prosthetic Titanium Rib (VEPTR) have been developed that allow curve progression to be prevented without definitive fusion (Sponseller et al. 2007). This is seen as advantageous for those who are skeletally immature because the negative consequences of early spinal fusion such as decreased trunk height, pulmonary restriction, crankshaft phenomenon and secondary curvatures can potentially be avoided (Vitale et al. 2008). These surgical methods can delay the timing of fusion until skeletal maturity is reached, without allowing the patient to reach Cobb angles that can significantly impair pulmonary function.

BOX 7.2 Current comprehensive care for scoliosis surgery

Time period	Clinical issue	Suggested strategies and actions
Prior to admission	Timing of surgery	Consider spinal surgery when the Cobb angle is 40–50° and time procedures to allow for maximal thoracic growth.
	Type of surgery	Taking into account the remaining predicted growth, determine the ability of the child to manage multiple surgeries with growing rods vs spinal fusion. Include pelvic fixation if child unable to walk.
	Family needs	Take family perspectives into account when making surgical plans.
Pre-operative	Poor growth	Assess body mass index, hemoglobin, electrolytes, albumin, and white cell count as markers of nutrition. Consider hyperalimentation via a nasogastric tube or gastrostomy if weight less than the 5th centile.
	Functional abilities	Assess physical skills and activities of daily living. Plan support needs for daily activities after surgery.
	Gastrointestinal function	Review symptoms and medications to minimize reflux and constipation.
	Anesthetic	Conduct ECG (potential for long QT interval) and assess altered breathing patterns alongside standard anesthetic review.
	Family needs	Provide full information about protocols and procedures.
During surgery	Anesthetic safety	Surgery should be performed at a specialist center given the high risk of anesthetic complications.
	Spinal cord damage	If a reliable signal can be obtained, use motor evoked potentials (MEPs) and/or somatosensory evoked potentials (SSEPs) to detect neurological injury.
	Blood loss	Consider using Amicar or other fibrinolytic inhibitor to reduce blood loss.
Post-operative	Risk of respiratory failure	Admit to high dependency unit/intensive care unit (HDU/ICU) postoperatively to support ventilation as necessary.
		Provide frequent and aggressive chest physiotherapy.
	Pain	Titrate analgesia carefully so that pain relief is adequate, sedation is minimized, and that respiratory effort is not compromised. Take into account increased sensitivity to some analgesic, sedative, and volatile anesthetics. Construct a clear pain management plan when the patient is transferred back to the ward.
	Restricted mobility	Log roll when moving in bed. Sit over the edge of the bed on the first postoperative day, transfer to a chair on the second, and walk (if possible) on the third postoperative day.
	GI function	Optimize nutritional status and treat proactively to reduce constipation.
	Neurological function	Check management of seizures as surgery may have altered metabolism and absorption of antiepileptic medications. Monitor for dystonia and adjust medications accordingly.
	Discharge home	Check able to sit in a chair or walk if previously able. Arrange therapy follow-up. Orthopedic review at 6 weeks and then every 2–3 months over the first year, annually thereafter.

Assessment time	Coronal observation	Antero-posterior X-ray	Coronal measures	Sagittal X-ray	Sagittal measures
Pre-operative			Main thoracic curve: T4–T11: 52°		Kyphosis: 46°
			Thoracolumbar curve: T11–L3: 60°		Lordosis: 96°
Six weeks after surgery			Proximal thoracic curve: T1–T5: 15°		Kyphosis: 38°
			Main thoracic curve: T5–T10: 17°		Lordosis: 54°

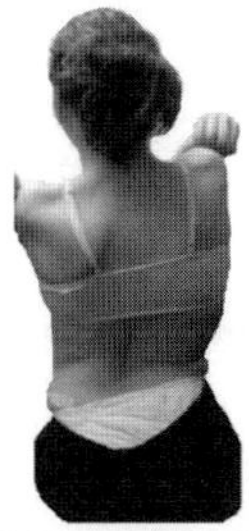

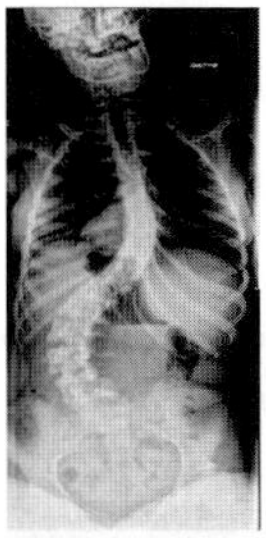

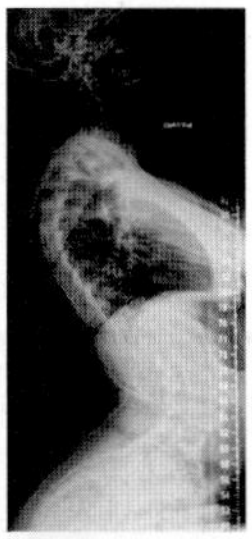

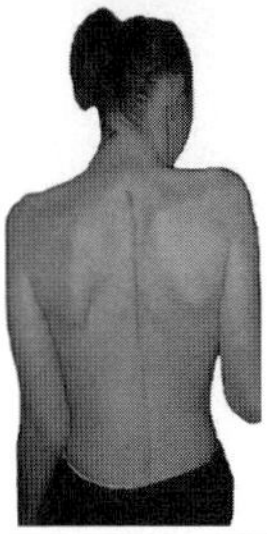

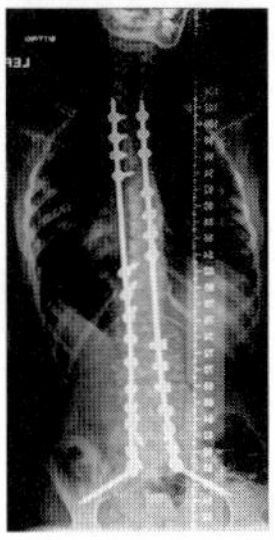

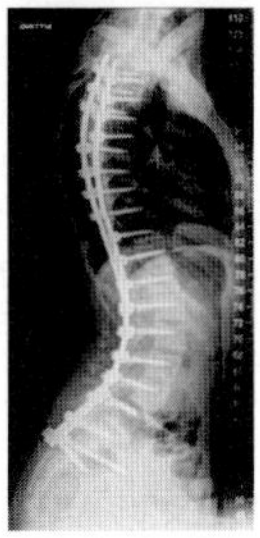

Fig. 7.1. Illustrations show a double scoliosis curve in a 15-year-old girl with RTT managed with a posterior segmental instrumentation and fusion from T2 to the sacrum. Walking skills improved compared with pre-operatively. A normal thoracic kyphosis is 10–40° and a normal lumbar lordosis is 40–60°.

These new growing techniques have brought into question whether it is better to 'grow' or fuse skeletally immature patients with a scoliosis. Consideration of these techniques is recommended for children under 9 years old with a large curve and in whom bracing has not reduced curve progression. Once a child is approximately 9 years old, the optimal surgical strategy is less clear. Variability among expert pediatric spinal surgeons regarding the decision as to whether to use growing techniques, or fuse a child with neuromuscular scoliosis of that age has been demonstrated (Corona et al. 2013). Our case study presented in Box 7.1 reflects clinical decision making and family involvement on this issue.

Severe scoliosis
In severe scoliosis where surgical intervention is not deemed appropriate, the management plan should consist of optimization of sitting posture, surveillance for and treatment of pressure sores, chest physiotherapy, influenza immunization, and a low threshold for antibiotic treatment in order to minimize the increased risks associated with restrictive lung disease (Downs et al. 2009).

Outcomes following surgery
There is growing evidence on outcomes following spinal fusion for progressive scoliosis in RTT. There can be immediate improvement in symmetry and sitting balance following surgery (Larsson et al. 2002), also illustrated in Figure 7.1. In a series of eight patients with

Positioning for X-ray	
• Accuracy and reproducibility requires specific positioning. • Antero-posterior pelvic X-ray is taken with legs in neutral abduction/adduction position (+ or − 6°). • Pelvic tilt is corrected with supports under the calves in those with hip flexion deformities to keep pelvis in the AP plane. This enables visualization of the triradiate cartilages in the hips (Wynter et al. 2008).	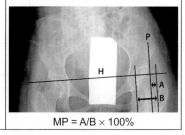
Measurement of the migration percentage (see right)	
• Migration percentage (MP) is measured as the proportion of ossified femoral head beyond the acetabular roof. • A line H is drawn between the most superior medial part of both triradiate cartilages. • A line P perpendicular to the first line is then drawn that passes through the lateral margin of the acetabulum. • The migration percentage is the proportion of the femoral head lateral to the second line, i.e. MP = A/B × 100%.	MP = A/B × 100%

Fig. 7.2. Radiographic measurement of the hip migration percentage to quantify the presence and development of hip dysplasia.

RTT undergoing PSIF, the average correction in Cobb angle was 63.5° with an average post-operative curve of 29° (Tay et al. 2010). A population-based qualitative study suggested that general wellness of the child was usually achieved by 6 months and that recovery of pre-operative sitting, standing and walking skills was usually achieved before 12 months (Marr et al. 2015). In a Swedish clinic series of 23 girls and young women with RTT, improved posture and balance as well as fewer daytime naps were reported at 12 months (Larsson et al. 2009). Nineteen of this latter sample were followed over 6 years and the earlier gains that had been observed at 12 months were maintained (Larsson et al. 2009). The individual described in Figure 8.1 demonstrated rapid improvement in ambulation after her spinal fusion. Longer-term outcomes have been investigated using data from the Australian Rett Syndrome Database and medical records at eight tertiary hospitals throughout Australia (Downs et al. 2016b). Mortality was reduced in those with severe scoliosis who underwent spinal fusion ($n = 98$) compared to those who were managed conservatively ($n = 42$). The effect was particularly evident for those with an earlier onset of scoliosis who also experienced a moderately reduced likelihood of later lower respiratory tract infections (Downs et al. 2016b).

Hip dysplasia

Hip dysplasia includes subluxation and dislocation, known complications in many types of neurodisability. Hip subluxation occurs when the femoral head migrates beyond the margins of the acetabulum and the hip is dislocated when the femoral head no longer articulates with the acetabulum. Hip subluxation measured by migration percentage is illustrated in Figure 7.2. This has been an area of intense study in children with cerebral palsy and robust surveillance and management guidelines have been adopted in many centers to prevent hip subluxation progressing to dislocation (Wynter et al. 2014); however, motor patterns are different in RTT to those in cerebral palsy and some girls may be ambulant but then lose this ability. The screening and treatment protocols that are well established in cerebral palsy may not be directly applicable to girls and women with RTT.

Hip dislocation typically results in pain, particularly with movement, and the resultant pelvic tilt is problematic for postural management with areas of undue pressure on the skin. Screening for hip subluxation and early intervention aims to prevent hip dislocation, which has the potential to detract from quality of life and add to the burden of care. Neither medical nor surgical management are particularly successful in treating hip pain and therefore, prevention is paramount.

PREVALENCE AND RISK FACTORS

Several orthopedic case series have described variable frequencies of hip subluxation or dislocation, with differences probably relating to the methods of case ascertainment. Either hip subluxation or dislocation have been described in 15/31 (Tay et al. 2010) and 1/9 (Guidera et al. 1991) girls with RTT in different studies. Hip dislocation on its own has been described in 4/31 (Tay et al. 2010) and 2/22 (Roberts and Conner 1988) girls with RTT whereas two series of nine (Guidera et al. 1991) and seven (Loder et al. 1989) patients did not report any dislocations. One of these studies ascertained participants from a clinic that serves the majority of the population in the state of Victoria, Australia (Tay et al. 2010). Even if none of the remaining individuals in Victoria had significant hip subluxation, and using the population figures from the Australian Rett Syndrome Database, the incidence in the Victorian population would be at least 37% (Tay et al. 2010), suggesting that hip dysplasia is more common than previously thought. Hip subluxation was present in our case study at the age of 7 years (Box 7.1), although there is no population study to date to give us reliable information about prevalence at different ages. Population-based studies are necessary to determine the true prevalence of hip dysplasia and their relationships to genotype in RTT.

The depth of the acetabulum, the shape of the femoral neck and head, and the effects of weight bearing and walking are thought to influence the development and progression of hip dysplasia. Increased tone in the adductor muscles may contribute to displacement of the femoral head, although subluxation and dislocation also occurs in individuals with low adductor tone. In cerebral palsy, there is a higher prevalence of hip displacement with decreasing ambulatory ability, irrespective of the nature of muscle tone (Soo et al. 2006). This has particular relevance to girls and women with RTT. In the series of 31 participants in the Victorian study, the youngest female to have a hip migration percentage of more than 30% was 11 years and the youngest to have a dislocated hip diagnosed was 14 years (Tay et al. 2010). Early ambulatory abilities could be protective of hip dysplasia with subluxation and dislocation occurring at older ages than in other conditions such as cerebral palsy. In addition, investigating the age of peak ambulatory ability and its decline may be important determinants of the risk for hip dysplasia in RTT and longitudinal studies are required.

Clinically, hip dysplasia is determined by observable asymmetry of the hips or the groin creases, and decreased range of hip movement (particularly hip abduction in flexion), and/ or the femoral head may be palpable at a distance from the acetabulum. In many cases, there are no apparent signs of hip dysplasia. While clinical assessment allows the clinician to determine if an individual may be at risk for hip subluxation or dislocation, radiographs are necessary to confirm their presence and quantify the extent of any subluxation.

Hip subluxation and dislocation are diagnosed by a pelvic radiograph performed with careful attention to standard positioning. Hip subluxation is quantified by the migration percentage or the amount of ossified femoral head that is not covered by ossified acetabular roof (Reimers 1980). A migration percentage of 30% or greater is considered at risk of dislocation and orthopedic referral is indicated (Reimers 1980). Figure 8.2 describes necessary positioning for the pelvic radiograph and how to measure the migration percentage.

Consistent with the principles established in cerebral palsy (Dobson et al. 2002) and until more systematically collected evidence for RTT becomes available, we propose a hip surveillance program with regular examinations and 12 monthly radiographs from an early age until skeletal maturity is achieved. Surveillance protocols for cerebral palsy begin at 18 months, but starting at a later age may be appropriate for RTT, given the apparently later onset of hip dysplasia (Tay et al. 2010). Longitudinal population-based studies would be desirable to determine the parameters of a hip surveillance system, balanced against the effects and costs of repeated radiological investigations, particularly in those at low risk (Mazrani et al. 2007). Meanwhile, clinical practice should be determined on a case by case basis with a low threshold for surveillance, particularly in those with clinically observable asymmetry and when losing the ability to walk.

SURGICAL INTERVENTION

Surgical treatment for hip subluxation and dislocation is guided by the principles established for individuals with cerebral palsy. When subluxation is diagnosed early, preventative surgery involving soft tissue releases (e.g. adductor tendonotomy) or later femoral varus derotation osteotomy (VDRO) is indicated. In cerebral palsy, VDRO is usually successful in preventing dislocation; however, if subluxation progresses to dislocation then reconstructive or salvage procedures are required, though these operations more frequently lead to suboptimal results. Data are lacking as to outcomes of these operations in girls and women with RTT.

Foot deformities

Foot deformities often develop in RTT (Hagberg and Romell 2002). The earliest manifestation of foot deformity is often that of increased plantarflexor tone followed shortly by the onset of toe walking. Over time, the feet may become dystonic with hyperflexed and plantar-deviated toe malpositions, which further restrict the ability to stand and walk (Hagberg and Romell 2002). Therefore, early mild lower limb spasticity is complicated by slowly progressive, distal dystonia and contracture. There is currently no information on the prevalence of foot deformities in RTT or relationships with genotype.

MANAGEMENT

An evidence-base for the management of foot deformity in RTT is currently lacking and the authors therefore recommend management algorithms based on their experience with other neuromuscular conditions such as cerebral palsy. There are two aspects of the clinical presentation to consider when deciding on treatment: (1) the etiology of the deformity in terms of altered muscle tone or contracture; and (2) the severity of the deformity in which increasingly invasive options are considered for greater and worsening pathology, taking into account functional skills. Currently, there are three tiers of management: physiotherapy and bracing (Cusick 1988; Figueiredo et al. 2008), use of botulinum neurotoxin type A (BoNT-A) (Lukban et al. 2009), and surgery (Salter 1999). Escalation to higher levels of intervention is dependent on the type and severity of deformity, as well as the judgment of the clinical team and family regarding the potential benefits of the treatment.

Altered muscle tone

Deformity caused by altered muscle tone usually presents in those who are younger or are less clinically severe. Physiotherapy is typically the first mode of intervention and focuses on regular stretching, plantargrade foot positioning to avoid long periods of time spent in equinus, and opportunities to practice standing and walking skills. Practice of these activities aims to maintain functional use of the foot so that ambulation is retained and worsening deformity is avoided. As an adjunct, ankle-foot orthoses (AFOs) maintain foot alignment in the plantargrade position and can assist with maintaining the ability to stand, which is important for overall muscle strength and bone health.

If these strategies are insufficient, judicious use of BoNT-A has become a commonly used management option in patients with neuromuscular-related spastic foot deformity. It is considered safe for use in children and has demonstrated efficacy in children with cerebral palsy, resulting in decreased muscle tone and improved gait (Lukban et al. 2009); however, treatment results are short term and there is no evidence of cumulative or persisting benefit from repeated BoNT-A treatments beyond one year (Moore et al. 2008). As such, it should be viewed as a temporary measure for the relief of lower limb spasticity. Foot deformity resulting from contracture will not respond to BoNT-A treatment and clinicians need to differentiate as to whether the muscle tightness results from altered muscle tone or contracture.

Contracture of soft tissues

Contracture-related foot deformity results from improper positioning over long periods of time and once developed, physiotherapy and bracing serve little use in correcting the deformity. Management choices for contracture-based foot pathology in RTT include the following: ignoring the deformity, bracing around the deformity, or surgical correction. For those who are severely involved and nonambulant, ignoring the deformity is a common option, especially when correcting the foot deformity is complicated and contributes little to quality of life or burden of care. Bracing around contracture-based foot deformity can provide some cosmetic improvement and help to maintain the current deformity, although once contracture has developed, progression is usually inevitable. Surgery is rarely utilized in those who are nonambulant.

Surgery may be considered for worsening foot deformity in those who are less severely affected. Before considering surgery, the authors recommend careful consideration of current ambulatory ability, potential gains from use of bracing, as well as future ambulation potential. If a consensus for surgery is determined by the clinicians and family, the goal of treatment is to achieve a plantigrade correction to allow for transfers, standing, and walking. The authors have experience with percutaneous tendo-achilles lengthening, tibialis posterior transfers and lengthening, and other soft tissue procedures in individuals with a neuromuscular disorder, and these may be indicated in RTT. Complex surgery is rarely indicated because patients with foot deformity to that extent are seldom still ambulatory. Nevertheless, foot surgery is performed, albeit infrequently, in this group. There are currently 16 of approximately 392 girls and women in the longitudinal Australian Rett Syndrome Database who have had foot surgery. Most were adolescents or young women when they underwent foot surgery and the most common procedure was tendo-achilles lengthening ($n = 18$ of 26 procedures).

Therefore, consideration of both the etiology and severity of the deformity is necessary when planning the management of foot deformity in RTT. Maintaining ambulation as far as possible has an important role in minimizing foot deformity and in general, management should be as conservative as possible, especially when ambulation is not possible.

Fracture

PREVALENCE AND RISK FACTORS

Girls and women with RTT are at an increased risk of osteoporosis (Leonard et al. 1999; Motil et al. 2008; Jefferson et al. 2011) and have four times the rate of fracture compared with females in the general population of a similar age (Downs et al. 2008). Osteopenia has been described in girls as young as 3 years (Budden and Gunness 2003; Motil et al. 2006) and long bones frequently fracture (Downs et al. 2008). The case study presented in Box 7.1 illustrates long bone fracture at a young age. There is a higher risk of fracture in those with a p.Arg168X or p.Arg270X mutation (Downs et al. 2008) and increased risk of fracture with the presence of epilepsy (Downs et al. 2008; Motil et al. 2008), particularly when the antiepileptic medication sodium valproate is used (Leonard et al. 2010). Other factors such as vitamin D insufficiency, physical inactivity, and muscle weakness contribute to decreased bone mineral density and susceptibility to fracture in the general population (Grossman 2011), and such factors are also relevant to RTT.

PREVENTION OF FRACTURE

General strategies to optimize bone health over the life span are important. A high dietary intake of calcium rich or calcium-fortified foods is recommended, and if levels are low, calcium supplements to meet the local recommended daily intake should be prescribed (Grossman 2011). The appropriate amount of safe sunlight exposure based on latitude, time of day, season, and skin type should be advised, and local protocols for the supplementation of vitamin D implemented if 25 hydroxyvitamin D levels are low (Motil et al. 2011; Thacher and Clarke 2011). Physical activity is recommended to increase muscle strength and endurance, including participation in as much walking as possible for those who are able to walk, and supported standing for those who are wheelchair-dependent. Where mobility is limited, body weight-supported treadmill walking may be useful to increase physical activity, but the optimal protocols are still unclear (Damiano and DeJong 2009). If menstrual suppression forms a part of medical management, avoiding use of progesterone-only medications will minimize adverse effect on bone mineral density (Lopez et al. 2007). Prevention of fracture avoids periods of immobilization and allows consistent participation in physical activity.

ASSESSMENT AND TREATMENT OF FRACTURE

Approximately two-thirds of parents in a population-based study reported that their daughter had decreased sensitivity to pain, apparent during decreased or delayed reactions to venipuncture and immunizations, or reduced responses to injuries such as burns and fracture (Downs et al. 2010). Therefore, a low threshold to clinical investigation of potential injuries such as fracture would appear justified.

Fracture management in RTT should focus on avoiding unnecessary mobility restrictions and encourage rapid return to weight bearing or functional use of fractured extremities. In the event of a displaced fracture, operative treatment should be strongly considered to provide stability and promote rapid rehabilitation.

Conclusion

Orthopedic problems occur commonly in girls and women with RTT and vigilance for the development of scoliosis, progressive hip instability, and foot deformity is necessary. Regular clinical review of these issues can help assure the best outcomes by allowing early diagnosis and appropriate intervention. Promoting physical activity is important as ambulation is protective against scoliosis and hip dysplasia, and is advantageous for bone health. Maintaining ambulation and physical activity levels also provide greater participation in life opportunities and a better quality of life, and such strategies should be sustained into adulthood as far as possible. Orthopedic surgery can successfully treat progressive scoliosis and correct hips at risk of dislocation.

There are still many areas where our knowledge is lacking in relation to orthopedic issues in RTT. Studies are needed that address the population-based incidence and genotype relationships with hip dysplasia and foot deformities. Longitudinal studies are required to provide important information on the modifying effects of ambulation and other conservative interventions on the development of deformity, and outcomes following surgical interventions. With increasing longevity of women with RTT, there are clear needs for longer-term follow-up of orthopedic comorbidities in terms of function and the impacts of previous treatments.

REFERENCES

Bassett GS, Tolo VT (1990) The incidence and natural history of scoliosis in Rett syndrome. *Dev Med Child Neurol* 32: 96–966.
Bebbington A, Anderson A, Ravine D et al. (2008) Investigating genotype-phenotype relationships in Rett syndrome using an international data set. *Neurology* 70: 868–875.

Bebbington A, Percy A, Christodoulou J et al. (2010) Updating the profile of C-terminal MECP2 deletions in Rett syndrome. *J Med Genet* 47: 242–248.

Budden S, Gunness M (2003) Possible mechanisms of osteopenia in Rett syndrome: Bone histomorphometric studies. *J Child Neurol* 18: 698–702.

Cass H, Reilly S, Owen L et al. (2003) Findings from a multidisciplinary clinical case series of females with Rett syndrome. *Dev Med Child Neurol* 45: 325–337.

Corona J, Miller DJ, Downs J et al. (2013) Evaluating the extent of clinical uncertainty among treatment options for patients with early-onset scoliosis. *J Bone Joint Surg Am* 95: e67.

Cusick BD (1988) Splints and casts. Managing foot deformity in children with neuromotor disorders. *Phys Ther* 68: 1903–1912.

Damiano D, DeJong S (2009) A systematic review of the effectiveness of treadmill training and body weight support in pediatric rehabilitation. *J Neurol Phys Ther* 33: 27–44.

Dobson F, Boyd RN, Parrott J, Nattrass GR, Graham HK (2002) Hip surveillance in children with cerebral palsy. Impact on the surgical management of spastic hip disease. *J Bone Joint Surg Briti Vol* 84: 720–726.

Downs J, Bebbington A, Woodhead H et al. (2008) Early determinants of fractures in Rett syndrome. *Pediatrics* 121: 540–546.

Downs J, Bergman A, Carter P et al. (2009) Guidelines for management of scoliosis in Rett syndrome patients based on expert consensus and clinical evidence. *Spine* 34: E607– E617.

Downs J, Granton S, Bebbington A et al. (2010) Linking MECP2 and pain sensitivity: The example of Rett syndrome. *Am J Med Genet A* 152A: 1197–1205.

Downs J, Torode I, Wong K et al. (2016a) The natural history of scoliosis in females with Rett syndrome. *Spine* 41(10): 856–863. doi: 10.1097/BRS.0000000000001399.

Downs J, Torode I, Wong K et al. (2016b) Surgical fusion of early onset severe scoliosis increases survival in Rett syndrome: A cohort study. *Dev Med Child Neurol* 58(6): 632–638. doi: 10.1111/dmcn.12984.

Fehr S, Bebbington A, Ellaway C, Rowe P, Leonard H, Downs J (2011) Altered attainment of developmental milestones influences the age of diagnosis of Rett syndrome. *J Child Neurol* 26(8): 980–987.

Figueiredo E, Ferreira G, Maia-Moreira R, Kirkwood R, Fetters L (2008) Efficacy of ankle-foot orthoses on gait of children with cerebral palsy: Systematic review of literature. *Pediatr Phys Ther* 20: 207–223.

FitzGerald PM, Jankovic J, Glaze DG, Schultz R, Percy AK (1990) Extrapyramidal involvement in Rett's syndrome. *Neurology* 40: 293–295.

Foley KR, Downs J, Bebbington A et al. (2011) Change in gross motor abilities of girls and women with Rett syndrome over a 3- to 4-year period. *J Child Neurol* 26: 1237–1245.

Fribourg D, Delgado E (2004) Occult spinal cord abnormalities in children referred for orthopedic complaints. *Am J Orthop* 33: 18–25.

Gabos P, Inan M, Thacker M, Borkhu B (2012) Spinal fusion for scoliosis in Rett syndrome with an emphasis on early postoperative complications. *Spine* 37: E90–E94.

Graham HK, Selber P (2003) Musculoskeletal aspects of cerebral palsy. *J Bone Joint Surg Brit Vol* 85: 157–166.

Grossman J (2011) Osteoporosis prevention. *Curr Opin Rheumatol* 23: 203–210.

Guidera KJ, Borrelli J, Raney E, Thompson-Rangel T, Ogden JA (1991) Orthopaedic manifestations of Rett syndrome. *J Pediatr Orthop* 11: 204–208.

Hagberg B (2002) Clinical manifestations and stages of Rett syndrome. *Ment Retard Dev Disabil Res Rev* 8: 61–65.

Hagberg B, Romell M (2002) Rett females: Patterns of characteristic side-asymmetric neuroimpairments at long-term follow-up. *Neuropediatrics* 33: 324–326.

Halbach NSJ, Smeets EEJ, Schrander-Stumpel CTRM et al. (2008) Aging in people with specific genetic syndromes: Rett syndrome. *Am J Med Gen A* 146A: 1925–1932.

Jefferson A, Woodhead H, Fyfe S et al. (2011) Bone mineral content and density in Rett syndrome and their contributing factors. *Pediatr Res* 69: 293–298.

Kerr A, Webb P, Prescott R, Milne Y (2003) Results of surgery for scoliosis in Rett syndrome. *J Child Neurol* 18: 703–708.

Larsson EL, Aaro S, Normelli H, Oberg B (2002) Weight distribution in the sitting position in patients with paralytic scoliosis: Pre- and post-operative evaluation. *Eur Spine* J 11: 94–99.

Larsson EL, Aaro S, Ahlinder P, Normelli H, Tropp H, Oberg B (2009) Long-term follow-up of functioning after spinal surgery in patients with Rett syndrome. *Eur Spine* J 18: 506–511.

Leonard H, Thomson MR, Glasson EJ et al. (1999) A population-based approach to the investigation of osteopenia in Rett syndrome. *Dev Med Child Neurol* 41: 323–328.

Leonard H, Downs J, Jian L et al. (2010) Valproate and risk of fracture in Rett syndrome. *Arch Dis Child* 95: 444–448.

Lidstrom J, Stokland E, Hagberg B (1994) Scoliosis in Rett syndrome. Clinical and biological aspects. *Spine* 19: 1632–1635.

Loder RT, Lee CL, Richards BS (1989) Orthopedic aspects of Rett syndrome: A multicenter review. *J Ped Orthop* 9: 557–562.

Lopez LM, Grimes DA, Schulz KF (2007) Steroidal contraceptives: Effect on carbohydrate metabolism in women without diabetes mellitus. *Cochrane Database Syst Rev* CD006133.

Lotan M, Merrick J, Carmeli E (2005) Managing scoliosis in a young child with Rett syndrome: A case study. *Scientific World Journal* 5: 264–273.

Lukban M, Rosales R, Dressler D (2009) Effectiveness of botulinum toxin A for upper and lower limb spasticity in children with cerebral palsy: A summary of evidence. *J Neural Transm* 116: 319–331.

Marr C, Leonard H, Torode I, Downs J (2015) Spinal fusion in girls with Rett syndrome: Post-operative recovery and family experiences. *Child Care Health Dev* 41(6): 1000–1009.

Mazrani W, McHugh K, Marsden PJ (2007) The radiation burden of radiological investigations. *Arch Dis Child* 92: 1127–1131.

Moore AP, Ade Hall RA, Smith CT et al. (2008) Two-year placebo-controlled trial of botulinum toxin A for leg spasticity in cerebral palsy. *Neurology* 71: 122–128.

Motil K, Schultz R, Abrams S, Ellis K, Glaze D (2006) Fractional calcium absorption is increased in girls with Rett syndrome. *J Pediatr Gastroenterol Nutri* 42: 419–426.

Motil K, Ellis K, Barrish J, Caeg E, Glaze D (2008) Bone mineral content and bone mineral density are lower in older than in younger females with Rett syndrome. *Pediatric Res* 64: 435–439.

Motil KJ, Barrish JO, Lane J et al. (2011) Vitamin D deficiency is prevalent in females with Rett syndrome. *J Pediatric Gastroenterol Nutr* 53(5): 569–574.

Musson R, Warren D, Bickle I, Connolly D, Griffiths P (2010) Imaging in childhood scoliosis: A pictorial review. *Postgrad Med J* 86: 419–427.

Neul JL, Fang P, Barrish J et al. (2008) Specific mutations in methyl-CpG-binding protein 2 confer different severity in Rett syndrome. *Neurology* 70: 1313–1321.

Neul JL, Kaufmann WE, Glaze DG (2010) Rett syndrome: Revised diagnostic criteria and nomenclature. *Ann Neurol* 68: 944–950.

Olafsson Y, Saraste H, al-Dabbagh Z (1999) Brace treatment in neuromuscular spine deformity. *J Pediatr Orthop* 19: 376–379.

Percy A, Lee H-S, Neul J et al. (2010) Profiling scoliosis in Rett syndrome. *Pediatr Res* 67: 435–439.

Reimers J (1980) The stability of the hip in children. A radiological study of the results of muscle surgery in cerebral palsy. *Acta Orthop Scand Supplementum* 184: 1–100.

Roberts AP, Conner AN (1988) Orthopaedic aspects of Rett's syndrome: Brief report. *J Bone Joint Surg Brit Vol* 70: 674.

Roussouly P, Nnadi C (2010) Sagittal plane deformity: An overview of interpretation and management. *Eur Spine J* 19: 1824–1836.

Salter RB (1999) Neuromuscular disorders. In: Salter RB, editor. *Textbook of Disorders and Injuries of the Musculoskeletal System*, 3rd ed. Philadelphia: Lippincott Williams and Wilkins, 303–315.

Soo B, Howard J, Boyd R et al. (2006) Hip displacement in cerebral palsy. *J Bone Joint Surg Am Vol* 88: 121–129.

Sponseller P, Yazici M, Demetracopoulos C, Emans J (2007) Evidence basis for management of spine and chest wall deformities in children. *Spine* 32: S81–S90.

Tay G, Graham H, Graham HK, Leonard H, Reddihough D, Baikie G (2010) Hip displacement and scoliosis in Rett syndrome – screening is required. *Dev Med Child Neurol* 52: 93–98.

Temudo T, Ramos E, Dias K et al. (2008) Movement disorders in Rett syndrome: An analysis of 60 patients with detected MECP2 mutation and correlation with mutation type. *Mov Disord* 23: 1384–1390.

Thacher T, Clarke B (2011) Vitamin D insufficiency. *Mayo Clin Proc* 86: 50–60.

Vitale M, Matsumoto H, Bye M et al. (2008) A retrospective cohort study of pulmonary function, radiographic measures, and quality of life in children with congenital scoliosis: An evaluation of patient outcomes after early spinal fusion. *Spine* 33: 1242–1249.

Vitale M, Gomez J, Matsumoto H, Roye D (2011) Variability of expert opinion in treatment of early-onset scoliosis. *Clin Orthop Relat Res* 469: 1317–1322.

Wazeka A, Dimaio M, Boachie Adjei O (2004) Outcome of pediatric patients with severe restrictive lung disease following reconstructive spine surgery. *Spine* 29: 528–534.

Wynter M, Gibson N, Kentish M, Love SC, Thomason P, Graham HK. (2014) *Australian Hip Surveillance Guidelines for Children with Cerebral Palsy*. Endorsed by the Australasian Academy of Cerebral Palsy and Developmental Medicine. Available at: www.ausacpdm.org.au/professionals/hip-surveillance.

8
SLEEP ISSUES IN RETT SYNDROME

Daniel G Glaze, Sarojini Budden, Yoshiko Nomura and Carolyn Ellaway

Introduction

Sleep problems occur commonly in Rett syndrome (RTT), affecting 70–80% of individuals, and become more evident between 18 months and 2 years of age (Young et al. 2007). The prevalence of sleep disturbance is significantly greater than the 20–40% reported for typically developed children (Owens et al. 2000a; Owens and Witmans 2004).

Females with RTT appear to have specific sleep-related problems, unlike those with other neurodevelopmental disabilities. They sleep longer during the day (Nomura et al. 1984), less at night, and have more total sleep time than their age-related peers (Piazza et al. 1990; Ellaway et al. 2001). Common sleep problems in RTT include insomnia characterized by difficulties initiating and maintaining sleep, prolonged night awakenings, and circadian sleep disorders with irregular sleep–wake patterns. Of the girls and women currently enrolled in the Natural History Study (in progress, current enrollment 1078; 828 with classic RTT) in the United States, 72% with classic RTT were reported to have sleep problems, which were reported across all age groups. Sixty-eight percent of children under 5 years of age and 89% of individuals over 21 years were reported to have sleep problems. Of those with sleep problems, over half (53%) experienced frequent night-time wakening and over a third (36%) experienced frequent daytime naps. The frequency of night wakening was similar across age groups, while daytime napping became more frequent with advancing age.

A prospective study evaluated the occurrence of sleep problems in general, and sleep disordered breathing and daytime sleepiness in female participants in the Natural History Study (Sultana et al. 2015). These individuals (*n* = 264) were age 19 years or less and had a clinical diagnosis of classical RTT and a disease causing *MECP2* mutation. A comparison group consisted of age-matched typically developing siblings (*n* = 322). At baseline, and at 1-year follow-up, four validated sleep questionnaires were completed by the parents for each participant: Sleep Related Breathing Disorder Scale (extracted from the Pediatric Sleep Questionnaire) (Chervin et al. 2000); Child's Sleep Habits Questionnaire (CHSQ) (Owens et al. 2000b); Pediatric Daytime Sleepiness Scale (Drake et al. 2003); Cleveland Adolescent Sleepiness Questionnaire (Spilsbury et al. 2007). At baseline, and at 1 year, caretakers endorsed more overall sleep problems, as well as more problems with sleep disordered breathing and excessive daytime sleepiness for the RTT participants than for the sibling comparisons. Though there was improvement in the scores on the CSHQ at 1 year, the mean score remained above 41, indicating persistence of sleep problems. In addition, there was no improvement demonstrated for the other scales and all scores were higher for the RTT participants at 1 year, indicating more significant problems than the sibling comparisons. These findings indicate that children and adolescents with RTT have more overall sleep problems, as well as sleep disordered breathing and excessive daytime sleepiness than typically developing age-matched children and adolescents, and that sleep problems in RTT are chronic.

In infancy, females with RTT are often described as quiet, placid babies who 'slept a lot and seldom cried' (Nomura et al. 1984; Nomura 2005). The change in sleep behavior may be due to the lack of neuromaturational changes, which occur as a result of altered *MECP2* expression in the brain, interfering with sleep regulation. It may also be related to regulatory disturbances (DeGangi and Breinbauer 1997). Parents and caregivers often report irregular sleep time, delayed onset of sleep, and periodic night-time awakenings with disruptive behavior, such as crying, screaming, laughter, or playing. Parents and teachers consistently report that girls fall asleep during the day at school. Whether this pattern reflects immature brain function, or becomes a physiological necessity in getting sufficient sleep during a 24-hour period, is not clear. Several studies have documented low levels of melatonin in RTT and other neurodevelopmental disorders, which may explain some of the disruptive sleep patterns (McArthur and Budden 1998). However, prolonged daytime sleep appears to be more commonly reported in RTT and unique to this condition (Nomura et al. 1984).

Other sleep disturbances, such as sleep disordered breathing (obstructive sleep apnea and central sleep apnea), and nocturnal events such as parasomnias and seizures, have been reported in RTT. A frequently reported nocturnal event is night-time laughter, which is most prevalent in younger girls and tends to decrease with age (Aldrich et al. 1990; D'Orsi et al. 2009). Night-time laughter was shown to be more prevalent in females with a large deletion of the *MECP2* gene (Wong et al. 2015). Nocturnal seizures and daytime napping appear to increase with age (McDougall et al. 2005). In comparison with age-matched comparison females, individuals with RTT do not show the age-related decrease in total and daytime sleep time (Nomura et al. 1984). They have significantly more total sleep time with less night-time sleep, and more daytime sleep. There are significant differences between the younger and the older RTT individuals, which include decreased night-time sleep and increased daytime sleep with increasing age (Segawa and Nomura 1990; Ellaway et al. 2001). These findings underscore the marked impairment in sleep–wake patterns and suggest the persistence of sleep dysfunction over time in RTT.

A study involving 83 Australian individuals with RTT, aged 4–40 years, used a sleep diary for seven consecutive days and nights and compared the data obtained with normative sleep data (Ellaway et al. 2001). The study showed that in contrast to typical children, total sleep time, including daytime sleep, did not decline with age. In the general population of children, the total number of hours slept in a 24-hour period decreases with age. Females with RTT did not show this decrease and the mean total sleep time did not vary significantly with age. Daytime sleep is rare after 4 years of age in the typical population. Excessive daytime sleep, however, was seen in the study cohort with a mean of 0.78 hours per day with no significant difference across age groups. The authors concluded that individuals with RTT demonstrated poor sleep compared with healthy children.

In a study using the Australian Rett Syndrome Database (Young et al. 2007), the prevalence of sleep disturbance in the RTT population was estimated at 80%. The most commonly reported specific sleep problems were night-time laughter and teeth grinding, followed by screaming episodes and seizures. Frequent daytime napping was reported in over 77% of cases. The prevalence of night-time laughter decreased with age and the prevalence of reported daytime napping increased with age. There appeared to be some variation with age and *MECP2* mutation type. The prevalence of sleep problems was highest in cases with a large deletion of the *MECP2* gene and in those with the p.Arg294X and p.Arg306Cys mutations. Sleep problems were least likely to be reported in cases with C-terminal deletions. Night-time laughing was the most common night-time behavior in individuals with a large deletion. Daytime napping was common in individuals with p.Arg270X, p.Arg255X, and p.Thr158Met mutations. For some sleep problems, such as night screaming and night seizures, there were no statistically significant relationships with mutation type (Young et al. 2007). Similar results, especially in relation to p.Arg294X have been reported in a larger cohort using the Australian Rett Syndrome Database (Wong et al. 2015) and in an international study using the InterRett Database (Boban et al. 2016).

The presence of sleep problems can impact significantly, not only on the individual with RTT, but also on their families and carers (McDougall et al. 2005). When sleep problems are significant, carers and families need additional support, especially as their child with RTT becomes an adult. Sleep problems may not diminish with age and those with some mutation types appear to be more likely to have a sleep problem than others. An assessment of the sleep pattern should be considered as part of the overall multidisciplinary management of females with RTT.

Pathophysiology of sleep
Typical development of sleep–wake rhythm (SWR) involves specific age-dependent changes. The daytime sleep decreases as a child gets older, with three epochs. The first epoch is the first 4 months, which is the critical age for the development of the circadian sleep–wake cycle synchronizing to a 24-hour day–night cycle (Parmelee and Stern 1972; Segawa 1999a, 2006). During the second epoch, from 4 months, the main sleep time begins to shift to night-time and daytime sleep decreases, taking the form of naps. In the third epoch, at age of 4–5 years, the biphasic sleep and wake pattern appears, completing the circadian sleep–wake cycle (Segawa 1999a, 2006). Disturbances of the development of each epoch of circadian rhythm suggest abnormalities in particular monoaminergic projections of the raphe nuclei and the locus ceruleus (Segawa 1999a, 2006). Thus, the disturbed SWR in RTT points to an abnormality in the second epoch, indicating possible dysfunction of aminergic neurons, responsible for the development of the SWR after 4 months of age (Segawa and Nomura 1990, 1992a; Nomura and Segawa 2001).

Each sleep component is controlled by the specific neurons of brainstem and mid-brain (McCarley and Hobson 1971; Hobson et al. 1975). Thus, analysis of sleep components can inform understanding of the underlying pathophysiology, particularly of brainstem and mid-brain. Rapid eye movement (REM) sleep consists of tonic components, atonia of axial muscles and desynchronization of EEG, and phasic components with rapid eye and body movements. The components of REM sleep are executed by the cholinergic neurons of the pons. In non-REM (NREM) sleep, aminergic neurons of the brainstem, particularly noradrenergic neurons of the locus coeruleus, increase activity. These suppress the REM sleep executive cholinergic neurons, and prevent the components of REM sleep in NREM sleep (Hobson and McCarley 1975). Body movements during sleep are also known to reflect particular neuronal systems, particularly the dopaminergic system (Segawa 1999a, 2006). REM sleep components mature at specific ages. The occurrence of rapid eye movements and muscle twitch movements in REM sleep are observed at around 28 gestational weeks, and atonia begins to appear being restricted exclusively to REM sleep at 4 months postnatal age (Parmelee and Stern 1972; Segawa 1999b).

The examination of body movements in RTT suggest that there is hypofunction of the dopaminergic system, which is followed by receptor supersensitivity of dopaminergic projection to the striatum (Segawa 1997; Segawa and Nomura 1990, 1992a; Nomura and Segawa 1986). The neuronal system underlying atonia of REM sleep is the same as the postural suppression pathway (Nomura 1986; Segawa 1997; Segawa and Nomura 1990, 1992a; Nomura and Segawa 2001). Atonia in REM sleep inhibits all reflex systems, including those of the autonomic nervous system. The leakage of atonia into NREM sleep has been postulated as one of the causes of sudden infant death syndrome, because it prevents augmentation of respiration in response to hypoxia due to hypoventilation during NREM sleep (Segawa 1992). Leakage of atonia into NREM sleep also leads to dysfunction initially of the pedunculopontine nucleus and subsequently the dopaminergic system. This is manifested in terms of synaptic supersensitivity in the projection to the basal ganglia. Clock dependent waking during the night suggests that this is a phenomenon of REM sleep. Waking during REM sleep is considered to be due to increased body movements caused by the dopaminergic receptor supersensitivity (Segawa 1997; Nomura and Segawa 2001).

Evaluation of sleep in Rett syndrome

Evaluation of sleep in RTT should include a detailed sleep history that characterizes the sleep problems, parental responses, interventions, sleep–wake pattern, co-existing medical problems, medications that may impact on sleep, as well as a 'sleep diary' over a 1- to 2-week period and objective investigations. The objective investigations include actigraphy; that is, a wrist watch-like device, worn for a period of time (days to weeks) that records activity. A computer program is used to determine sleep–wake patterns using a paradigm in which activity equals wake state and inactivity equals sleep state. Another assessment tool is the overnight polysomnogram (PSG) or sleep study; that is, a multichannel recording of EEG, airflow, and respiratory effort, as well as oxygen levels, electrocardiogram, extremity movement, and video recording to identify nocturnal events. These parameters are recorded continuously over the duration of sleep allowing for the characterization of sleep staging, breathing, and motor activities. Nocturnal events such as seizures may be precisely characterized (Glaze et al. 1987a).

The study of sleep in RTT has identified several consistent findings including abnormalities in NREM sleep and REM sleep, evidence of autonomic dysfunction, and breathing abnormalities (Glaze et al. 1987b). A characteristic feature of the EEG in RTT, in addition to slowing and epileptiform abnormalities, is the loss after 2 years of age of expected sleep characteristics, such as sleep spindles and K-sleep complexes, which are the identifying features of NREM sleep (Weese-Mayer et al. 2008). These features may reappear in adulthood. In addition, epileptiform abnormalities appear to occur more frequently during sleep and during Stages 1 and 2 of NREM sleep (Weese-Mayer et al. 2008).

Overnight studies of breathing and heart rate have been performed to characterize autonomic dysfunction. Weese-Mayer and associates performed in-home continuous recordings of breathing, determined by inductance plethysmography and electrocardiogram in 47 girls with RTT aged 2–7 years with a mutation in the *MECP2* gene and 47 aged-matched female comparisons. It was found that girls with RTT demonstrated irregularities in breathing and heart rate during the night and day. During night-time recordings their breathing was more irregular, with an increase in breathing frequency and irregularity, mean amplitude of respiratory inductance plethysmography sum, and heart rate. These investigators concluded that there was an uncoupling of the measures of breathing and heart rate control indicating dysregulation in the autonomic nervous system during the day and night (Weese-Mayer et al. 2008).

The characteristic breathing disturbances in RTT such as hyperventilation and breath holding episodes mainly occur during wakefulness. Autonomic dysregulation may contribute to the occurrence of apnea, shallow breathing, hypoventilation, tachycardia, and bradycardia. These abnormalities occur during wakefulness and sleep, but episodes of bradycardia are more prominent during sleep; however, central apnea, characterized by absence of effort and airflow, and obstructive sleep apnea, characterized by respiratory effort with no or diminished air flow, are also observed in RTT (Glaze et al. 1987b; Marcus et al. 1994; Rohdin et al. 2007). These findings are similar to typical children and adults and are distinct from the wake breathing dysrhythmias of RTT. Individuals with RTT may be at increased risk for sleep disordered breathing because of contributing factors which include autonomic dysregulation as described above, alterations in central (brainstem) control of breathing, alterations in muscle tone, and tonsillar-adenoidal hypertrophy commonly occurring in young children.

In summary, objective evaluation of sleep in RTT demonstrates abnormal sleep characteristics and sleep–wake patterns. Autonomic dysfunction involving breathing and cardiac rhythm is present, while awake and during sleep. While the characteristic breathing dysrhythmia is evident during wakefulness, other breathing abnormalities including hypoventilation and central and obstructive apnea are also recorded in some females with RTT.

Management of sleep problems in Rett syndrome

Sleep plays an important role in restoring the body by allowing and supporting metabolic pathways and stimulating brain protein synthesis (Adams 1980). When an individual experiences sleep problems, everyday functioning and learning are compromised.

Managing sleep disorders requires a clear understanding of the child's patterns and rhythm of sleep, precipitating factors, and methods used to cope. Clinicians should request a daily 'sleep diary' (see Box 8.1).

BOX 8.1 A sleep diary should document and address the following questions:

- What time does the child or adult go to bed?
- What is the bedtime routine?
- Is the household noisy with TV, loud music, etc.?
- Are foods and drinks given before bedtime? Do they contain caffeine?
- Is the child on medications that may disrupt sleep?
- Does the she need holding, music, lights, rocking, or swinging movement?
- What is the frequency of night awakenings and does this disturb the family?
- How do caregivers respond to awakenings?
- Does the girl have inappropriate laughter?
- Is she awake and playing?
- Does she cry and scream for no apparent reason?
- Are there possible seizures?
- Does she snore or have sleep apnea?
- Does she cough, gag, choke, or vomit?
- Does she have excessive bruxism?
- Does she have dystonic spasms, or muscle cramps?
- If ambulatory, does she wake up and walk about the house?
- Is daytime sleep related to any specific time of day or activity?

Before recommendations for sleep hygiene and behavioral management are considered it is essential to identify co-existing medical conditions which may cause children to wake. A thorough history and clinical examination should include ruling out simple treatable conditions (see Box 8.2).

If sleep disorders, for example snoring or witnessed apnea, suggest occurrence of sleep disordered breathing or if other medical problems are suspected, diagnostic testing and evaluation, including an overnight sleep study (polysomnography), should be considered (see Box 8.3).

BOX 8.2 Co-existing medical problems to consider when evaluating sleep disturbance in RTT

- Pain
- Dental problems
- Ear infections
- Enlarged tonsils and adenoids causing obstructive apnea
- Gastroesophageal reflux is commonly reported in RTT and may result in dental caries
- Silent aspiration
- Chronic sinus infections
- Severe constipation
- Gallbladder colic often related to meal times and excessive flatulence
- Epilepsy
- Marked dystonic spasms especially seen in older females
- Rhythmic movement disorder in young children and restless leg syndrome
- Anxiety, night terrors or nightmares
- Premenstrual cramps which are often cyclical
- Unrecognized bone fracture which can occur without significant trauma

---

BOX 8.3 Diagnostic studies to be performed if clinically indicated

- Polysomnography (overnight sleep study) is indicated to evaluate breathing and unusual nocturnal events including seizures
- Electroencephalogram with 24-hour video telemetry

If periodic limb movements are suspected or recorded:

- Full blood count, ferritin, vitamin B12 for investigation of anemia

If sleep disordered breathing is suspected or documented:

- Dental evaluation
- ENT evaluation
- Lateral X-ray of neck and face
- Overnight oximetry

If gastrointestinal problems are suspected:

- Ph probe, barium swallow and upper gastrointestinal series for investigation of gastroesophageal reflux (GER) disease. Endoscopy may be necessary
- Plain X-ray abdomen to diagnose constipation and fecal impaction
- Abdominal ultrasound for suspected gall stones or renal stones

---

Treatment of sleep disturbance in Rett syndrome

Specific treatment for identified medical conditions will provide an expected response.

Nonmedical interventions

Sleep hygiene and behavioral approaches emphasize consistency in intervention. Parents should be instructed to practice a regular bedtime routine (see Box 8.4).

BOX 8.4 Steps for parents to improve sleep hygiene

- Always put the girl or woman to bed at the same time.
- Put her to bed where she normally sleeps, not, for example, in the parent's bed or on the living room sofa. If she wakes up she needs to know that she is in the same bed where she started to sleep.
- Feed large meals during the day and do not overfeed before bedtime.
- Avoid caffeinated foods, drinks, and medications at least 6 hours before bedtime.
- Identify factors that help early onset of sleep, such as avoiding day time naps, exercise, and outdoor activities during the day.
- A warm bath before bedtime promotes sleep.
- Many girls respond well to deep pressure massage after a warm bath.
- Avoid a stimulating environment such as loud music and television.
- Provide a room with low lighting and a comfortable bed. Some parents have used a vibrating mattress or a weighted blanket and claim that it helps.
- If the girl wakes during the night and wants to play, provide a safe environment. Place a gate at her bedroom door.
- Some girls are soothed by music.
- If the girl wakes up and is playing without disturbing the family, LEAVE HER ALONE as she may go back to sleep. If, however, she is awake and screaming and you hold her, change her diaper, and position her so that she may fall asleep.

MEDICAL MANAGEMENT

A behavioral approach using the steps outlined in Box 8.4 to improve the quality of sleep should be the first approach to the management of sleep problems. However, this approach may not be effective when used as the only treatment for sleep problems in individuals with neurological disorders such as RTT. For this reason, and because the sleep problems may have a significant negative impact on the quality of life of the individual as well as her family, the use of medication may be warranted. Moreover, while behavior approaches are effective treatment of sleep problems in typically developing children, there is no established evidence base for the use of these in children with developmental disorders, including RTT.

For adults with sleep problems, such as insomnia, there are several approved medications including benzodiazepines such as temazepam and non-benzodiazepines such as zolpidem, eszopiclone, and melatonin receptor agonists such as ramelteon. There are no approved medications with an indication for insomnia in children; however, a variety of medications with primary indications for non-sleep problems, but with sleep inducing properties, are frequently used for children in general and RTT specifically for difficulty initiating and maintaining sleep. A recent systematic review of the literature (Hollway and Aman 2011) identified 25 randomized, double-blind, placebo-controlled trials in typically developing children and children with developmental disabilities. There are none for RTT. To paraphrase the conclusion of these authors, there is a lack of empirical evidence on which to base decisions concerning the choice of hypnotics for girls with RTT experiencing sleep problems.

Of the potential candidates for use as a hypnotic, melatonin appears to be the 'best' studied. There are a number of randomized controlled trials of exogenous melatonin in children with developmental disabilities. In general, these studies demonstrated positive effects, including shortening of sleep onset latency and total sleep time; however, the mechanism of action for the hypnotic effect of melatonin is not well established. There is a paucity of information regarding the circadian profile and the levels of endogenous melatonin in RTT.

If the child with RTT has difficulty initiating sleep and staying asleep, melatonin has been reported to be effective (McArthur and Budden 1998). The dose is based on the child's age. Melatonin should be given approximately 30 minutes before anticipated sleep time. Doses of up to 10 mg have been used in blind children with no ill effects (Jan et al. 1994). Melatonin can be obtained from a health food store, but this preparation may not be the pure form and the desired response may not be observed.

Another commonly used medication is clonidine, an alpha-2 noradrenergic agonist used in adults for hypertension. Its use as a hypnotic in children has not been adequately established. There are currently only a few uncontrolled studies suggesting safety and efficacy of clonidine. Studies in adults have demonstrated reduction of REM sleep. The medication should be given 30 minutes before bedtime. An ECG should be performed before initiating this treatment and the child's blood pressure monitored because of the potential for lowering blood pressure. Nevertheless, it is an effective medication in managing pediatric insomnia (Owens et al. 2005).

Controlled studies in adults have demonstrated efficacy and safety of certain benzodi-azepines in adults. Uncontrolled studies of small sample size, which have been performed in children with other sleep disorders, such as parasomnias, support the safety and efficacy of clonazepam for use in children with sleep problems. This group of drugs is not used consistently, although one of the authors has found that diazepam or clonazepam may be effective in children who wake up with spasms due to rigidity. Clonazepam may also be effective in girls who are very irritable (Hollway and Aman 2011).

Certain antidepressants have significant sedating or sleep-inducing side effects and have been used to manage difficulties with initiating and maintaining sleep experienced by females with RTT. These include trazodone and quetiapine, which have an indication for management of insomnia in adults. Chloral hydrate can also be effective in initiating sleep; however, there is the potential for obstructive sleep apnea and loss of effectiveness with time.

Diphenhydramine has been evaluated in drug trials in children with developmental disabilities. Most of these studies have demonstrated no benefit of this medication and no differences when compared to placebo. However, in some of our clinical experience, this medication appears to be effective. Its effectiveness may wane over time and cause daytime drowsiness. In addition, some children may react paradoxically with irritability and agitation.

Effective management of sleep disorders in RTT requires a clear understanding of co-existing medical problems such as gastroesophageal reflux and nocturnal seizures, as well as, medications, which may precipitate recurrent awakenings. Additionally, sleep problems such as sleep disordered breathing and parasomnias should be appropriately addressed and managed. If these issues are successfully addressed and sleep problems persist then the use of behavioral approaches, possibly combined with the judicious use of medication, may resolve or improve the sleep problems with a positive secondary impact on daytime functioning for the girl or woman with RTT and quality of life for her family.

Conclusion

An arrest of brain development has been hypothesized in RTT. The immature sleep pattern demonstrated in several studies, without an age-related decrease in sleep time and exces-sive daytime sleep, may be a consequence of arrested brain development. An important area for future research is the extent to which the sleep dysfunction is amenable to pharma-cological or behavioral intervention. While studies comparing RTT to aged-matched com-parisons appear to establish the occurrence of autonomic dysfunction awake and asleep in RTT, studies characterizing sleep architecture in RTT are based on small sample sizes without the use of a matched comparison group or consideration of phenotype–genotype relationships. There is a need for studies to further characterize sleep architecture in RTT in large, well characterized RTT cohorts of all ages in order to develop appropriate treatment strategies.

The frequency of sleep problems in RTT and the potential negative impact on cognition, behavior, and quality of life of the individual and her family underscore the need for the development of effective and safe treatment strategies to address these sleep problems. In addition, characterization of sleep architecture and sleep problems in RTT, and development of safe and efficacious treatment strategies will depend on well-designed and powered trials of behavioral strategies and pharmacological agents.

Case study illustrating some sleep issues commonly seen in RTT

History and early development

BL was born at term after a normal pregnancy and delivery. In retrospect, shortly after birth her mother felt that there was something wrong. Feeds were difficult to establish and she suffered with significant gastroesophageal reflux. BL rolled at 10 months and walked at 18 months. BL lost previously acquired fine motor skills at approximately 2 years of age. At 12 months of age BL could say 'mum mum', 'dad dad' which she subsequently stopped saying. From approximately 2.5 to 3 years of age BL was noted to have mid-line hand clasping and clapping movements. She was diagnosed with Rett syndrome and found to have a mutation of the *MECP2* gene, p.Arg133Cys. BL always seemed to have a very disturbed sleep pattern. From 5 years of age she would not fall asleep until after 11 pm and often wake again at 4 am. This was very disruptive for the entire family as she would get out of bed and disturb other family members. On most days she had a 30 minute nap during the day. BL had a seizure disorder which was well controlled with carbemazepine. BL had a good appetite, however she enjoyed drinking a large amount of fruit juice each day. It was difficult for her parents to brush her teeth and she had dental caries. At 12 years of age her menstrual cycle started, which was heavy and caused her some discomfort.

Clinical assessment

On examination at 13 years of age BL appeared in good health. Her weight was 56.5 kg (78th centile) and height was 147 cm (4th centile). She was very active and walked about the consultation room. BL demonstrated mid-line hand clasping, hand wringing, and hand to mouth movements. She was able to finger feed herself. She vocalized and said 'mum' during the consultation. BL was in Stage 4 of breast and pubic hair development. Her muscle mass and general muscle tone were normal. There were no contractures. Her deep tendon reflexes were brisk and symmetrical. Her back was straight. Decay was noted on several of her teeth. There was no associated facial swelling, tenderness, or lymphadenopathy.

Baseline investigations

Evaluation included serum ferritin and vitamin B12 levels. The vitamin B12 level was low 17 pmol/L (normal >35 pmol/L) consistent with vitamin B12 deficiency. The ferritin was borderline low 12 ug/L (10–150 ug/L). The remainder of the investigations were normal.

Management

- Vitamin B12 and oral iron supplementation commenced
- Referral to pediatric dietician
- Referral to pediatric gynecologist, for management of her menstrual cycle
- Referral to dentist for assessment and management of dental caries
- Treatment with melatonin commenced

Outcomes

Coexisting medical issues were addressed and appropriately managed.

   Melatonin treatment led to a significant reduction in sleep latency. She fell asleep within 30 minutes of administration. With an improvement of night-time sleep she stopped napping during the day.

100

REFERENCES

Adams K (1980) Sleep as a restorative process and theory to explain why. *Prog Brain Res* 53: 289–325.

Aldrich M, Garofalo E, Drury I (1990) Epileptiform abnormalities during sleep in Rett syndrome. *Electroenceph Clin Neurophysiol* 75: 365–370.

Boban S, Wong K, Epstein A et al. (2016) Determinants of sleep disturbances in Rett syndrome: Novel findings in relation to genotype. *Am J Med Genet A* 170(9): 2292–2300.

Chervin RD, Hedger H, Dillon JE (2000) Pediatric Sleep Questionnaire: Validity and reliability of scales for sleep disordered breathing, snoring, sleepiness, and behavioral problems. *Sleep Med* 1: 21–32.

DeGangi GA, Breinbauer C (1997) The symptomatology of infants and toddlers with regulatory disorders. *J Dev Learn Disord* 1: 183–215.

D'Orsi G, Demaio V, Scapelli F et al. (2009) Central sleep apnoea in Rett syndrome. *Neurol Sci* 30: 389–391.

Drake C, Nickel C, Burduvali E, Roth T, Jefferson C, Pietro B (2003) The pediatric daytime sleepiness scale (PDSS): sleep habits and school outcomes in middle-school children. *Sleep* 26(4): 455–458.

Ellaway C, Peat J, Leonard H, Christodoulou J (2001) Sleep dysfunction in Rett syndrome: Lack of age related decrease in sleep duration. *Brain Dev* 23(Suppl. 1): S101–S103.

Glaze DG, Frost JD, Zoghbi HY, Percy AH (1987a) Rett's syndrome: Correlation of electroencephalogram characteristics with clinical staging. *Arch Neurol* 44: 1053–1056.

Glaze DG, Frost JD, Zoghbi HY, Percy AK (1987b) Rett's syndrome: Characteristics of respiratory patterns and sleep. *Ann Neurol* 21: 377–382.

Hobson JA, McCarley RW, Wyzinski PW (1975) Sleep cycle oscillation: Reciprocal discharge by two brainstem neuronal groups. *Science* 189: 55–58.

Hollway JA, Aman MG (2011) Pharmacological treatment of sleep disturbance in developmental disabilities: A review of the literature. *Res Dev Disabil* 32: 939–962.

Jan JE, Espezel H, Appleion RE (1994) The treatment of sleep disorders with melatonin. *Dev Med Child Neurol* 36: 97–107.

Marcus CL, Carroll JL, McColley SA et al. (1994) Polysomnographic characteristics of patients with Rett syndrome. *J Pediatr* 125: 218–224.

McCarley RW, Hobson JA (1971) Single unit activity in cat gigantocellular tegmental field: Selectivity of discharge in desynchronized sleep. *Science* 174: 1250–1252.

McArthur AJ, Budden SS (1998) Sleep dysfunction in Rett syndrome: A trial of exogenous melatonin treatment. *Dev Med Child Neurol* 40: 186–190.

McDougall A, Kerr A, Espie C (2005) Sleep disturbance in children with Rett syndrome: A qualitative investigation of the parental experience. *J Appl Res Intell Disab* 18: 201–215.

Nomura Y (2005) Early behavior characteristics and sleep disturbance in Rett syndrome. *Brain Dev* 27(Suppl 1): S35–S42.

Nomura Y, Segawa M (1986) Anatomy of Rett syndrome. *Am J Med Genet* Suppl. 1: 289–303.

Nomura Y, Segawa M (2001) The monoamine hypothesis in Rett syndrome. In: Kerr A, Engerström IW, editors. *Rett Disorder and the Developing Brain*. New York: Oxford University Press, 205–225.

Nomura Y, Segawa M, Hasegawa M (1984) Rett syndrome – clinical studies and pathophysiological consideration *Brain Dev* 6(5): 475–486.

Nomura Y, Segawa M, Higurashi M (1985) Rett syndrome – an early catecholamine and indolamine deficient disorder? *Brain Dev* 7(3): 334–341.

Owens JA, Witmans M (2004) Sleep problems. *Curr Probl Pediatr Adolesc Health Care* 34(4): 154–179.

Owens JA, Spirito A, McGuinn M, Nobile C (2000a) Sleep habits and sleep disturbance in elementary school-aged children. *J Dev Behav Pediatr* 21(1): 27–36.

Owens JA, Spirito A, McGuinn M (2000b) The Children's Sleep Habits Questionnaire (CSHQ): Psychometric properties of a survey instrument for school-aged children. *Sleep* 23(8): 1043–1051.

Owens JA, Babcock D, Blumer J et al. (2005) The use of pharmacotherapy in the treatment of pediatric insomnia in primary care; rational approaches. A consensus meeting summary. *J Clin Sleep Med* 1(1): 49–59.

Parmelee AH, Stern E (1972) Development of states in infants. In: Clement CD, Purpura DP, Mayer FE, editors. *Sleep and the Maturing Nervous System*. New York: Academic Press, 199–228.

Piazza CC, Fisher W, Kiesewetter K, Bowman L, Moser H (1990) Aberrant sleep patterns in children with the Rett syndrome. *Brain Dev* 12: 488–493.

Rohdin M, Fernell, E, Eriksson M, Albage M, Lagercrantz H, Katz-Salamon M (2007) Ng day disturbances in cardiorespiratory function during day and night in the Rett syndrome. *Pediatr Neurol* 37: 338–344.

Segawa M (1992) Sudden infant death syndrome. *Shinkei Kenkyu no Shinpo* 36: 1029–1040 (in Japanese).

Segawa M (1997) Pathophysiology of Rett syndrome from the standpoint of early catecholamine disturbance. *Review Eur Child Adolesc Psychiatry* 6(Suppl 1): 56–60.

Segawa M (1999a) Modulation of sleep in early childhood. In: Torii S, editor. *Sleep Ecology*. Tokyo: Asakura, 110–123 (in Japanese).

Segawa M (1999b) Ontogenesis of REM sleep. In: Mallick BN, Inoue S, editors. *Rapid Eye Movement Sleep*. New Delhi, India: Narosa Publishing House, 39–50.

Segawa M (2006) Epochs of development of the sleep-wake cycle reflect the modulation of the higher cortical function particular for each epoch. *Sleep Biol Rhyth* 4(1): 4–15.

Segawa M, Nomura, Y (1990) The pathophysiology of the Rett syndrome from the standpoint of polysomnography. *Brain Dev* 12: 55–60.

Segawa M, Nomura Y (1992) Polysomnography in the Rett syndrome. *Brain Dev* 14(Suppl): S46–S54.

Spilsbury JC, Drotar D, Rosen CL, Redline S (2007) The Cleveland adolescent sleepiness questionnaire: a new measure to assess excessive daytime sleepiness in adolescents. *J Clin Sleep Med* 15(6): 603–612.

Sultana R, Knight A, Lee HS, Glaze DG (2015) Prevalence of sleep problems in children with neuro-developmental disorders: A follow-up study. Abstract SLEEP Association Professional Sleep Society, June 2015.

Weese-Mayer DE, Lieske SP, Booyhby CM, Kenny AS, Bennett HL, Ramirez JM (2008) Autonomic dysfunction in young girls with Rett syndrome during nighttime in-home recordings. *Pediatr Pulmonol* 43: 1045–1060.

Wong K, Leonard H, Jacoby P, Ellaway C, Downs J (2015) The trajectories of sleep disturbances in Rett syndrome. *J Sleep Res* 24: 223–233.

Young D, Nagarajan L, de Klerk N, et al. (2007) Sleep problems in Rett syndrome. *Brain Dev* 29: 609–616.

9
Epilepsy in Rett Syndrome

Andreea Nissenkorn, Maria Pintaudi, Daniel G Glaze and Bruria Ben-Zeev

Introduction

Seizures are the major comorbidity in Rett syndrome (RTT) and significantly influence individuals' well-being and functioning. Although included in previous iterations (Hagberg et al. 2002), epilepsy is missing from the current diagnostic criteria (Neul et al. 2010), but still present in all functional scales grading disease severity (Colvin et al. 2003). The prevalence of epilepsy is high and reports range between 60–90% (Cooper et al. 1998; Steffenburg and Hagberg 2001; Jian et al. 2006, 2007; Huppke et al. 2007; Moser et al. 2007; Nissenkorn et al. 2010, 2015; Pintaudi et al. 2010; Cardoza et al. 2011), but may be affected by study design and the underlying population and its distribution. Moreover, these rates might be overestimated, since nonepileptic paroxysmal events in RTT are frequent and most studies are based on reporting of seizure semiology by caregivers or physicians and not on actual demonstration of ictal activity on EEG. Recent data suggest that frequency of epileptic seizures might be lower, about 48% (Glaze et al. 2010). Epilepsy may also be more prevalent among those without a proven mutation in the *MECP2* gene (Glaze et al. 2010), probably because of inclusion of the early epileptic variant, now known to be caused by a mutation in the *CDKL5* gene (Fehr et al. 2013). Some series have found relationships between presence of epilepsy and general severity, impairment of ambulation, and hand use (Jian et al. 2007; Glaze et al. 2010).

NATURAL HISTORY
Traditionally, seizures were described after regression (Stage 3), at about 4 years of age, based on research measuring the mean age of individuals at onset of epilepsy (Steffenburg and Hagberg 2001; Moser et al. 2007) or median age using time-to-event analysis (Jian et al. 2006; Nissenkorn et al. 2015). Recent accumulating data suggest that mean age of individuals at onset of epilepsy may be slightly younger (Nissenkorn et al. 2010; Pintaudi et al. 2010). Epilepsy appears earlier in nonambulatory patients and in those with abnormal development in the first 10 months of life (Jian et al. 2007). Mutation type and location (Charman et al. 2005; Jian et al. 2006; Nectoux et al. 2008), as well as brain derived neurotrophic factor (*BDNF*) polymorphisms may also influence age at onset of epilepsy (Ben Zeev et al. 2009; Nectoux et al. 2008; Nissenkorn et al. 2010). Among individuals with a classic presentation, onset of epilepsy before 5 years of age has been shown to predict seizure intractability and severity (Nissenkorn et al. 2010, 2015; Pintaudi et al. 2010).

Seizure frequency and severity peak is usually during the postregression period, while the seizures become easier to manage during the second decade of life (Jian et al. 2006; Ben Zeev Ghidoni 2007). Occasionally epilepsy may start in the second decade of life (Nissenkorn et al. 2015). Data regarding the natural history of epileptic seizures into adulthood are sparse, but a Dutch cohort, based on caregiver questionnaires of 53 adult participants showed no reduction with age in seizure prevalence (Halbach et al. 2008). This is in contrast to an earlier study by Hagberg et al. (2001) and international cross-sectional data (Bao et al. 2013), as well as our own clinical impression based on continuous clinic follow up into adulthood; there appears to be a reduction of both frequency and severity of seizures from the end of the second decade of life (Hagberg et al. 2001). Girls who are seizure free and show relatively 'quiet' sleep and awake EEG recordings for several years may have their anticonvulsant treatment cautiously tapered off.

All kinds of seizure types have been reported (Hagberg 1992; Cooper et al. 1998; Steffenburg and Hagberg 2001; Ben Zeev Ghidoni 2007; Nissenkorn et al. 2010; Cardoza et al. 2011) with no specific presenting seizure. Generalized tonic–clonic seizures, simple, and partial complex seizures are more frequent than atypical absences and myoclonic seizures (Nissenkorn et al. 2015). Tonic seizures and drop attacks have not been reported. Multiple seizure types may be present in the same patient. Fever related seizures have been shown to be over-represented and may be the first seizure type (Nissenkorn et al. 2010). Although infantile spasms and hypsarrhythmia are the hallmark of *CDKL5* gene mutations, there are sporadic reports of girls with this early epileptic variant with *MECP2* mutations. Status epilepticus is not uncommon and includes generalized tonic–clonic status and non-convulsive status epilepticus. Transient deterioration in motor skills may be observed in girls following status epilepticus. Girls with onset of epilepsy before 5 years of age are particularly prone to develop electrical status epilepticus during slow wave sleep (ESES) that may evolve into awake nonconvulsive status (Nissenkorn et al. 2010). The presence of ESES negatively affects child alertness, communication, and motor skills.

Myoclonus may represent either an epileptic event or a subcortical movement disorder (Guerrini 1998) and clinical discrimination between them may be difficult; however, accurate diagnosis is important whenever it evolves into epileptic myoclonic status (d'Orsi et al. 2009). Lately, reflex seizures triggered by food intake or proprioception were described in three individuals although other seizures started at an early age the reflex seizures appeared at adolescence (Roche Martínez 2011). Interestingly, the self-induced 'pressure' triggered attacks were influenced by stress and excitement.

A unique phenomenon of awake, rhythmic, continuous hand tapping synchronous to contralateral central spikes have been noticed and may be under-recognized. Despite the 'ictal-like' EEG appearance, this phenomenon is considered by us as nonepileptic, most probably representing evoked potentials in a hyperexcitable cortex and therefore not requiring treatment (Nissenkorn and Ben Zeev 2013). In addition, one should be aware of the variety of paroxysmal nonepileptic events characteristic of RTT, which may be difficult to diagnose without an ictal video-EEG (Glaze et al. 1998).

The severity of epilepsy and resistance to antiepileptic treatment varies between different series, ranging from 16%, a rate that is comparable to the general epilepsy population (Huppke et al. 2007; Buoni et al. 2008), up to frequent drug resistant epilepsy in 30–50% of cases (Steffenburg and Hagberg 2001; Nissenkorn et al. 2010, 2015; Pintaudi et al. 2010, 2015; Bao et al. 2013).

GENOTYPE–PHENOTYPE EPIGENETICS AND RISK FACTORS

In several studies the rate of epilepsy was found to be higher in participants with RTT without *MECP2* mutations and seizures tended to occur earlier. For example, seizures in the first year of life occurred only in 4% of all girls with RTT studied but only 20% of them carried a *MECP2* mutation (Charman et al. 2005). The rarity of *MECP2* mutations in girls with seizure onset at the first year of life was confirmed also by Jian et al. (2006).

MECP2 mutations are spread over the gene and can be described according to the specific protein function related to their location. Although there are more than 300 different mutations described so far in the *MECP2* gene, 60% of the classic cases carry one of eight hot-spot mutations. The most prevalent in most cohorts are p.Thr158Met and p.Arg168X. Most studies investigating genotype–phenotype relationships in RTT compare differences among those with specific hot-spot mutations, and rarely relate to the other less common mutations. Few studies take into account mutation location in relation to the protein functional regions. Severe mutations [large deletions, early truncating, and missense in the methyl binding domain (MBD) or the nuclear localizing segment (NLS)] were found to present with earlier or more severe epilepsy, while a milder mutation (late truncating or C terminal deletions) had a protective effect on epilepsy onset (Jian et al. 2006, 2007; Nectoux et al. 2008; Pintaudi et al. 2010). However, no relationships between genotype and phenotype were found in large international, Italian, Israeli, and British studies (Buoni et al. 2008; Bebbington et al. 2008; Nissenkorn et al. 2010; Cardoza et al. 2011), but the results could have been negatively influenced by the relatively small case numbers in some analyses.

Recently, four different large studies examining genotype–phenotype relationships for epilepsy were published, with contradictory results (Glaze et al. 2010; Bao et al. 2013; Cuddapah et al. 2014; Nissenkorn et al. 2015). A tendency to a higher prevalence of epilepsy or to increased severity of epilepsy was present in all four studies for the p.Thr158Met mutation (Glaze et al. 2010; Bao et al. 2013; Cuddapah et al. 2014; Nissenkorn et al. 2015). The localization of this missense mutation in the MBD region, affecting interaction with chromatin, might explain its severe effect on the general phenotype, including epilepsy (Charman et al. 2005; Jian et al. 2006; Buoni et al. 2008; Nectoux et al. 2008; Glaze et al. 2010); however, there was no agreement in these studies about the effect of other mutations. The p.Arg255X mutation, associated with a severe RTT phenotype, was less associated with epilepsy in one study (Glaze et al. 2010), while being associated with more severe epilepsy in two others (Cuddapah et al. 2014; Nissenkorn et al. 2015). The p.Arg133Cys, usually associated with the preserved speech variant (PSV) form, was less associated with epilepsy by Bao et al. (2013), while being associated with increased frequency of epilepsy, which was relatively easily managed by Nissenkorn et al. (2015). Contradictory results were also found regarding the tendency towards epilepsy in the p.Arg306Cys mutation (Glaze et al. 2010; Cuddapah et al. 2014; Nissenkorn et al. 2015). C terminal deletions, which are associated with a general milder disease severity, were related to decreased frequency of epilepsy

(Nissenkorn et al. 2015). Conversely, large deletions, which are associated with a more severe phenotype, were associated with more severe epilepsy in three studies (Bebbington et al. 2012; Pintaudi et al. 2010; Bao et al. 2013), but onset of seizures was later than in other mutations in one study (Pintaudi et al. 2010).

The discrepancies between different studies in relation to the effect of specific mutations on epilepsy outcomes might well be due to their methodological differences or associated with the different X inactivation status in individuals with similar mutations. The relationship between X inactivation patterns in the brain and lymphocytes is unclear, but since brain tissue is unavailable, studies have used the lymphocyte X inactivation ratios when examining phenotype–genotype relationships. Skewed inactivation was a protective factor for early seizure onset and seizure rate in two studies based on the Australian database (Jian et al. 2006, 2007).

Polymorphisms in the *BDNF* gene have been shown to associate independently with epilepsy in RTT (Nectoux et al. 2008; Ben Zeev et al. 2009; Buoni et al. 2010; Nissenkorn et al. 2010). BDNF has a special role in the pathophysiology of RTT, since it is one of the major genes up-regulated by MeCP2 (Charcour et al. 2008). Increasing BDNF levels in *Mecp2* mutant mice were shown to improve disease phenotype (Ogier et al. 2007; Larimore et al. 2009). Therefore, it is not surprising that the Val/Val polymorphism, present in 20% of the general population and responsible for higher BDNF synaptic secretion, was associated with overall decreased disease severity and later seizure onset in a large Australian–Israeli cohort of girls with the p.Arg168X mutation (Ben Zeev et al. 2009). In the Israeli cohort of individuals with RTT, this polymorphism was found as the only parameter influencing seizure onset in participants with different mutations (Nissenkorn et al. 2010). The findings are in contrast to those presented from a French cohort using different statistical methods (Nectoux et al. 2008), but are supported by those for an Italian cohort investigating the Zappella/PSV variant (Buoni et al. 2010).

EEG

The first description of an abnormally slow background on EEG recording was by Andreas Rett himself in his initial description of RTT in 1966 (Rett 1966), and confirmed by Hagberg in 1983 (Hagberg et al. 1983). Niedermeyer further delineated EEG abnormalities in 1986 in a review of 230 recordings of EEG in 44 individuals with clinical RTT and described monotonous rhythmic slowing of background in the delta wave range in wakefulness and drowsiness and bilateral slow spike and wave accentuated in sleep with abolishment of the physiological sleep pattern (Niedermeyer et al. 1986) (Fig. 9.1). Most prominent abnormalities were observed between 3 and 10 years of age.

Glaze et al. (1987) emphasized the correlation between EEG features and disease stage: in Stage 1 EEG is usually normal or shows minimal slowing; in Stage 2, slowing of the occipital dominant rhythm becomes more prominent, nonREM sleep physiologic features (sleep spindles, vertex waves, and K complexes) tend to disappear, and focal spikes and sharp waves are noticed, first during nonREM sleep and then during wakefulness. At Stage 3, there is aggravation of generalized slowing and multifocal and generalized epileptiform discharges appear during sleep and awake state. Prominent rhythmic theta activity may be

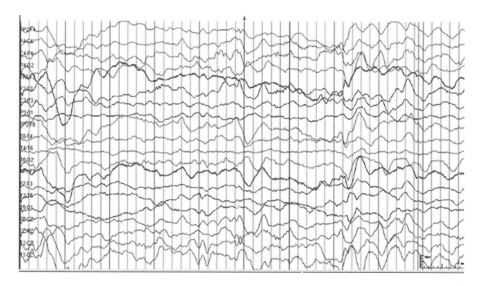

Fig. 9.1. Slow disorganized sleep pattern in a 10-year-old girl.

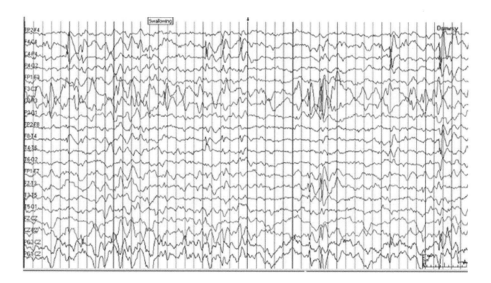

Fig. 9.2. Characteristic bilateral independent centrotemporal 'rolandic' spikes in a 4-year-old girl.

present in central regions. Stage 4 is characterized by diffuse delta activity and multifocal epileptic discharges during wakefulness. The centro-temporal 'rolandic' location and morphology of the spikes was first mentioned by Hagne et al. (1989), emphasizing their prominence and consistency in patients already at Stage 2 (Hagne et al. 1989) (Fig. 9.2). Variability in EEG patterns of background and epileptiform activity is characteristic of Stages 3 and 4.

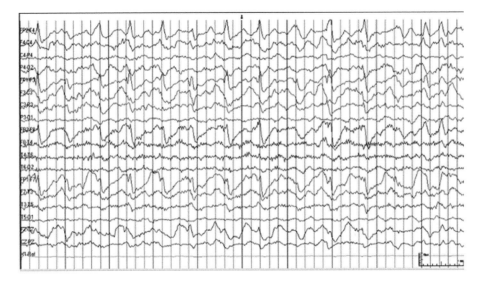

Fig. 9.3. Slow spike and wave EEG pattern resembling Angelman syndrome in a 3-year-old girl.

More up to date longitudinal studies on EEG features in large cohorts of individuals with RTT are lacking. Further emphasis should be given to the centro-temporal spikes aggravated during sleep as an almost pathognomonic EEG feature for RTT, although occasionally patients have rhythmic slow spike and wave pattern, 'Angelman-like' at an early clinical stage (Stages 2 and 3) (Fig. 9.3). These frequent centro-temporal spikes precede clinical seizures by 1 year and in some patients evolve gradually from sporadic spikes during sleep into a full blown electrical status epilepticus during slow wave sleep (ESES) pattern (Nissenkorn et al. 2010) (Fig. 9.4). The frequency of ESES may be as high as 23.4% in girls with onset of epilepsy before 5 years of age. The incidence of this phenomenon is at least as common in individuals with PSV (Zappella) variant, which may lead to misdiagnosis of these girls as having idiopathic Landau Kleffner syndrome (Nissenkorn et al. 2010; Al Keilani et al. 2011).

In the studies where it has been investigated, no clear relationship to date has been found between severity of epilepsy and drug resistance, and extent of epileptic activity on EEG (Moser et al. 2007; Buoni et al. 2008).

Treatment

There is considerable debate in the literature concerning the preferred antiepileptic drug treatment in RTT-related epilepsy. No clear guidelines exist in relation to the optimal first line anticonvulsant to be used, and personal experience of the epileptologist plays a major role in the decision-making process. The choice should be influenced by the type of seizures, the characteristics of the epileptiform activity on EEG, and other unrelated symptoms (e.g. appetite, sleep quality, drooling, tone, hyperventilation, and hyperkinetic activity). Response to treatment is difficult to evaluate because of the wide variability in seizure types

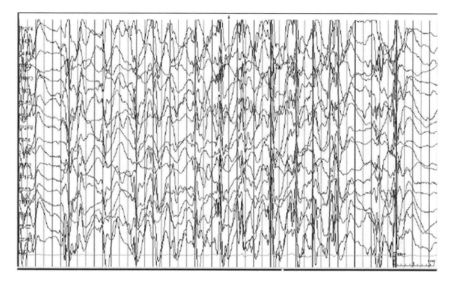

Fig. 9.4. Abundant epileptiform activity during sleep evolving into epilepticus during slow wave sleep in a 7-year-old girl.

and nonepileptic paroxysmal events, as well as high variability amongst patients, and even in the same patient. This is probably the reason why there are so few studies that compare the efficacy of antiepileptic drugs in individuals with RTT and none of them is a prospective controlled study (Jian et al. 2007; Huppke et al. 2007; Krajnc et al. 2011; Pintaudi et al. 2010, 2015).

According to the majority of authors, valproic acid is usually the first antiepileptic drug used with patients (Jian et al. 2007; Nissenkorn et al. 2010; Krajnc et al. 2011; Pintaudi et al. 2015). The advantage of valproic acid is in its broad spectrum of efficacy (effective in generalized, partial, absences, and myoclonic seizures), as well as its positive influence on the interictal EEG epileptiform activity (Nissenkorn et al. 2010). It probably should be chosen as a first line in younger individuals with abundant interictal activity during sleep and those with ESES (Nissenkorn et al. 2010). Since valproic acid is a histone deacetylase (HDAC) inhibitor, theoretically it could worsen disease symptoms by amplifying the effect of MeCP2 defect on transcription repression (Huppke et al. 2007). However, disease severity scores in patients treated with valproic acid were similar to those on different antiepileptic treatment in a large Israeli cohort (Nissenkorn et al. 2010). There have been concerns raised about the effect of valproic acid on bone metabolism in individuals with RTT who are already prone to osteoporosis (Leonard et al. 2010). Carbamazepine is a good alternative as a first line antiepileptic treatment (Huppke et al. 2007; Jian et al. 2007; Kranjc et al. 2011; Pintaudi et al. 2015), but one should be aware of the possible aggravation of generalized spike and wave discharges, absences, and myoclonic seizures (Nissenkorn et al. 2010). Sulthiame, which is a popular drug for benign epilepsies in some countries, while being almost unknown in others, has been found to be effective in one study (Huppke et al. 2007). Topiramate is an appealing alternative, since it is effective against all seizure types, as well as against respiratory dysregulation (Goyal et al. 2004); however, anorexia and drowsiness may limit dosage elevation. Lamotrigine was found in several studies to be as effective as monotherapy, as well as add-on therapy (Uldall et al. 1993; Stenbom et al. 1998; Krajnc et al. 2011). It has less effect on alertness, and may be especially of benefit in adolescents in whom epilepsy starts later and in generalized seizures (Pintaudi et al. 2015). Newer antiepileptic drugs such as levetiracetam also may be used with success in drug resistant seizures (Specchio et al. 2010).

Our guidelines would be to use valproic acid or lamotrigine as a first line treatment. Carbamazepine is a good alternative in older girls without abundant spike and wave epileptiform activity on EEG. In girls with concurrent hyperventilation episodes, topiramate should be considered as the first drug of choice. Since epilepsy is severe in RTT, many individuals require polytherapy. Lamotrigine, topiramate, or levetiracetam could be added as a second line. Benzodiazepines are especially useful as add-on therapy at low dosage in patients with RTT, paying attention to their sedative effect. Phenobarbitone should be avoided since it is less effective and causes severe drowsiness. Some individuals are especially resistant to antiepileptic drug therapy, but may respond to a ketogenic diet (Haas et al. 1986; Liebhaber et al. 2003), or vagal nerve stimulation (Wilfong et al. 2006).

One should avoid overzealous treatment of seizures in RTT. Breakthrough seizures are frequent, and treatment adjustment should not be carried out as long as seizures are not prolonged, do not endanger the patient, or do not lower the patient's or family's well-being. In individuals with infrequent absences or rare sporadic myoclonic events only, there is probably no need for 'aggressive' treatment if low-dose benzodiazepines have failed. Epileptiform activity without documented clinical seizures does not require treatment (Huppke et al. 2007; Krajnc et al. 2011). With regard to ESES, treatment with valproic acid or levetiracetam should be attempted, but more aggressive treatments such as high dose steroids should be avoided (Nissenkorn et al. 2010).

Pathophysiology

Epilepsy is a frequent comorbidity in children with developmental disability; however, the high rate of epilepsy and even higher rate of interictal epileptiform activity in the face of normal gross brain structure in individuals with RTT suggests an intrinsic role of MeCP2 in pathophysiology of epilepsy. Calfa et al. (2011), using sophisticated in vitro techniques, studied the amplitude and neuronal depolarization in hipoccampal slices from male symptomatic *Mecp2* mutant knockouts and revealed that both CA1 and CA3 regions are highly excitable. Interestingly, when isolating the CA1 slices and investigating them separately, no hyperexcitability was detected, while recording from the CA3 pyramidal neurons revealed higher spontaneous firing rate. Therefore, the hyperactive CA3 pyramidal neurons might be responsible for the dysfunction of the hippocampal network leading to limbic seizures. The hyperexcitablilty of the hippocampal circuitry was reduced by application of adenosine, a brain endogenous neuromodulator, opening up interesting avenues for intervention (Calfa et al. 2011).

The underlying mechanism of synaptic dysfunction in the hippocampus is still unclear. Several aberrations in neurotransmitters may be responsible, including abnormal glutamate clearance by astrocytes (Okabe et al. 2012), abnormal BDNF levels (Ogier et al. 2007), aberrant GABAergic neurons (Chao et al. 2010), or abnormal perinatal expression of ion channels related to epilepsy (Bedogni et al. 2016).

Rett variants

Early epileptic variant (Hanefeld variant) and *CDKL5*

Almost 2 decades after Andreas Rett described the first clinical cases of RTT (Rett 1966), Hanefeld described females with atypical RTT and infantile spasms with hypsarrhythmia during the first year of life (Hanefeld 1985). The phenotype was widened by Goutières and Aicardi (1985) to include early seizures of any kind and was entitled Hanefeld variant. Patients with the early epileptic variant have onset of seizures during the first 3 months of life; usually the seizures are partial, myoclonic, tonic, or generalized, and infantile spasms also occur. Seizures are drug resistant and often remain refractory. In contrast to classic RTT, development is delayed from the first month of life, but hand stereoypies and decreased hand usage appear during the second year of life. A unique feature of these girls is poor eye contact and cortical blindness (Huppke et al. 2003; Nissenkorn et al. 2010).

While mutations in the *MECP2* gene may be found in 20–50% of RTT variants, in the Hanefeld variant they are rare (Rajaei et al. 2011). Mutations in other genes could be responsible for this phenotype, but at the present time the only known gene is *CDKL5*. Initially associated with hypsarrhythmia without features of RTT (Kalscheuer et al. 2003), mutations in *CDKL5* have been subsequently described in the Hanefeld variant (Evans et al. 2005; Scala et al. 2005). The RTT like features are considered to be due to the common molecular pathway of CDKL5 and MeCP2 (Mari et al. 2005), but they are not mandatory in the CDKL5 phenotype (Fehr et al. 2013); however, several features are characteristic of epilepsy in CDKL5 syndrome (Bahi Buisson et al. 2008). Seizures appear during the first 3 months of life; tonic generalized spasms, autonomic or myoclonic, while interictal EEG is still characteristically normal. Later on, infantile spasms with hypsarrhythmia develop in a portion of cases. Occasionally, after the early seizures, there may be a honeymoon period, followed by the development of epilepsy with tonic and myoclonic seizures. While seizures might be refractory to treatment, the EEG has surprisingly scarce epileptic activity. Juvenile spasms are a peculiar type of seizure, characteristic for CDKL5 (Klein et al. 2011).

Preserved speech variant (Zappella variant)

Patients with the Zappella variant have higher functional scores in speech as well as hand functioning domains; therefore, one might instinctively infer that epilepsy would be milder. However, not all studies show a difference in age at onset or severity of epilepsy in this milder variant (Nissenkorn et al. 2010, 2015). A study of 16 girls with the Zappella variant found lower prevalence of epilepsy (37.5%) (Buoni et al. 2010). The authors found that girls with higher functioning (true PSV, that is, with words and sentences and higher hand functioning such as drawing), had occasional seizures, centrotemporal spikes on EEG, but no slowing of the background. By comparison, lower functioning girls (single words and no preservation of hand functioning), had frequent daily seizures, multifocal epileptiform activity with slowing of the background on EEG. The difference between the two groups was not related to missense versus nonsense mutation, but to the BDNF polymorphism (Buoni et al. 2010).

One should be aware of the possibility of language regression in a girl with PSV, along with abundant epileptiform activity during sleep, and not confuse it with Landau-Kleffner syndrome, but consider aggressive intervention (Nissenkorn et al. 2010).

DUPLICATIONS IN MECP2

In several small series of males with MECP2 duplications, epilepsy was a major symptom with both partial and generalized seizures, as well as myoclonic astatic epilepsy (Echenne 2009; Ramoki et al. 2010). In most cases, epilepsy was intractable and coincides with developmental regression. Interestingly, the most prominent EEG feature was generalized slowing of the background, rather than abundant spike and wave activity characteristic of classic RTT (Vignoli et al. 2012). Prevalence of epilepsy in symptomatic females with MECP2 duplications is probably much lower (Bijlsma et al. 2012).

Conclusion

Epilepsy is a frequent comorbidity in RTT, affecting as many as 50–70% of individuals with the disorder Epilepsy appears at around 3–4 years of age and may recede during the second decade of life. While all types of seizures may be present, special attention should be paid to fever-induced seizures. Electroencephalographic features are almost pathognomonic for this syndrome, with centrotemporal spikes accentuating in sleep and slowing of the background. The abundant epileptic activity during sleep may evolve into electrical status epilepticus during slow sleep (ESES). Special caution should be made to differentiate epileptic seizures from nonepileptic paroxysmal and autonomic events, which are frequent in RTT.

Seizures may be difficult to treat with a 30% rate of drug-resistant epilepsy. Girls with earlier onset of epilepsy have a tendency towards more severe epilepsy. While some studies failed to identify any genotype–phenotype relationships, others found that individuals carrying the p.Thr158Met or p.Arg106Trp mutations are more likely to have epilepsy than the ones with p.Arg255X or p.Arg306Cys. In addition, the val/val polymorphism in the *BDNF* gene, causing higher synaptic secretion of BDNF, is associated with a milder epilepsy course.

Treatment of epilepsy should be adjusted to seizure type and severity, but overtreatment should be avoided. Valproic acid and lamotrigine should be used as first line drugs, with carbamazepine being reserved for older individuals without abundant spike and wave activity on EEG. Topiramate, levetiracetam, or low dose benzodiazepines may be added as a second line.

Early diagnosis and rational treatment of epilepsy are fundamental for the quality of life in individuals with RTT and their families.

REFERENCES

Al Keilani MA, Carlier S, Groswasser J, Dan B, Deconinck N (2011) Rett syndrome associated with continuous spikes and waves during sleep. *Acta Neurol Belg* 111(4): 328–332.

Bahi-Buisson N, Kaminska A, Boddaert N et al. (2008) The three stages of epilepsy in patients with CDKL5 mutations. *Epilepsia* 49: 1027–1037.

Bao X, Downs J, Wong K, Williams S, Leonard H (2013) Using a large international sample to investigate epilepsy in Rett syndrome. *Dev Med Child Neurol* 55(6): 553–558.

Bebbington A, Anderson A, Ravine D et al. (2008) Investigating genotype-phenotype relationships in Rett syndrome using an international data set. *Neurology* 70: 868–875.

Bebbington A, Downs J, Percy A et al. (2012) The phenotype associated with a large deletion on MECP2. *Eur J Hum Genet*: 20(9): 921–927.

Bedogni F, Cobolli Gigli C, Pozzi D et al. (2016) Defects during Mecp2 null embryonic cortex development precede the onset of overt neurological symptoms. *Cereb Cortex* 26: 2517–2529.

Ben Zeev Ghidoni, B (2007) Rett syndrome. *Child Adolesc Psychiatr Clin N Am* 16: 723–743.

Ben Zeev B, Bebbington A, Ho G et al. (2009) The common BDNF polymorphism may be a modifier of disease severity in Rett syndrome. *Neurology* 2(14): 1242–1247.

Bijlsma EK, Collins A, Papa FT et al. (2012) Xq28 duplications including MECP2 in five females: Expanding the phenotype to severe mental retardation. *Eur J Med Genet* 55(6–7): 404–413.

Buoni S, Zanolli R, De Felice C et al. (2008) Drug-resistant epilepsy and epileptic phenotype-EEG association on MeCP2 mutated Rett syndrome. *Clin Neurophysiol* 119: 2455–2458.

Buoni S, Zannolli R, De Felice C et al. (2010) EEG features and epilepsy in MECP2-mutated patients with the Zappella variant of Rett syndrome. *Clin Neurophysiol* 121: 652–657.

Calfa G, Hablitz JJ, Pozzo-Miller L (2011) Network hyperexcitability in hippocampal slices from Mecp2 mutant mice revealed by voltage-sensitive dye imaging. *J Neurophysiol* 105(4): 1768–1784.

Cardoza B, Clarke A, Wilcox J et al. (2011) Epilepsy in Rett syndrome: Association between phenotype and genotype, and implications for practice. *Seizure* 20: 646–649.

Chao HT, Chen H, Samaco RC et al. (2010) Dysfunction in GABA signalling mediates autism-like stereotypies and Rett syndrome phenotypes. *Nature* 468(7321): 263–269.

Charcour M, Jung SY, Shaw C et al. (2008) MeCP2, a key contributor to neurological disease, activates and represses transcription. *Science* 320: 1224–1229.

Charman T, Neilson TC, Mash V et al. (2005) Dimensional phenotypic analysis and functional categorisation of mutations reveal novel genotype-phenotype associations in Rett syndrome. *Eur J Hum Genet* 13(10): 1121–1130.

Cooper RA, Kerr AM, Amos PA (1998) Rett syndrome: Clinical examination of clinical features, serial EEG and video-monitoring in understanding and management. *Eur J Pediatr Neurol* 2: 127–135.

Colvin, Fyfe S, Leonard S et al. (2003) Describing the phenotype in Rett syndrome using a population database. *Arch Dis Child* 88: 38–43.

Cuddapah VA, Pillai RB, Shekar KV et al. (2014) Methyl-CpG-binding protein 2 (MECP2) mutation type is associated with disease severity in Rett syndrome. *J Med Genet* 51(3): 152–158.

d'Orsi G, Demaio V, Minervini MG. (2009) Myoclonic status misdiagnosed as movement disorders in Rett syndrome: A video-polygraphic study. *Epilepsy Behav* 15(2): 260–262.

Echenne B, Roubertie A, Lugtenberg D et al. (2009) Neurologic aspects of MECP2 gene duplication in male patients. *Pediatr Neurol* 41(3): 187–191.

Evans JC, Archer HL, Colley JP et al. (2005) Early onset seizures and Rett-like features associated with mutations in CDKL5. *Eur J Hum Genet* 13(10): 1113–1120.

Fehr S, Wilson M, Downs J et al. (2013) The CDKL5 disorder is an independent clinical entity associated with early-onset encephalopathy. *Eur J Hum Genet* 21(3): 266–273.

Glaze DG, Frost JD Jr, Zoghbi HY, Percy AK (1987) Rett's syndrome. Correlation of electroencephalographic characteristics with clinical staging. *Arch Neurol* 44(10): 1053–1056.

Glaze DG, Schultz RJ, Frost JD (1998) Rett syndrome: Characterization of seizures versus non-seizures) *Electroencephalogr Clin Neurophysiol* 106(1): 79–83.

Glaze DG, Percy AK, Skinner S et al. (2010) Epilepsy and the natural history of Rett syndrome. *Neurology* 74: 909–912.

Goutières F, Aicardi J (1985) Rett syndrome: Clinical presentation and laboratory investigations in 12 further French patients. *Brain Dev* 7(3): 305–306.

Goyal M, O'Riordan MA, Wiznitzer M (2004) Effect of topiramate on seizures and respiratory dysrhythmia in Rett syndrome. *J Child Neurol* 19: 588–591.

Guerrini R, Bonanni P, Parmeggiani L, Santucci M, Parmeggiani A, Sartucci F (1998) Cortical reflex myoclonus in Rett syndrome. *Ann Neurol* 43(4): 472–479.

Haas RH, Rice MA, Trauner DA, Merritt TA. (1986) Therapeutic effects of a ketogenic diet in Rett syndrome. *Am J Med Genet* Suppl. 1: 225–246.

Hagberg B (1992) *Rett Syndrome: Clinical and Biologic Aspects*. London: Mac Keith Press.

Hagberg B, Aicardi J, Dias K, Ramos O (1983) A progressive syndrome of autism, dementia, ataxia, and loss of purposeful hand use in girls: Rett's syndrome: Report of 35 cases. *Ann Neurol* 14(4): 471–479.

Hagberg B, Berg M, Steffenburg U (2001) Three decades of sociomedical experiences from West Swedish Rett females 4–60 years of age. *Brain Dev* 23(Suppl 1): S28–S31.

Hagberg B, Hanefeld F, Percy A, Skjeldal O (2002) An update on clinically applicable diagnostic criteria in Rett syndrome. Comments to Rett Syndrome Clinical Criteria Consensus Panel Satellite to European Paediatric Neurology Society Meeting, Baden Baden, Germany, 11 September 2001. *Eur J Paediatr Neurol* 6(5): 293–297.

Hagne I, Witt-Engerström I, Hagberg B (1989) EEG development in Rett syndrome. A study of 30 cases. *Electroencephalogr Clin Neurophysiol* 72(1): 1–6.

Halbach NS, Smeets EE, Schrander-Stumpel CT et al. (2008) Aging in people with specific genetic syndromes: Rett syndrome. *Am J Med Genet* 146A(15): 1925–1932.

Hanefeld F (1985) The clinical pattern of the Rett syndrome. *Brain Dev* 7(3): 320–325.

Huppke P, Held M, Laccone F, Hanefeld F (2003) The spectrum of phenotypes in females with Rett Syndrome. *Brain Dev* 25(5): 346–351.

Huppke P, Kohler K, Brockmann K, Stettner GM, Gartner J (2007) Treatment of epilepsy in Rett syndrome. *Eur J Paediatr Neurol* 11: 10–16.

Jian L, Nagarajan L, De Klerk N et al. (2006) Predictors of seizure onset in Rett syndrome. *J Pediatr* 149: 542–547.

Jian L, Nagarajan L, De Klerk N, Ravine D, Christodoulou J, Leonard H (2007) Seizures in Rett syndrome: An overview from a one-year calendar study. *Eur J Paediatr Neurol* 11: 310–317.

Kalscheuer VM, Tao J, Donnelly A et al. (2003) Disruption of the serine/threonine kinase 9 gene causes severe X-linked infantile spasms and mental retardation. *Am J Hum Genet* 72(6): 1401–1411.

Klein KM, Yendle SC, Harvey AS et al. (2011) A distinctive seizure type in patients with CDKL5 mutations: Hypermotor-tonic-spasms sequence. *Neurology* 76(16): 1436–1438.

Krajnc N, Župančič N, Oražem J. (2011) Epilepsy treatment in Rett syndrome. *J Child Neurol* 6(11): 1429–1433.

Larimore JL, Chapleau CA, Kudo S, Theibert A, Percy AK, Pozzo-Miller L (2009) Bdnf overexpression in hippocampal neurons prevents dendritic atrophy caused by Rett associated MECP2 mutations. *Neurobiol Dis* 34(2): 199–211.

Leonard H, Downs J, Jian L et al. (2010) Valproate and risk of fracture in Rett syndrome. *Arch Dis Child* 95(6): 444–448.

Liebhaber GM, Riemann E, Baumeister FA (2003) Ketogenic diet in Rett syndrome. *J Child Neurol* 18: 74–75.

Mari F, Azimonti S, Bertani I et al. (2005) CDKL5 belongs to the same molecular pathway of MeCP2 and it is responsible for the early-onset seizure variant of Rett syndrome. *Hum Mol Genet* 14(14): 1935–1946.

Moser SJ, Weber P, Lutschg J (2007) Rett syndrome: Clinical and electrophysiological aspects. *Pediatr Neurol* 36(2): 95–100.

Nectoux P, Bahi-Buisson N, Guellec I et al. (2008) The p.Val66Met polymorphism in the BDNF gene protects against early seizures in Rett syndrome. *Neurology* 70(Pt 2): 3145–3151.

Neul JL, Kaufmann WE, Glaze DG et al. (2010) Rett syndrome: Revised diagnostic criteria and nomenclature. *Ann Neurol* 68(6): 944–950.

Niedermeyer E, Rett A, Renner H, Murphy M, Naidu S (1986) Rett syndrome and the electroencephalogram. *Am J Med Genet* Suppl. 1: 195–199.

Nissenkorn A, Ben Zeev B (2015) Hand stereotypies or reflex motor seizures? – A newly described phenomenon in Rett syndrome. *J Child Neurol* 28(10): 1210–1214.

Nissenkorn A, Gak E, Vecsler M, Reznik H, Menascu S, Ben Zeev B (2010) Epilepsy in Rett syndrome – the experience of the National Rett Center. *Epilepsia* 51: 1252–1258.

Nissenkorn A, Levy-Drummer RS, Bondi O et al. (2015) Epilepsy in Rett syndrome-lessons from the Rett networked database. *Epilepsia* 56(4): 569–576.

Ogier M, Wang H, Hong E, Wang Q, Greenberg ME, Katz DM. (2007) Brain-derived neurotrophic factor expression and respiratory function improve after ampakine treatment in a mouse model of Rett syndrome. *J Neurosci* 27: 10912–10917.

Okabe Y, Takahashi T, Mitsumasu C, Kosai K, Tanaka E, Matsuishi T (2012) Alterations of gene expression and glutamate clearance in astrocytes derived from an MeCP2-null mouse model of Rett syndrome. *PLoS One* 7(4): e35354.

Pintaudi M, Calevo MG, Vignoli A et al. (2010) Epilepsy in Rett syndrome: Clinical and genetic features. *Epilepsy Behav* 19(3): 296–300.

Pintaudi M, Calevo MG, Vignoli A et al. (2015) Antiepileptic drugs in Rett Syndrome. *Eur J Paediatr Neurol* 19: 446–452.

Rajaei S, Erlandson A, Kyllerman M (2011) Early infantile onset "congenital" Rett syndrome variants: Swedish experience through four decades and mutation analysis. *J Child Neurol* 26(1): 65–71.

Ramocki MB, Tavyev YJ, Peters SU (2010) The MECP2 duplication syndrome. *Am J Med Genet* 52A(5): 1079–1088.

Rett A (1966) [On a unusual brain atrophy syndrome in hyperammonemia in childhood]. *Wien Med Wochenschr* 116(37): 723–726.

Roche Martínez A, Alonso Colmenero MI, Gomes Pereira A, Sanmartí Vilaplana FX, Armstrong Morón J, Pineda Marfa M (2011) Reflex seizures in Rett syndrome. *Epileptic Disord* 13(4): 389–393.

Scala E, Ariani F, Mari F et al. (2005) CDKL5/STK9 is mutated in Rett syndrome variant with infantile spasms. *J Med Genet* 42(2): 103–107.

Specchio N, Balestri M, Striano P et al. (2010) Efficacy of levetiracetam in the treatment of drug-resistant Rett syndrome. *Epilepsy Res* 88(2–3): 112–117.

Steffenburg U, Hagberg G, Hagberg B (2001) Epilepsy in a representative series of Rett syndrome. *Acta Paediatr* 90: 34–39.

Stenbom Y, Tonnby B, Hagberg B (1998) Lamotrigine in Rett syndrome: Treatment experience from a pilot study. *Eur Child Adolesc Psychiatry* 7: 49–52.

Uldall P, Hansen FJ, Tonnby B (1993) Lamotrigine in Rett syndrome. *Neuropediatrics* 24: 339–340.

Vignoli A, Borgatti R, Peron A et al. (2012) Electroclinical pattern in MECP2 duplication syndrome: Eight new reported cases and review of literature. *Epilepsia* 53(7): 1146–1155.

Wilfong AA, Schultz RJ (2006) Vagus nerve stimulation for treatment of epilepsy in Rett syndrome. *Dev Med Child Neurol* 48(8): 683–686.

10
BREATHING ABNORMALITIES IN RETT SYNDROME

Jan Marino Ramirez, Christopher Scott Ward and Jeffrey L Neul

Introduction

Abnormalities in breathing is one of the common features associated with the neurode-velopmental disorder, Rett syndrome (RTT), with studies reporting different prevalences of people displaying bouts of either or both hyperventilation and hypoventilation (Amir et al. 2000; Julu et al. 2001). Because of the variability in their presentation, the bouts of breathing abnormalities have been categorized across studies as periods of forced breath-ing, deep breathing, hyperventilation (rapid shallow breathing), hypoventilation, apneas, apneustic breathing, Valsalva's maneuvers, Biot's breathing, periodic breathing, and breath-holds (Julu et al. 2001; Weese-Mayer et al. 2008). Additionally, many of the breathing dis-turbances are associated with dysregulation in cardiorespiratory coupling (Julu et al. 2001; Weese-Mayer et al. 2008).

Assessing the degree and prevalence of breathing disturbances in RTT has been dif-ficult, in part due to inconsistency in fitting the observed anomalies into the pre-defined categories described above. Thus, the same disturbance may be classified as Valsalva maneu-ver by some authors, and apnea or breath-holds by others. Another complicating factor is that the occurrence of breathing disturbances shows a high degree of both inter- and intra-patient variability. Some people with RTT seem to gain or lose these disturbances over the course of development, and many can go for several days with normal breathing between episodes of marked disruption with normal breathing leading into hyperventilation (Southall et al. 1988). Also contributing to the variability is the apparent interaction between the individual's breathing and emotional state. These children can become easily agitated and often hyperactive, making it difficult to characterize their breathing in clinical settings. Furthermore, the fact that agitation can trigger episodes of abnormal breathing in the individuals with RTT and that these episodes were originally thought to be absent during sleep, led to early belief that breathing disturbances are in large part 'behavioral', that is a consequence of agitation (Southall et al. 1988). However, although somewhat diminished, breathing abnormalities still persist during sleep, and data from mouse models of the disease suggest impairments in the central control of breathing (Stettner et al. 2007; Weese-Mayer et al. 2008; Mironov et al. 2011). The complexity of breathing in RTT, like many other phenotypes associated with the disease, is also likely to be related to differences in the underlying genotype, the specific types of mutation, and the degree of X-chromosome inactivation (Amir et al. 2000).

As will be discussed in this chapter, the complexity of breathing disturbances is also partly the result of the diversity of neuronal mechanisms that contribute to the different dysfunctions. These neuronal mechanisms include imbalances in synaptic transmission, the diversity of neuromodulatory alterations that may in part explain the characteristic state-dependency of these breathing disorders, as well as developmental and compensatory mechanisms that can partly explain why the breathing irregularities can come and go during the development of a child. In this context, it will be important to discriminate between mechanisms that directly cause certain breathing irregularities from those mechanisms that can indirectly be affected by these breathing abnormalities. For example, it is very likely that during a child's development some of the breathing disturbances will evoke compensatory responses which could be adaptive and improve breathing in some children, while in others they may lead to a vicious cycle of detrimental responses which may in fact worsen the breathing irregularities. For example, similar to individuals with obstructive sleep apnea, a child who exhibits recurrent apneas and breath-holds will be exposed to oxidative and hypoxic stress, which is known to be detrimental to neuronal functions. Among individuals with RTT, marks of oxidative stress have been observed (De Felice et al. 2009). As already mentioned, agitation and other behavioral aspects of the disease may also play a role in exaggerating the breathing irregularities, as was suspected early on (Southall et al. 1988).

Thus, in trying to understand the etiology of the breathing phenotype in RTT it will be important to consider not only direct mechanisms, but also indirect responses that may contribute to the large catalog of disturbances. Although the complexity of the breathing phenotype in RTT may seem discouraging to some, animal models of RTT, in which it was possible to fully or partly reverse the breathing phenotype, raised hope that one day it may be possible to treat, control, and potentially cure this detrimental phenotype in humans (Abdala et al. 2010; Derecki et al. 2012). Although large systematic clinical trials offer no reliable treatments that consistently improve the breathing disturbances in individuals with RTT, some successes have been found in smaller trials and case reports (Andancki et al. 2005).

Breathing patterns in individuals with Rett syndrome

Characterizations of breathing in individuals with RTT reveal two distinct breathing disturbances: (1) disturbances in the timing of ongoing breathing, which is reflected in breath-to-breath irregularities and an increased breathing frequency (hyperventilation); and (2) intermittent disturbances in the initiation or completion of individual breaths (often referred to as apneas or breath-holds), which frequently occur during ongoing breathing and are associated with dramatic autonomic dysregulation and significant hypoxia (Southall et al. 1988; Weese-Mayer et al. 2008). The breath-to-breath analyses by Weese-Mayer et al. (2008) in which breath-holds were analyzed separately from consecutive 'normal' breaths that occurred at least five breaths before or after a breath-hold, provided an unbiased characterization in a small series of girls with RTT and confirmed *MECP2* mutations. These characterizations suggested that the mechanisms underlying disturbances in 'ongoing breathing' are different from those underlying 'breath-holds'. For this reason, this chapter will describe their characteristics separately.

DISTURBANCES IN 'ONGOING BREATHING'

'Hyperventilation' is one of the most documented breathing abnormalities in individuals with RTT (Southall et al. 1988; Weese-Mayer et al. 2008). Southall et al. (1988) observed that hyperventilation was not preceded by hypoxemia, suggesting that it is a primary deficit and not secondary to hypercapnia or hypoxemia as a result of apnea and irregular breathing. Also, breath-to-breath analysis indicates that the timing of both inspiratory and expiratory activity is decreased (Weese-Mayer et al. 2008). The effects on the timing of breathing are likely to be caused by a disturbance in central respiratory mechanisms, and as will be discussed later in this chapter, this conclusion is consistent with studies using animal models.

While inspiratory timing was reduced by approximately 10%, a more dramatic reduction of approximately 25% was noted for the time spent in exhalation (Weese-Mayer et al. 2008). This significant shortening of expiratory timing has important mechanistic implications, because expiratory timing is neuronally determined by two distinct phases: (1) The initial expiratory phase is also referred to as 'post-inspiration'. During this phase phrenic nerve activity is neuronally activated in a decrementing manner. This decrementing activation leads to the passive exhalation of air from the lungs. (2) The secondary phase of expiration is also referred to as 'active expiration'. During active expiration, intercostal muscles are activated which leads to the active exhalation of air (Richter 1982; Weese-Mayer et al. 2008). The data obtained for individuals with RTT are therefore inconsistent with data obtained in so called 'in situ' mouse preparations which suggest that postinspiration is prolonged (Stettner et al. 2007). In individuals with RTT, the depth of the breaths is also affected. The mean amplitude that is reached during inspiration is enhanced in individuals with RTT and so is the associated amplitude irregularity. Thus, the breath-to-breath characterizations indicate that on average breaths are deeper, faster, and more irregular in amplitude and timing (Weese-Mayer et al. 2008). However, the degree of these disturbances can vary from individual to individual, which probably explains why some authors subdivide the breathing phenotype of RTT individuals into subgroups on the basis of severity and the predominant breathing disturbances present in the individual (i.e. feeble vs forceful breathers) (Southall et al. 1988; Julu et al. 2001). However, whether there are indeed distinct phenotypic subtypes among individuals with RTT, or whether they represent extremes of a continuum of breathing disturbances has not been quantitatively assessed by any study. Moreover, it is inherently difficult to define the abnormality based on the existing methodology. Thus, without recording phrenic nerve activity, it remains uncertain whether some of the breathing disturbances indeed reflect prolonged inspiratory activation leading to 'apneustic breathing'.

One of the most consistent findings is that individuals with RTT hyperventilate most dramatically during active wakefulness, that is, during the day. Despite earlier beliefs that breathing was normal during sleep in individuals with RTT, there is increasing evidence that breathing is also disturbed during the night (Southall et al. 1988; Weese-Mayer et al. 2008).

Indeed, quantitative breath-to-breath characterization revealed that during the night, breathing in individuals with RTT is significantly faster and more irregular when compared with age-matched controls (Weese-Mayer et al. 2008). The state-dependency of breathing in RTT is one of the hallmarks of this phenotype, and mechanistic studies are needed to explain this dependency.

BREATH-HOLDS OR 'APNEIC EVENTS' IN RETT SYNDROME

Among the most consistent disturbances in RTT are episodes of 'breathing cessation' (Weese-Mayer et al. 2008). Yet, defining these events has generated considerable uncertainty in the field. These relatively long-lasting breathing events seem to be specific to RTT, and the existing terms may not adequately describe these disturbances. It is possible (and very likely), that the frequently observed breathing cessation is indeed the same type of disturbance that some authors call 'breath-hold', 'apnea', or 'Valsalva maneuver'(Julu et al. 2001; Weese-Mayer et al. 2008). Moreover, investigation of cardiovascular function during these 'breath cessation' events provides further evidence of impaired integration of breathing with other autonomic functions.

'Apneas' are generally defined as 'cessation of breathing' and are usually associated with the absence of inspiratory activity as opposed to 'apneusis' during which respiratory activity is centrally maintained in inspiration. Typically the lungs are deflated during apnea, which is typically not the case in girls with RTT. In these children, the lungs remain inflated during these events, which is typical for 'breath-holds' apparent in published raw traces (Southall et al. 1988; Weese-Mayer et al. 2008). Interestingly, breath-holds in healthy individuals are characterized by an initial drop in heart rate, whereas in girls with RTT the heart rate displays an initial drop followed by an increase to above the baseline heart rate (Weese-Mayer et al. 2008). A somewhat similar biphasic response in the heart rate is characteristic of 'Valsalva maneuvers' (Elisberg 1963). Yet, Valsalva maneuvers are typically generated voluntarily in healthy individuals and the changes in thoracic and abdominal pressure cause biphasic changes in blood pressure, and are thought to result in biphasic changes in the heart rate via the activation of the baroreflex. As a consequence of the reflexive nature of this heart rate response, the heart rate may exhibit a reflex bradycardia and return to baseline shortly after cessation of the Valsalva maneuver, that is upon resumption of normal breathing (Elisberg 1963). By contrast, girls and women with RTT sometimes have heart rates that remain elevated as they resume breathing (Weese-Mayer et al. 2008). Indeed, the increased heart rate occurring during the breath-holds is very regular and exhibits very little beat-to-beat variability, even as breathing resumes. These data suggest the biphasic heartrate change may primarily be caused by central dysautonomia, rather than a physiological response to changes in blood pressure that are generated during the breath-hold. Of course, these considerations do not rule out the possibility that an activated baroreflex also contributes to the observed breathing disturbance. From the above considerations, it can be concluded that the cessation of breathing in RTT seems to be specific for this disorder and it may not be simply classified as 'breath-hold', 'apnea', or Valsalva maneuver, even though aspects of this disturbance have clear resemblance with similar types of breathing events as characterized in healthy individuals. The occurrence of these events in RTT is periodic, as these events occur frequently interspersed by periods of normal breaths (Southall et al. 1988; Julu et al. 2001; Weese-Mayer et al. 2008).

Mouse models of Rett syndrome

Genetically engineered mice have been developed to model the disorder by disrupting MeCP2 function. In particular, the laboratories of Rudolph Jaenisch and Adrian Bird have developed mouse lines in which *Mecp2* can be conditionally knocked-out: *Mecp2*^{TM1Jae} and *Mecp2*^{TM1Bird} (Chen et al. 2001; Guy et al. 2001). Initial characterization of breathing abnormalities was performed using null alleles of *Mecp2* derived from the aforementioned conditional alleles: *Mecp2*$^{TM1.1Jae}$ and *Mecp2*$^{TM1.1Bird}$. More recently, Adrian Bird's laboratory developed an allele allowing conditional rescue of *Mecp2*: *Mecp2*^{TM2Bird}. These mouse lines have been used to test both neuroanatomic origins of MeCP2 dependent phenotypes as well as preclinical therapies to treat them. Among the breathing abnormalities described in these models were the occurrence of hyperventilation, apnea, and increased variability in breath frequency (Ogier et al. 2007; Voituron et al. 2009, 2010). In contrast to the breath cessation' events that are typically observed in humans with inflated lungs, the 'breath cessation' events that have been described in the mice typically show an exhalation before the pause and inhalation immediately following it, suggesting that they occur with the lungs deflated and are akin to either central or obstructive apneas (Ogier et al. 2007; Voituron et al. 2009, 2010).

PROGRESSIVE 'ACQUISITION' OF BREATHING ABNORMALITIES IN MOUSE MODELS OF RETT SYNDROME
Although apnea has been identified in both male and female mice possessing either of the null alleles of *Mecp2*, hyperventilation has been most often attributed to mice possessing the *Mecp2*^{TM1Jae} allele. However, this distinction has since been overruled, the previously observed difference between the alleles was likely to be due to differences in methodology, restrained versus unrestrained plethysmography, as well as the genetic background used for the mice. *Mecp2*$^{TM1.1Jae}$ mice were often studied on a mixed 129S6, C57BL/6, and BALBC background while *Mecp2*$^{TM1.1Bird}$ mice were typically studied back-crossed to C57BL/6 (Voituron et al. 2009, 2010; Ward et al. 2011). Characterization of male *Mecp2*$^{TM1.1Bird/Y}$ mice across their lifespan has identified relatively normal breathing with regard to apneas, until the mice approach adulthood and begin to display apneic and bradypneic breathing patterns that progressively worsen until the end of life (Viemari et al. 2005; Voituron et al. 2009). However, by challenging the mice with decreased oxygen or increased carbon dioxide these irregularities can be observed in younger mice several weeks before they are overtly symptomatic as adults. Furthermore, allowing mice to mature to adulthood before removing Mecp2 function still results in progression of RTT associated phenotypes in mice, including disrupted breathing (Cheval et al. 2012). Conversely, restoration of Mecp2 function in symptomatic adults is capable of ameliorating breathing dysfunction (Robinson et al. 2012). The ability to induce or ameliorate breathing abnormalities in the adult mouse suggests that the aberrations caused by lack of Mecp2 are not due to deficits in establishing the respiratory circuitry, but reflect a role for Mecp2 in their maintenance.

Further characterization of the breathing abnormalities beyond hyperventilation and apnea in mice lacking Mecp2 function has uncovered additional insights and parallels to the human phenotype. Similar to the improvement in breathing regularity during sleep observed in humans light anesthesia of *Mecp2$^{TM1.1Bird}$* mice improves their breathing regularity (Viemari et al. 2005). Also, in addition to hypoxic or hypercapnic challenges uncovering latent abnormalities in breathing, the homeostatic breathing responses to these challenges also appear to be impaired by the absence of Mecp2. In particular, *Mecp2$^{TM1.1Bird/Y}$* mice exhibit a blunted response to mild hypercapnia, failing to raise their breathing frequency and tidal volume in response to increasing levels, up to 3%, of carbon dioxide (Zhang et al. 2011). Conversely, *Mecp2$^{TM1.1Bird/Y}$* mice also possess an increased and persistent response to acute moderate hypoxia (8–10% oxygen), exhibiting an increased level of ventilation and breathing rate that fails to undergo normal hypoxic ventilatory decline observed in adult mice (Voituron et al. 2009; Ward et al. 2011). Given the apparent deficits in homeostatic breathing responses alongside the progressive nature of the hyperventilation and apnea, the development of breathing abnormalities is likely to represent a progressive loss of breathing circuit function that first manifests as diminished homeostatic capacity.

NEUROANATOMIC ORIGINS OF BREATHING ABNORMALITIES IN RETT SYNDROME

Our understanding of the components of the respiratory network disrupted by the loss of MeCP2 function has been helped through the use of the conditional alleles of *Mecp2* as well as in vitro experiments examining the neurophysiological consequences within the brainstem from the absence of MeCP2. In particular, although restoration of MeCP2 to regions in the medulla and caudal pons is sufficient to restore a normal hypoxic breathing response, it was insufficient to prevent hyperventilation associated with loss of MeCP2, suggesting contributions from rostral brain regions may influence this phenotype, corroborating the strong association between behavioral and emotional state and hyperventilation (Ward et al. 2011). Furthermore, absence of MeCP2 reduces norepinephrine, dopamine, serotonin, gamma aminobutyric acid (GABA), and brain derived neurotrophic factor (BDNF) levels within the brain, and this decrease can be traced to a specific requirement of MeCP2 within the neurons that produce them (Viemari et al. 2005; Chao et al. 2010). Dopaminergic and noradrenergic neurons can be defined by the expression of tyrosine hydroxylase, the enzyme controlling the rate-limiting step of their biosynthesis. Investigation of the requirement of MeCP2 within tyrosine hydroxylase expressing neurons, identified a decline with age in *Mecp2$^{TM1.1Bird}$* mice with regard to tyrosine hydroxylase expression, norepinephrine, and dopamine levels within the brain (Viemari et al. 2005). Furthermore, the loss of tyrosine hydroxylase expression in the brains of mice lacking Mecp2 is due to some regions that decrease cellular tyrosine hydroxylase expression and other regions that decrease the number of tyrosine hydroxylase expressing cells. This loss of tyrosine hydroxylase expressing cells occurs without a decrease in neuron number or signs of neuronal death, and may represent a common neuropathology with several populations of neurons losing their cellular identity and disrupting their circuit function (Viemari et al. 2005). In addition, removal of Mecp2 from GABAergic neurons leads to an increased occurrence of apnea (Chao et al. 2010).

Despite delayed onset of breathing abnormalities in mice with null alleles of *Mecp2*, cellular and circuit level abnormalities can be found preceding the onset of overt breathing symptoms. In particular, inhibitory action of GABAergic neurons in the ventrolateral medulla is impaired as early as postnatal day 7 in *Mecp2*[TMI.1Bird/Y] mice, manifesting as decreased amplitude and frequency of spontaneous inhibitory synaptic currents (sIPSC), and increased amplitude and frequency of spontaneous excitatory synaptic currents (sEPSC) (Medrihan et al. 2008). Furthermore, Mironov and colleagues (2011) tested slice cultures taken from the medullas of 3-day-old *Mecp2*[TMI.1Bird/Y] and wild type mice and observed several deficits in the respiratory pace-maker neurons of the pre-Botzinger complex in mice lacking Mecp2: decreased resting cyclic adenosine monophosphate (cAMP) levels, diminished cAMP production in response to stimulation, and slow arrhythmic bursting measured by Ca^{+2} imaging and whole cell recordings (Mironov et al. 2011). Additionally, slice cultured neurons located within the pre-Botzinger complex from mice lacking Mecp2 also were less interconnected compared to wild type littermates, a deficit that is predictive of network instability. This lack of connectivity progressively worsened from p3 to p20; supplementation of the slices with BDNF ameliorated this deficit (Mironov et al. 2005). An additional role of BDNF regarding control of breathing is suggested in the nucleus of the tractus solitarious (NTS), a key relay center responsible for matching peripheral inputs, including blood oxygen and lung inflation status, to the appropriate autonomic control circuitry to maintain homeostasis. The expression of BDNF localized to the NTS is drastically reduced by the absence of MeCP2 and correlates with excitatory/inhibitory imbalance defined by an increase in amplitude and frequency of sEPSCs recorded from medial NTS neurons (Kline et al. 2010).

The use of a working heart-brainstem preparation (WHBP), allowing simultaneous in vitro recording from the phrenic and central vagus nerves, provided additional evidence that the respiratory network is less stable in the absence of MeCP2. Respiratory cycle times, measured by phrenic nerve discharge rates, and intracycle phases, including inspiration, postinspiration, and late-expiration from *Mecp2*[TMI.1Bird/Y] samples, showed greater irregularity in duration, a propensity for central apnea, and an increased duration of the postinspiratory phase during breathing. Increased postinspiratory duration is linked to excitatory inputs from the Kolliker-Fuse, a region involved in coordinating upper airway function and glottal position during breathing. Furthermore, by examining clusters of glutamate micro-injections into the rostral brainstem that were sufficient to induce central apnea in mice, as well as the duration of those evoked apneas in wild type and *Mecp2*[TMI.1Bird/Y] mice, the Kolliker-Fuse nucleus emerged as a region of importance regarding MeCP2 function, with *Mecp2*[TMI.1Bird/Y] mice demonstrating an increased sensitivity and apnea duration during glutamate-induced signaling from the Kolliker-Fuse nucleus (Stettner et al. 2007). Consistent with the importance of the Kolliker-Fuse nucleus, synchronous plethysmography measurements of nasal/oral airflow and the chest movements driving it led to the identification of two different types of apnea in *Mecp2*[-Bird] mice, central apneas due to a failure to initiate inspiration, and obstructive apneas due to transient upper airway obstruction identified by chest movements in the absence of airflow through the nose or mouth (Voituron et al. 2010). The obstructive apneas are consistent with hypotheses put forward suggesting poor coordination of glottal closure mediated via the Kolliker-Fuse nucleus during breathing.

PRECLINICAL TREATMENTS FOR BREATHING ABNORMALITIES

Several attempts have been made to test both pharmacological and less traditional therapies for efficacy at improving the breathing abnormalities in mice. Given the aforementioned deficits in GABAergic and serotoninergic signaling, several groups have attempted preclinical experiments to pharmacologically upregulate these systems via enhancing GABA-A receptor signaling via benzodiazepines, targeting the serotoninergic 5HT1a receptor with agonists, or trying to upregulate BDNF signaling, which is known to also be down regulated in mice lacking Mecp2. Treatments targeting GABAergic, serotoninergic, and BDNF signaling have shown promise in the various mouse models (Ogier et al. 2007; Abdala et al. 2010).

Conclusion

Breathing abnormalities in individuals with RTT contribute to a compromised quality of life, are indicative of central dysautonomia that can be modified by the individual's emotional and behavioral state, and may aggravate additional pathologies in the disease. We are arriving at a better understanding of the pleiotropic nature of the deficits caused by the loss of MeCP2, including diminished function across several neural signaling systems and excitatory/inhibitory imbalance across several circuits. Although promising preclinical data in the mouse models and anecdotal case reports in individuals have found success when targeting GABAergic and serotoninergic systems as well as BDNF signaling, several considerations would benefit the field. In particular, better understanding is needed regarding genetic, environmental, and temporal consequences on primary breathing dysfunction and the secondary effects of that dysfunction. Genetic background plays a significant role in the expression of breathing abnormalities in mice, and future studies should ensure that observed differences in breathing parameters are not simply due to inherent differences between mouse strains or identify potential strain-specific modifiers of breathing dysfunction. Furthermore, effects of fear, anxiety, or other stresses believed to impact the occurrence of episodes of marked breathing abnormality in individuals with RTT have yet to be studied in a rigorously controlled manner in humans or mouse models. Longitudinal studies are also needed to determine the degree to which the breathing abnormalities worsen or are ameliorated over an individual's lifetime. Lastly, it is unknown whether the progressive nature of the breathing abnormalities and other pathologies of RTT solely reflect the decline in neuronal control as a consequence of lacking MeCP2, or whether consequences from episodes of irregular breathing lead to neuronal injury and maladaptive changes contributing to disease progression.

REFERENCES

Abdala AP, Dutschmann M, Bissonnette JM, Paton JF (2010) Correction of respiratory disorders in a mouse model of Rett syndrome. *Proc Natl Acad Sci USA* 107(42): 18208–18213.
Amir RE, Van den Veyver IB, Schultz R et al. (2000) Influence of mutation type and X chromosome inactivation on Rett syndrome phenotypes. *Ann Neurol* 47(5): 670–679.

Andaku DK, Mercadante MT, Schwartzman JS (2005) Buspirone in Rett syndrome respiratory dysfunction. *Brain Dev* 27(6): 437–438.

Chao HT, Chen H, Samaco RC et al. (2010) Dysfunction in GABA signalling mediates autism-like stereotypies and Rett syndrome phenotypes. *Nature* 468(7321): 263–269.

Chen RZ, Akbarian S, Tudor M, Jaenisch R (2001) Deficiency of methyl-CpG binding protein-2 in CNS neurons results in a Rett-like phenotype in mice. *Nat Genet* 27(3): 327–331.

Cheval H, Guy J, Merusi C, De Sousa D, Selfridge J, Bird A (2012) Postnatal inactivation reveals enhanced requirement for Mecp2 at distinct age windows. *Hum Mol Genet* 21(17): 3806–3814.

De Felice C, Ciccoli L, Leoncini S et al. (2009) Systemic oxidative stress in classic Rett syndrome. *Free Radic Biol Med* 47(4): 440–448.

Elisberg EI (1963) Heart rate response to the Valsalva maneuver as a test of circulatory integrity. *JAMA* 186: 200–205.

Guy J, Hendrich B, Holmes M, Martin JE, Bird A (2001) A mouse Mecp2-null mutation causes neurological symptoms that mimic Rett syndrome. *Nat Genet* 27(3): 322–326.

Julu PO, Kerr AM, Apartopoulos F et al. (2001) Characterisation of breathing and associated central autonomic dysfunction in the Rett disorder. *Arch Dis Child* 85(1): 29–37.

Kline DD, Ogier M, Kunze DL, Katz DM (2010) Exogenous brain-derived neurotrophic factor rescues synaptic dysfunction in Mecp2-null mice. *J Neurosci* 30(15): 5303–5310.

Medrihan L, Tantalaki E, Aramuni G et al. (2008) Early defects of GABAergic synapses in the brain stem of a MeCP2 mouse model of Rett syndrome. *J Neurophysiol* 99(1): 112–121.

Mironov SL, Skorova E, Hartelt N, Mironova LA, Hasan MT, Kügler S (2009) Remodelling of the respiratory network in a mouse model of Rett syndrome depends on brain-derived neurotrophic factor regulated slow calcium buffering. *J Physiol* 587(Pt 11): 2473–2485.

Mironov SL, Skorova EY, Kugler S (2011) Epac-mediated cAMP-signalling in the mouse model of Rett syndrome. *Neuropharmacology* 60(6): 869–877.

Ogier M1, Wang H, Hong E, Wang Q, Greenberg ME, Katz DM (2007) Brain-derived neurotrophic factor expression and respiratory function improve after ampakine treatment in a mouse model of Rett syndrome. *J Neurosci* 27(40): 10912–10917.

Richter DW (1982) Generation and maintenance of the respiratory rhythm. *J Exp Biol* 100: 93–107.

Robinson L, Guy J, MacKay L et al. (2012) Morphological and functional reversal of phenotypes in a mouse model of Rett syndrome. *Brain* 135(9): 2699–2710.

Southall DP, Kerr AM, Tirosh E, Amos P, Lang MH, Stephenson JB (1988) Hyperventilation in the awake state: Potentially treatable component of Rett syndrome. *Arch Dis Child* 63(9): 1039–1048.

Stettner GM, Huppke P, Brendel C, Richter DW, Gärtner J, Dutschmann M (2007) Breathing dysfunctions associated with impaired control of postinspiratory activity in Mecp2-/y knockout mice. *J Physiol* 579(Pt 3): 863–876.

Viemari JC, Roux JC, Tryba AK et al. (2005) Mecp2 deficiency disrupts norepinephrine and respiratory systems in mice. *J Neurosci* 25(50): 11521–11530.

Voituron N, Zanella S, Menuet C, Dutschmann M, Hilaire G (2009) Early breathing defects after moderate hypoxia or hypercapnia in a mouse model of Rett syndrome. *Respir Physiol Neurobiol* 168(1–2): 109–118.

Voituron N, Menuet C, Dutschmann M, Hilaire G. (2010) Physiological definition of upper airway obstructions in mouse model for Rett syndrome. *Respir Physiol Neurobiol* 173(2): 146–156.

Ward CS, Arvide EM, Huang TW, Yoo J, Noebels JL, Neul JL (2011) MeCP2 is critical within HoxB1-derived tissues of mice for normal lifespan. *J Neurosci* 31(28): 10359–10370.

Weese-Mayer DE, Lieske SP, Boothby CM, Kenny AS, Bennett HL, Ramirez JM (2008) Autonomic dysregulation in young girls with Rett Syndrome during nighttime in-home recordings. *Pediatr Pulmonol* 43(11): 1045–1060.

Zhang X, Su J, Cui N, Gai H, Wu Z, Jiang C (2011) The disruption of central CO2 chemosensitivity in a mouse model of Rett syndrome. *Am J Physiol Cell Physiol* 301(3): C729–C738.

11
GROWTH, FEEDING AND NUTRITION, AND BONE HEALTH IN RETT SYNDROME

Kathleen J Motil

Introduction

Although seizures, breathing abnormalities, and autonomic dysfunction represent over-arching concerns in Rett syndrome (RTT), impaired growth, altered nutritional status, oral pharyngeal dysfunction, and disturbed bone health contribute significantly to heightened morbidity and mortality in this disorder. This chapter will focus on the nutritional aspects of RTT, including the clinical features, diagnostic considerations, and therapeutic interventions related to growth and body composition, oral motor and pharyngeal function, and bone health. A better understanding of these challenging aspects of RTT will improve the quality of life of individuals affected with this disorder.

Underweight, growth failure, overweight

CLINICAL FEATURES OF IMPAIRED GROWTH AND NUTRITIONAL STATUS

Impaired linear growth and altered nutritional status are characteristic features of RTT (Schultz et al. 1993; Motil et al. 2008; Tarquinio et al. 2012). Height-for-age and weight-for-age, but not body mass index (BMI)-for-age, z-scores are lower in females with RTT than in reference populations (Schultz et al. 1993; Tarquinio et al. 2012). The average rate of growth for head circumference, length, and weight in females with classic RTT deviates below the reference population at 1 month, 17 months, and 6 months of age respectively (Tarquinio et al. 2012). Pubertal increases in height and weight are absent in classic RTT (Tarquinio et al. 2012). *MECP2* mutations may adversely affect linear growth even in the absence of under-nutrition, particularly during adolescence. As a consequence, linear growth failure may not be corrected completely by nutritional interventions (Motil et al. 2009).

Females with RTT have less lean body mass and greater body fat deposition throughout childhood and early adolescence than that observed in reference groups (Motil et al. 2008). Leptin, a peptide hormone that is proportional to the fat mass of the body, has been reported to be higher in females with RTT than in unaffected girls, despite similarities in weight (Blardi et al. 2009). Nevertheless, progressive weight deficits in the presence of continued linear growth during adolescence may result in lower BMI and worsening undernutrition (Motil et al. 2012). Although females with RTT usually are shorter and weigh less than unaffected individuals, a small proportion may be overweight based on weight-for-height or BMI criteria (Motil et al. 2012). The prevalence of overweight may be underestimated because weight-for-height gains are overlooked in the presence of small body size or an aberrant distribution of body fat. Weight-for-height comparisons may be monitored less frequently than weight alone because of the difficulty obtaining accurate height measurements.

PREVALENCE

The true prevalence of growth failure and underweight or overweight in RTT is unknown. Growth failure, defined as a height z-score more than two standard deviations below the reference mean, has been reported in 45% of affected individuals, whereas underweight, defined as a BMI-for-age less than the 5th centile, and overweight, defined as a BMI-for-age greater than the 85th centile, has been documented in 38% and 9%, respectively (Motil et al. 2012). Gastrostomy placement for nutritional support has been documented in 20–28% of large RTT cohorts, providing further evidence for undernutrition in affected individuals (Oddy et al. 2007; Motil et al. 2012).

PATHOPHYSIOLOGY

Genetic factors may be associated with the growth abnormalities in RTT. Growth failure in females with classic RTT has been associated with more severe developmental delay, higher disease severity, and certain *MECP2* mutations, notably early truncation, large deletion, and specific mutations including p.Thr158Met, p.Arg168X, p.Arg255X, and p.Arg270X (Tarquinio et al. 2012). C-terminal deletions are more likely to be associated with normal head circumference and body weight measurements (Bebbington et al. 2010).

Endocrine dysfunction does not explain growth retardation in RTT. Bone age may be delayed or accelerated in some, but not all females with RTT (Leonard et al. 1999a; Huppke et al. 2001; Motil et al. 2008). Insulin-like growth factor (IGF)-1 may be low; however, IGF-binding protein, insulin, and arginine-stimulated growth hormone secretion are normal, indicating normal growth hormone secretion in the majority of females with RTT (Huppke et al. 2001). Age-appropriate plasma levels are found for thyroid hormones, estradiol, and prolactin (Huppke et al. 2001). Morning cortisol levels are normal, but afternoon levels may not decline and urinary excretion of cortisol is higher in females with RTT than in unaffected girls (Huppke et al. 2001; Motil et al. 2006). Although a neural-mediated abnormality cannot be excluded, it is unlikely that a disturbance in hypothalamic control accounts for growth failure in RTT.

The role of hormones such as ghrelin, leptin, and adiponectin on growth and body composition in RTT remains speculative. Ghrelin is involved in the stimulation of growth hormone secretion and the modulation of energy metabolism. Plasma ghrelin levels are lower in females with RTT than in unaffected females and do not demonstrate the expected inverse relation with height, weight, and BMI in affected individuals (Hara et al. 2011). Leptin and adiponectin are involved in the regulation of body fat and weight. Plasma leptin and adiponectin levels are higher in females with RTT than in unaffected girls (Blardi et al. 2009). Leptin concentrations increase and adiponectin levels decrease over time, but neither appears to influence weight centiles of females with RTT (Blardi et al. 2009).

Altered nutritional status explains 10–15% of the variability in linear growth in children with neurological disabilities (Marchand et al. 2006). The altered growth patterns and nutritional status of females with RTT may be explained in part by inappropriate dietary nutrient intake, oral and pharyngeal motor dysfunction, increased nutrient loss, altered energy expenditure, or a combination of these factors (Motil et al. 1994, 1998, 1999).

Inappropriate dietary intake
Inappropriate dietary energy intake relative to metabolic needs is the primary cause of underweight and overweight in females with RTT. Because the task of feeding is difficult and time consuming, females with RTT consume less dietary energy than unaffected individuals (Motil et al. 1998). Females with RTT may be unable to communicate hunger, food preferences, or satiety, leaving caregivers responsible for regulating their dietary intake. When adequate dietary energy is provided by gastrostomy feedings, nutritional therapy leads to weight gain and linear growth (Motil et al. 2009). Careful monitoring may be necessary to avoid overfeeding, and consequently, overweight in these individuals.

Oral motor and pharyngeal dysfunction
Although 84% of parents report their daughters have excellent appetites, parents perceive mealtime as a stressful, unpleasant experience because of associated feeding problems (Reilly and Cass 2001; Cass et al. 2003). Parents' perceptions are important because the majority of females with RTT depend on a caregiver for their nutrition. Dependency on a caregiver and inefficiency of the feeding process, including the amount of food ingested or spilled and the time required for feeding, influence the child's nutritional status (Marchand et al. 2006; Oddy et al. 2007).

Prevalence
Feeding problems due to oral and pharyngeal motor dysfunction are reported in 81% of a large sample of females with RTT (Motil et al. 2012). Chewing and swallowing difficulties are reported by 56% and 43% of parents, respectively; choking and gagging with feedings are reported by 27%, and prolonged feeding times of 30–60 minutes per meal are reported by 62% of families (Motil et al. 2012). Others have documented parental concerns related to feeding in 52–87% of smaller groups of families (Reilly and Cass 2001; Oddy et al. 2007).

The Schedule for Oral Motor Assessment, a standardized approach to feeding, has been used to assess oral feeding patterns in RTT (Reilly and Cass 2001). Using this method, 64% of females with RTT have feeding patterns characterized by moderate to severe oral motor dysfunction that does not vary with age (Reilly and Cass 2001; Cass et al. 2003). Difficulty with solid, semi-solid, and pureed foods and liquids is observed in 53%, 36%, 26%, and 17%, respectively, of affected individuals (Reilly and Cass 2001; Cass et al. 2003). Parents report difficulty with liquids in 28% of their daughters (Cass et al. 2003). Others note an inability to ingest solid or soft food and difficulty drinking liquid in 81%, 46%, and 19%, respectively, of females with RTT (Oddy et al. 2007). As a result, 93% of families engage in special food preparation (Oddy et al. 2007). Sixty percent of females with RTT require chopped, mashed, or pureed foods, 20–32% consume supplemental enteral formulas, 9% use liquid thickeners, and 55% receive multivitamin and mineral supplements (Oddy et al. 2007; Motil et al. 2012). Gastrostomy placement has been documented in 20–28% of large RTT cohorts (Oddy et al. 2007; Motil et al. 2012). Individuals with late-truncating mutations require less enteral nutrition than those with other mutations, and hand use is retained by more than 85% of individuals with C-terminal truncation, p.Arg294X, or p.Arg133Cys mutations (Oddy et al. 2007; Neul et al. 2008).

Other factors that interfere with feeding, including inability to self-feed in 92%, involuntary movements throughout the meal in 100%, bruxism in 82%, hyperventilation in 60%, breath holding in 41%, gastroesophageal reflux in 29%, and constipation in 41% have been identified in females with RTT (Rebeiro et al. 1997; Motil et al. 1999; Reilly and Cass 2001; Cass et al. 2003; Isaacs et al. 2003; Schwartzman et al. 2008). Low plasma ghrelin levels may serve as a marker of central nervous system dysfunction in individuals who have eating difficulties (Hara et al. 2011).

Pathophysiology

Oral motor and pharyngeal dysfunction contributes to the pathogenesis of undernutrition in RTT (Morton et al. 1997a, b; Motil et al. 1999). Oral motor impairments characterized visually during therapy include poor lip closure in 62%, poor tongue mobility in 69%, decreased oral transit because of delayed initiation of swallowing in 31%, and coughing or choking with liquids and solids in 31% and 23%, respectively, all of which lead to prolonged feeding time in 92% of affected females (Motil et al. 1999). Oral and pharyngeal impairments characterized by videofluoroscopy demonstrate poor lateralization of the anterior tongue, resulting in poor food bolus formation and inadequate compression of the posterior tongue onto the palate, leading to piecemeal deglutition and delayed transit time in moving food from mouth to pharynx during the oral phase of feeding (Morton et al. 1997a, b; Motil et al. 1999). In the pharyngeal phase, the initiation of the swallow reflex may be delayed, resulting in food and liquid accumulation in the valleculae or pyriform sinuses (Morton et al. 1997a, b; Motil et al. 1999). Poor clearance of the pharynx may result in laryngeal penetration or frank aspiration of liquids and solids. Females with RTT show significant delay between the end of spoon contact and the first swallow with solid foods and liquids (Morton et al. 1997b). The direct correlation of time to first swallow with increasing age implies a gradual deterioration in oral motor and pharyngeal function in RTT (Morton et al. 1997b). Early, persistent, and severe feeding difficulties are markers of subsequent poor growth and identify individuals who may benefit from gastrostomy feedings (Marchand et al. 2006).

Increased nutrient losses

Inadequate lip closure, drooling, and tongue thrust or involuntary movements of the tongue are associated with food and liquid loss through spillage. Spillage of food may occur in individuals who feed themselves because of poor hand-to-mouth coordination. Gastroesophageal reflux and gastroparesis, found in 39% and 14%, respectively, of females with RTT, may result in a loss of nutrients because of frequent emesis (Motil et al. 2012).

Intestinal malabsorption does not occur in RTT in the absence of underlying gastrointestinal disease (Motil et al. 1994).

Energy requirements

Total daily energy expenditure, measured by the doubly-labeled water ($^2H_2^{18}O$) technique, is lower by 43% in females with RTT than in unaffected girls, because of the deficits in lean body mass (Motil et al. 1998). The proportion of time that females with RTT spend in repetitive motion does not represent a significant energy loss (Motil et al. 1998). Sleeping and quietly awake metabolic rates, measured by indirect calorimetry, also are lower by 23% in females with RTT than in unaffected girls, even when adjusted for differences in lean body mass (Motil et al. 1994). However, resting metabolic rates are higher in females with RTT than in girls with developmental delay (Platte et al. 2011). Females with RTT demonstrate linear growth and weight gain with energy intakes that approximate 60% of the Dietary Reference Intake (DRI) for age and sex. The DRI for energy in healthy children overestimates the energy needs of females with RTT in whom a value of 110% of age-appropriate basal energy expenditure (BEE) may be sufficient (USDA 2012). Energy needs for females with RTT who have protein-energy malnutrition may approximate 150% of age-appropriate BEE.

Micronutrients

METHYLATION FACTORS

Methylation diets have been proposed as part of the prevention and treatment strategies for RTT (Van den Veyver 2002). Folic acid, betaine, or its precursor, choline, and other nutrients influence methylation processes by affecting dietary levels of methyl-donor components. However, a placebo-controlled trial designed to increase DNA methylation using betaine and folate supplementation did not improve functional outcomes in females with RTT (Glaze et al. 2009). Similarly, a double-blind, randomized trial using folinic acid supplementation increased 5-methyltetrahydrofolate levels, but did not clinically improve affected individuals (Hagebeuk et al. 2012). Choline supplementation improved behavioral and neuroanatomical symptoms in a mouse model of RTT (Ward et al. 2009). An open-label trial of L-carnitine, a trimethylated amino acid similar to choline, improved sleep efficiency, energy level, and communication skills in females with RTT (Ellaway et al. 2001).

OMEGA-3-POLYUNSATURATED FATTY ACIDS

Omega-3-polyunsaturated fatty acids (ω-3-PUFA), primarily docosahexaenoic acid (DHA) and eicosapentaenoic acid (EPA), have been proposed as an alternative treatment strategy for neuronal membrane protection in RTT (Leoncini et al. 2011; De Felice et al. 2012). Oxidative stress and lipid peroxidation are thought to contribute to the pathophysiology of RTT. Membrane lipids containing long-chain PUFA are primary targets for reactive oxygen species. A placebo-controlled trial of fish oil containing high doses of DHA and EPA improved the clinical severity score of a small group of girls with RTT, affecting primarily their motor sitting skills, hand use, nonverbal communication, and respiratory dysfunction (De Felice et al. 2012). ω-3-PUFA supplementation improved biventricular myocardial systolic function in girls with RTT, an outcome thought to be mediated in part through the regulation of the redox balance (Maffei et al. 2014). ω-3-PUFA supplementation also improved ω-6/ω-3 PUFA ratios and lipid profiles, decreased PUFA peroxidation end-products, normalized biochemical markers of inflammation, and reduced bone hypodensity in these individuals (Signorini et al. 2014; De Felice et al. 2013).

Nutritional assessment

Nutritional assessment of females with RTT includes a thorough medical, nutritional, growth, and social history; accurate growth measurements; a complete physical examination; meal observation; and selected diagnostic studies (Leonard et al. 2013).

MEDICAL HISTORY

The medical history includes information about the severity of neurological impairment and its expected course. Periodic reassessment throughout childhood is necessary because the manifestation of the disorder may change over time. A review of medications is important because drugs prescribed for gastroesophageal reflux, constipation, and seizures may influence the child's eating pattern. Gastric acid inhibitors and laxatives may minimize abdominal discomfort and reverse feeding refusal. Valproic acid, gabapentin, topiramate, zonisamide, and felbamate may affect appetite and result in weight gain or loss. Many anticonvulsants impact the level of consciousness and have a secondary effect on oral motor skills and airway protection. The review of systems is important because respiratory and gastrointestinal symptoms impact all aspects of nutritional support.

NUTRITIONAL HISTORY

An assessment of the child's ability to feed independently and the efficiency of the feeding process may reveal obvious reasons for poor weight gain. An occupational or speech therapist may identify functional deficits in oral motor and swallowing skills during meals. A registered dietitian may identify restricted eating patterns related to texture intolerance or reduced nutrient intake due to poor oral ability to manage food. A 24-hour recall of habitual food intake or a 3-day record of actual food consumption may be used to assess dietary energy and nutrient intakes.

GROWTH HISTORY

Birthweight and length, as well as previous length or height and weight measurements, may be compared with those in a reference population to determine if genetic downsizing or abnormal weight gain or loss has occurred (Centers for Disease Control and Prevention 2012; Tarquinio et al. 2012). The interpretation of historical data may be flawed because accurate growth measurements, particularly standing heights, may be difficult to obtain in females with RTT.

SOCIAL HISTORY

All individuals involved in care-giving and all settings in which feeding occurs require inquiry to ensure that nutritional interventions can be integrated into family or institutional routines. Financial issues, medical insurance, and the availability of home care require exploration.

GROWTH MEASUREMENTS

Growth measurements are the most important components of the nutritional assessment. Accurate measurements of height or length (without shoes and orthotics), or a proxy when these measures are not reliable, and weight are obtained using standardized techniques and equipment at every medical encounter. Length is obtained supine in females younger than 2 years or in older females unable to stand. Weight is measured on the same scale with the individual wearing little or no clothing. BMI is calculated from height and weight measurements of females 2 years of age and older, and weight-for-length is estimated for females less than 2 years of age. Height or length, weight, BMI, and weight-for-length are plotted on reference growth charts and compared with previous measurements and reference standards (Centers for Disease Control and Prevention 2012). BMI or weight-for-length values below the 5th centile require nutritional intervention throughout childhood and adolescence. Once pubertal growth is completed, BMI values in the lower ranges are better tolerated.

PHYSICAL EXAMINATION

Physical examination focuses on signs of underweight, linear stunting, overweight, and specific nutrient deficiencies. Abnormal breath sounds may be suggestive of chronic respiratory problems associated with aspiration. Abdominal distention alone or in conjunction with palpable masses suggests aerophagia or constipation. Contractures and scoliosis are noteworthy for positioning during meals. Muscle mass, body fat stores, and activity level are relevant because they influence dietary energy needs. Pallor, smooth tongue, decubitus ulcers, or pedal edema may suggest other macro- or micronutrient deficiencies.

MEAL OBSERVATION

Meal observation may be useful because of the variable feeding patterns in females with RTT. Classification systems based on eating efficiency and oral motor feeding skills may be helpful to assess the effectiveness of oral feeding interventions (Reilly and Cass 2001; Marchand et al. 2006).

DIAGNOSTIC STUDIES

Although isolated nutrient deficiencies may be present in females with RTT, extensive laboratory evaluation generally is not necessary. A complete blood count and 25-hydroxyvitamin D level may document iron deficiency anemia or vitamin D deficiency. Blood urea nitrogen may reflect hydration status, but may be low because of poor protein intake and low muscle mass.

Radiographic or radionuclide studies may be helpful, depending on symptoms. A videofluoroscopic assessment of swallowing function using different food and beverage textures determines the degree of oral and pharyngeal motor dysfunction, as well as risk of aspiration, and provides guidance for appropriate food textures and therapeutic feeding techniques. An upper gastrointestinal series, gastric emptying scan, or chest radiograph may provide supportive evidence for gastroesophageal reflux, gastroparesis, or aspiration, and may aid in the management of these disorders.

Nutritional support

Nutritional support is essential for the care of females with RTT. Evidence of oral motor feeding difficulties, underweight, growth faltering unrelated to genetic downsizing, overweight, or individual nutrient deficiencies indicate the need for nutritional intervention. Nutritional support is provided enterally rather than parenterally, assuming competency of the gastrointestinal tract. Energy-dense complementary foods and commercial formulas may be used to supplement oral feedings. Enteral tube feedings are mandatory for those who cannot meet their energy and nutrient needs by the oral route alone. Many families find the idea of enteral tube feedings difficult to accept. Although medical opinions generally prevail, parental wishes need to be considered and respected.

Nutritional requirements

Energy requirements of females with RTT vary with the severity of their disability, the presence of feeding difficulties, and their mobility. Dietary energy can be estimated from DRI standards for basal energy expenditure for age (USDA 2012). The best way to determine the adequacy of the diet is to monitor the rate of weight gain and BMI in response to daily food and beverage consumption. Supplemental protein, vitamins, and calcium are mandatory when dietary energy intake is reduced to obtain the desired weight. In the absence of evidence-based nutrient allowances for females with RTT, the DRI for protein, vitamins, and minerals in healthy children is recommended (USDA 2012). Judicious use of multivitamin and mineral supplements, particularly vitamin D, 600 international units daily, is prudent for those who rely on table foods and beverages alone for their daily dietary intake (USDA 2012).

Specialized diets

The gluten-free, casein-free diet has been advocated for RTT based on the theory that gluteo- and casomorphines adversely affect brain maturation and function. Currently, there is no evidence to support the use of this diet unless celiac disease has been diagnosed. Consultation with a nutritionist is imperative if the diet is instituted because of associated micronutrient deficiencies. Similarly, there is no evidence to support the use of the phenylalanine (PKU) diet, which is inadequate in protein-containing foods, or the specific carbohydrate (grain-, lactose-, fructose-free) diet (SCD), which is inadequate in carbohydrates and micronutrients. Both diets are deficient in meeting nutrient needs for growth and functional outcomes.

The ketogenic diet is used to treat intractable seizures that do not respond to anticonvulsant drugs (Kossoff et al. 2011). The diet is high in fat and balanced by weight with protein and carbohydrate in a 2:1 or 3:1 ratio. The diet can be difficult to implement without a gastrostomy because of poor taste acceptance. Adverse consequences, including poor growth, bone mineral deficits, and renal stones, have been associated with the diet.

Positioning and oral therapy

The occupational or speech therapist can assist with oral feeding skills, correct positioning of the child, and use of appropriate chairs and adapted utensils during meals. Guided feeding techniques may improve oral motor coordination and participation in the eating process (Qvarfordt et al. 1997). Therapy to improve oral motor skills may enhance oral motor function, but may not promote feeding efficiency and weight gain (Marchand et al. 2006). VitalStim (DJO Global, Vista, CA, USA), a device that administers electrical stimulation to the musculature of the neck, may be used to treat swallowing dysfunction, but the efficacy of this treatment in RTT has not been documented (Marchand et al. 2006).

ALTERNATIVE FEEDING METHODS

Oral feedings can be maintained in females with adequate oral motor skills who have a low risk of aspiration. Adequate positioning and adjusting food consistency with thickening agents may improve feeding efficiency. Increasing the energy density of food maximizes energy intake. If oral intake is insufficient to promote weight gain, linear growth, and adequate hydration, if aspiration is a risk, or if parents request assistance with feeding and medication administration, enteral feedings may be considered. The type of enteral access selected will depend on the nutritional and clinical status of the child. Parents will be concerned about the child's loss of oral feeding skills and the risks and benefits of enteral tube feeding.

Nasogastric tube feeding is a minimally invasive method that may be used for short-term nutritional support in underweight individuals whose parents refuse surgical intervention or in those with severe acid reflux and aspiration who are awaiting gastrostomy placement. Nasogastric tubes are not used long-term because they may be dislodged easily, may stiffen and cause intestinal perforation, or may result in nasal congestion, sinusitis, otitis media, or skin and mucosal irritation. A gastrostomy 'button' is recommended for long-term enteral nutrition because it is more comfortable for the individual and is less easily dislodged. Gastrostomy feedings promote weight gain and linear growth, improve the child's health, and reduce the time spent feeding the individual (Motil et al. 2009). The type of gastrostomy placement, whether by percutaneous endoscopy, laparoscopic or open surgical technique, or image-guided, retrograde or antegrade methods, is decided on a case-by-case basis between the physician and family. Gastrojejunal tubes may be recommended in the setting of intractable gastroesophageal reflux disease in the absence of a gastric fundoplication.

The choice of enteral formula depends on the child's age, energy requirement, and nutrient sensitivity. Standard casein-based protein formulas are administered routinely. Whey-based protein formulas may be better tolerated because they enhance gastric emptying (Marchand et al. 2006). Protein hydrolysate or amino acid formulas are reserved for individuals who have milk protein sensitivity. Adult formulas may prevent hypoalbuminemia during periods of rapid catch-up growth, but care should be taken to avoid iron, calcium, phosphorus, or vitamin D deficiency (Marchand et al. 2006). High energy density formulas may be used when volume and energy are limiting factors; however, monitoring hydration status and protein and micronutrient intake may be necessary. Enteral formulas provide adequate amounts of micronutrients only when volumes consumed meet the age-appropriate DRI for energy (USDA 2012). Because many females with RTT require lower energy intakes, their micro-nutrient intakes are correspondingly lower. Replacement therapy reverses these deficits. A fiber-containing formula may ameliorate constipation, but may aggravate abdominal bloating.

Bolus formula feedings are preferred because they mimic the physiological responses associated with meals and allow a more flexible feeding schedule. Continuous infusions of formula may be used throughout the day or night for individuals who do not tolerate bolus feeds or have formula administered directly into the jejunum. A combination of both methods can be used if large volumes of formula are required.

Bone health

CLINICAL FEATURES OF LOW BONE MASS

Low bone mass, defined as low areal or volumetric bone mineral content (BMC) and bone mineral density (BMD), is a common feature of RTT (Haas et al. 1997; Motil et al. 2006, 2008; Shapiro et al. 2010; Jefferson et al. 2011; Roende et al. 2011a). Total body BMC and BMD, as well as spine, hip or femoral neck, and radius BMD, standardized for height, weight, and race and/or ethnicity, have been measured using dual-energy X-ray absorptiometry (DXA) in US, Australian, Danish, and Italian RTT cohorts (Haas et al. 1997; Cepollaro et al. 2001; Motil et al. 2006, 2008; Shapiro et al. 2010; Jefferson et al. 2011; Roende et al. 2011a). Total body BMC and BMD z-scores average –2.2 and –1.7, respectively, in females 15 years of age, whereas total body BMC z-scores average –1.5 in females 8.5 years of age (Motil et al. 2006, 2008). Bone mineral deficits are present at an early age in females with RTT. Total body BMC and BMD increase with age in most RTT cohorts (Haas et al. 1997; Motil et al. 2008; Shapiro et al. 2010; Roende et al. 2011a); however, the rate of bone mineral accretion is slower in females with RTT than in unaffected individuals (Haas et al. 1997; Motil et al. 2006, 2008; Shapiro et al. 2010; Roende et al. 2011a) and parallels the slower rate of accretion of lean body mass (Motil et al. 2008). The difference in total body BMC and BMD between RTT cohorts and unaffected individuals increases with age in most studies (Haas et al. 1997; Motil et al. 2006, 2008). Similar patterns of bone mineral deficits have been described using alternative methods, including cortical bone thickness of metatarsal bones from hand radiographs and qualitative ultrasound of the distal phalanxes of the hand (Leonard et al. 1999b; Cepollaro et al. 2001; Gonnelli et al. 2008).

PREVALENCE

The true prevalence of low bone mass in RTT is unknown. The prevalence of total body BMC 1 standard deviation and 2 standard deviation below the population mean is 84% and 59%, respectively, whereas the prevalence of total body BMD 1 standard deviation and 2 standard deviation below the population mean is 76% and 45%, respectively, across a broad range of ages in a US RTT cohort (Motil et al. 2008). The prevalence of lumbar spine BMD 2 standard deviation below the population mean is 49% in another US cohort (Shapiro et al. 2010). In contrast, the prevalence of total body BMC 1 standard deviation below the population mean is 45% in an Australian RTT cohort (Jefferson et al. 2011). The prevalence of BMD of the lumbosacral spine and femoral neck more than 1 standard deviation below the population mean is 41% and 78%, respectively, in this same group (Jefferson et al. 2011). Cortical bone thickness is severely reduced in 25%, moderately reduced in 44%, and mildly reduced in 15% in the Australian RTT cohort (Leonard et al. 2011).

Bone morphology
The mechanisms that account for bone mineral deficits in females with RTT have not been determined. The ultrastructure and density of bone, as well as its biochemical properties, have been examined in *Mecp2* mouse models (O'Connor et al. 2009; Blue et al. 2015; Kamal et al. 2015). Mice without the functional Mecp2 protein show decreased numbers of osteoblasts, abnormal growth plates with irregularly shaped chondrocytes and decreased cortical, trabecular, and calvarial bone, suggesting that the lack of Mecp2 protein may reduce bone density through osteoblast dysfunction (O'Connor et al. 2009). Partial or complete silencing of Mecp2 results in reductions in cortical bone stiffness, microhardness, and tensile modulus, all of which can be reversed with unsilencing of the *Mecp2* gene (Blue et al. 2015; Kamal et al. 2015). Bone histomorphometry, determined by double tetracyline labeling, demonstrates decreased bone volume due to decreased numbers of thin trabeculae and low bone formation rates in females with RTT (Budden and Gunness 2001).

Bone biomarkers
Bone metabolism, characterized by bone formation, resorption, mineralization, and turn-over, has not been uniformly studied in RTT. Biomarkers of bone formation, both osteo-calcin and the N-terminal propeptides of collagen type 1, are lower, while bone alkaline phosphatase is higher, across a broad age range of females with RTT compared with respective control groups (Motil et al. 2014; Roende et al. 2014). C-terminal telopeptide crosslinks, biomarkers of bone resorption, are lower in some affected females (Roende et al. 2014). However, bone mineral metabolites, bone biomarkers, and hormones involved in the regula-tion of bone mineral metabolism, including 25-hydroxyvitamin D, 1,25-dihydroxyvitamin D, parathyroid hormone, and ghrelin do not differ between females with RTT and unaffected individuals in several studies (Cepollaro et al. 2001; Motil et al. 2006, 2008, 2014; Gonnelli et al. 2008; Shapiro et al. 2010; Roende et al. 2011a; Caffarelli et al. 2012). Bone biomark-ers, including bone alkaline phosphatase, osteocalcin, and C-telopeptide, and hormones, including 25-hydroxyvitamin D; 1,25-dihydroxyvitamin D; parathyroid hormone, ghrelin, and urinary cortisol excretion do not demonstrate an association with measures of age- and height-adjusted bone mass in most studies (Cepollaro et al. 2001; Motil et al. 2006, 2014; Gonnelli et al. 2008; Shapiro et al. 2010; Caffarelli et al. 2012).

Risk factors for bone mineral deficits
Bone mass may be influenced by genetic predisposition, body size, dietary factors, hor-monal factors, anticonvulsant medications, and weight-bearing physical activity. However, associations between these factors and measures of bone mass demonstrate variability because of different methods used to characterize bone mass, the choice of bone sites mea-sured, and differences in classification of factors. *MECP2* genotype is associated with poor bone mineralization in some, but not all RTT cohorts (Motil et al. 2008; Shapiro et al. 2010; Jefferson et al. 2011; Roende et al. 2011a). Individuals with p.Arg168X or p.Thr158Met mutations have lower height-adjusted total body BMC than individuals with other muta-tions (Jefferson et al. 2011). X-chromosome inactivation (XCI) skewing has not been shown

to affect measures of bone mineralization (Roende et al. 2011a). Body size, measured as age-adjusted heights and weights, but not body mass index, is associated with total body BMC and BMD in some RTT cohorts (Haas et al. 1997; Gonnelli et al. 2008; Motil et al. 2008; Shapiro et al. 2010). The smaller size of the lean body mass, but not body fat, also parallels slower BMC accretion (Motil et al. 2008).

Dietary calcium, phosphorus, and protein intakes, estimated from 3-day food records, are associated with measures of bone mass (Motil et al. 2014). However, dietary calcium intakes, estimated by food frequency or 24-hour recall, do not meet the DRI for age in 30–40% of females with RTT (Haas et al. 1997; Motil et al. 2006, 2014). Fractional calcium absorption shows a compensatory increase in the presence of adequate dietary calcium intakes, mild hypercalcuria, and bone mineral deficits in females with RTT (Haas et al. 1997; Leonard et al. 1999b; Motil et al. 2006). Fractional calcium absorption is greater in affected than in unaffected females, but does not demonstrate an association with total body BMC, osteocalcin, or regulatory hormones including 25-hydroxyvitamin D, 1,25-dihydroxyvitamin D, or parathyroid hormone (Motil et al. 2006). Preliminary data suggest that supplemental dietary calcium increases biomarkers of bone formation in prepubertal girls with RTT (Motil KJ, unpublished observations).

Vitamin D deficiency, defined as serum 25-hydroxyvitamin D levels less than 50 nmol/L, is reported in 20% of females in a US RTT cohort; lower numbers are reported in a smaller group of individuals (Shapiro et al. 2010; Motil et al. 2011). Values less than 22.5 nmol/L are reported in 24% of an Italian RTT cohort (Gonnelli et al. 2008). Risk factors that may contribute to vitamin D deficiency include inadequate dietary consumption of vitamin D, reduced sunlight exposure, and the use of anticonvulsant medications. Multivitamin supplements and vitamin D fortified milk and commercial formulas are consumed by 40%, 52%, and 54%, respectively, of females with RTT (Motil et al. 2011). The use of vitamin supplements or vitamin D-fortified formula favorably influences serum 25-hydroxyvitamin D concentrations in females with RTT (Motil et al. 2011). Whether higher levels of serum 25-hydroxyvitamin D protects against fractures in females with RTT is unknown.

Seizures and the use of anticonvulsant medications have been associated with deficits in bone mineralization in some, but not all, RTT cohorts (Leonard et al. 1999b; Cepollaro et al. 2001; Motil et al. 2006, 2008; Gonnelli et al. 2008; Shapiro et al. 2010; Jefferson et al. 2011; Roende et al. 2011a). Better mobility is associated with higher measures of BMC and BMD in many, but not all studies (Haas et al. 1997; Leonard et al. 1999b; Cepollaro et al. 2001; Motil et al. 2008; Shapiro et al. 2010; Roende et al. 2011a; Jefferson et al. 2015). The presence of scoliosis is associated with decreased cortical bone thickness and low total body, but not lumbar, BMD (Leonard et al. 1999b; Motil et al. 2008; Shapiro et al. 2010).

Fractures

Low bone mass is important because of its association with bone fractures (Motil et al. 2008; Roende et al. 2011a). Females with RTT have nearly a four-fold increased risk of fractures compared with the general population (Downs et al. 2008; Motil et al. 2008). Fractures are more common in females with RTT who have moderate or severe reductions in cortical bone thickness or low BMC and BMD compared with unaffected children (Haas et al. 1997; Leonard et al. 1999b; Cepollaro et al. 2001; Motil et al. 2006, 2008; Gonnelli et al. 2008; Roende et al. 2011a). BMC and BMD are lower in affected females who have fractures than in affected individuals without fractures (Motil et al. 2008; Roende et al. 2011a). Females with RTT sustain more spontaneous fractures from an early age compared with unaffected individuals, even though overall fracture occurrence is not different between groups (Roende et al. 2011b). The maximum number of fractures in any individual is five, the most common site being the lower limb (Leonard et al. 1999b; Roende et al. 2011b).

Prevalence

The prevalence of bone fractures ranges between 15% and 35% in Danish, US, and Australian RTT cohorts (Leonard et al. 1999b; Downs et al. 2008; Motil et al. 2008, 2012; Jefferson et al. 2011; Roende et al. 2011a).

Pathophysiology

Fractures are associated with specific *MECP2* mutations, including p.Arg270X and p.Arg168X, in one study (Downs et al. 2008; Roende et al. 2011b). Fractures also are associated with less mobility and lack of ambulation in some studies, but the strength of the association is less clear in others (Leonard et al. 1999b; Downs et al. 2008; Roende et al. 2011b). Individuals with seizures who received anticonvulsant medications, especially valproic acid, are more likely to sustain a fracture in some, but not all studies (Leonard et al. 1999b, 2010; Downs et al. 2008; Roende et al. 2011b).

Bone mineral assessment

Standard radiographs may be used in the clinical setting to characterize osteopenia, a qualitative deficit in BMC, in females with RTT. Hand radiographs have been used in the research setting to describe quantitative measures of cortical bone thickness in RTT (Leonard et al. 1999b). This technique has limitations in that the interpretation of bone mineral status is derived from a relatively small portion of actual bone mass.

DXA is the standard method used to assess quantitatively total body, spine, and hip or femoral neck BMC and BMD in females with RTT. This test is difficult to perform because of stereotypies and involuntary movements which lead to motion artifact. Limited DXA scans of the spine and hip can be obtained in individuals who have minimal movement and do not have metal replacements in bone. Conscious sedation for DXA scans has been reserved primarily for research studies (Motil et al. 2006, 2008, 2014; Caffarelli et al. 2012).

Quantitative ultrasound has been used for the non-invasive assessment of bone mass in RTT; however, this technique has not been standardized across a broad range of individuals (Cepollaro et al. 2001; Gonnelli et al. 2008). One study suggests that the performance of quantitative ultrasound of the phalanges may be comparable to areal BMD obtained by the DXA technique in these individuals (Caffarelli et al. 2014).

The adequacy of dietary calcium and vitamin D consumption is determined using three-day food records or food frequency questionnaires with particular attention to the number of servings of dairy products and the use of multivitamin and mineral supplements. The adequacy of vitamin D also is determined from serum 25-hydroxyvitamin D levels; values of 50 nmol/L or greater are considered normal, although data in adults suggest a reduction in fracture rates when values are greater than 100 nmol/L (Bischoff-Ferrari et al. 2006; USDA 2012). Bone mineral metabolites, including serum calcium and phosphorus; bone biomarkers including osteocalcin, bone alkaline phosphatase, and C-telopeptide; and selected hormones, including 1,25-dihydroxyvitamin D and parathyroid hormone may be ordered through standard clinical laboratories, but generally do not alter the plan of care.

Bone mineral support

Few guidelines currently exist for the treatment of bone mineral deficits in RTT. Dietary interventions are the mainstay of therapy for bone mineral deficits. The DRI for calcium is age dependent; children 1–3 years, 4–8 years, and 9–18 years require daily calcium intakes of 700 mg, 1000 mg, and 1300 mg, respectively, while adults older than 18 years require 1000 mg daily (USDA 2012). The Institute of Medicine recommends that all children more than 1 year of age receive 600 international units of vitamin D daily to maintain serum 25-hydroxyvitamin D levels greater than 50 nmol/L. Sunlight exposure, vitamin D fortified dairy products, and commercially available formulas and vitamin supplements are good sources of vitamin D.

Physical activity, carried out as weight-bearing or ambulatory activities, should be encouraged. Although treadmill therapy improves stamina in females with RTT, the effect of this intervention on bone mineral status has not been studied (Lotan et al. 2004). Low magnitude mechanical stimulation increased spine mineral density in a small number of individuals (Afzal et al. 2014).

Bis-phosphonate therapies may have a limited role in the treatment of bone mineral deficits in RTT based on studies in mice and measures of biomarkers in females with RTT (O'Connor et al. 2009; Motil et al. 2014; Roende et al. 2014). The relation between bisphosphonates and fracture risk in females with RTT is unknown. The use of bisphosphonates generally is limited because their indications in childhood diseases are not well defined and their long-term effects on bone remodeling and atypical fracture rates are unknown (Meier et al. 2012).

Recommendations for the management of feeding and nutrition in Rett syndrome

- Accurate assessment of height, weight, and BMI are essential at each clinical encounter.
- Supplemental oral feedings are encouraged when a BMI less than the 5th centile is observed.
- Dietary energy intakes for weight maintenance and gain approximate age-appropriate basal energy expenditure by factors of 110% and 150%, respectively.
- Oral motor interventions, proper positioning during meals, and thickening of liquids or pureed food textures may provide additional support during feedings.

- Alternative enteral feeding methods are considered when oral intake is insufficient to promote weight gain, linear growth, or adequate hydration; aspiration is a risk; or parents request assistance with feeding and medication administration.
- Radiographic studies, such as a swallowing function study or upper gastrointestinal series, may identify clinical features that interfere with feeding.
- Milk and dairy products are encouraged to provide sufficient elemental calcium to meet recommended dietary intakes for age; calcium supplements may be added when dietary intakes are insufficient.
- Milk or fortified milk-based formulas are encouraged to ensure an adequate intake of vitamin D, 600 international units daily; multivitamin supplements may be added when dietary intakes or sunlight exposure are insufficient.
- Serum 25-hydroxyvitamin D measurements may be obtained to assess vitamin D status; supplements are considered for serum 25-hydroxyvitamin D levels less than 50 nmol/L.
- Radiographic studies such as DXA scans may identify clinical features consistent with low bone mass and bone mineral deficits.

REFERENCES

Afzal SY, Wender AR, Jones MD, Fung EB, Pico EL (2014) The effect of low magnitude mechanical stimulation (LMMS) on bone density in patients with Rett syndrome: A pilot and feasibility study. *J Pediatr Rehabil Med* 7: 167–178.

Bebbington A, Percy A, Christodoulou J et al. (2010) Updating the profile of C-terminal *MECP2* deletions in Rett syndrome. *J Med Genet* 47: 242–248.

Bischoff-Ferrari HA, Giovannucci E, Willett WC, Dietrich T, Dawson-Hughes B (2006) Estimation of optimal serum concentrations of 25-hydroxydivatmin D for multiple health outcomes. *Am J Clin Nutr* 84: 18–28.

Blardi P, de Lalla A, D'Ambrogio T et al. (2009) Long-term plasma levels of leptin and adiponectin in Rett syndrome. *Clin Endocrinol (Oxf)* 70: 706–709.

Blue ME, Boskey AL, Doty SB, Fedarko NS, Hossain MA, Shapiro JR (2015) Osteoblast function and bone histomorphometry in a murine model of Rett syndrome. *Bone* 76: 23–30.

Budden SS, Gunness ME (2001) Bone histotmorphometry in three females with Rett syndrome. *Brain Dev* 23: S133–S137.

Caffarelli C, Gonnelli S, Tanzilli L (2012) The relationship between serum ghrelin and body composition with bone mineral density and QUS parameters in subjects with Rett syndrome. *Bone* 50: 830–835.

Caffarelli C, Hayek J, Pitinca T, Nuti R, Gonnelli S (2014) A comparative study of dual-X-ray absorptiometry and quantitative ultrasonography for the evaluating bone status in subjects with Rett syndrome. *Calcif Tissue Int* 95: 248–256.

Cass H, Reilly S, Owen L (2003) Findings from a multidisciplinary clinical case series of females with Rett syndrome. *Dev Med Child Neurol* 45: 327–337.

Centers for Disease Control and Prevention (2012) www.cdc.gov/growthcharts/clinical_charts.htm (accessed 30 June 2012).

Cepollaro C, Gonnelli S, Bruni D (2001) Dual x-ray absorptiometry and bone ultrasonography in patients with Rett syndrome. *Calcif Tissue Int* 69: 259–262.

De Felice C, Signorini C, Durand T et al. (2012) Partial rescue of Rett syndrome by ω-3-polyunsaturated fatty acids (PUFAs) oil. *Genes Nutr* 7: 447–458.

De Felice C, Cortelazzo A, Signorini C et al. (2013) Effects of w-3 polyunsaturated fatty acids on plama proteome in Rett syndrome. *Mediators Inflamm* 723269. doi: 10.1155/2013/723269. Epub 9 December 2013.

Downs J, Bebbington A, Woodhead H et al. (2008) Early determinants of fractures in Rett syndrome. *Pediatrics* 121: 540–546.

Ellaway CJ, Peat J, Williams K, Leonard H, Christodoulou J (2001) Medium-term open label trial of L-carnitine in Rett syndrome. *Brain Dev* 23: S85–S89.

Glaze DG, Percy AK, Motil KJ et al. (2009) A study of the treatment of Rett syndrome with folate and betaine. *J Child Neurol* 24: 551–556.

Gonnelli S, Caffarelli C, Hayek J et al. (2008) Bone ultrasonography at phalanxes in patients with Rett syndrome: A 3-year longitudinal study. *Bone* 42: 737–742.

Haas RH, Dixon SD, Sartoris DJ, Hennessy MJ (1997) Osteopenia in Rett syndrome. *J Pediatr* 131: 771–774.

Hara M, Nishi Y, Yamashita Y et al. (2011) Ghrelin levels are reduced in Rett syndrome patients with eating difficulties. *Int J Dev Neurosci* 29: 899–902.

Hagebeuk EE, Duran M, Koelman JH, Abeling NG, Vyth A, Poll-The BT (2012) Folinic acid supplementation in Rett syndrome patients does not influence the course of the disease: A randomized study. *J Child Neurol*; 27: 304–309.

Huppke P, Roth C, Christen HJ, Brockmann K, Hanefeld F (2001) Endocrinological study on growth retardation in Rett syndrome. *Acta Paediatr* 90: 1257–1261.

Isaacs JS, Murdock M, Lane J, Percy AK (2003) Eating difficulties in girls with Rett syndrome compared with other developmental disabilities. *J Am Diet Assoc* 103: 224–230.

Jefferson AL, Woodhead HJ, Fyfe S et al. (2011) Bone mineral content and density in Rett syndrome and their contributing factors. *Pediatr Res* 69: 293–298.

Jefferson A, Fyfe S, Downs J, Woodhead H, Jacoby P, Leonard H (2015) Longitudinal bone mineral content and density in Rett syndrome and their contributing factors. *Bone* 74: 191–198.

Kamal B, Russell D, Payne A et al. (2015) Biomechanical properties of bone in a mouse model of Rett syndrome. *Bone* 71: 106–114.

Kossoff EH, Freeman JM, Turner Z, Rubenstein JE (2011) *Ketogenic Diets: Treatments for Epilepsy and Other Disorders*, 5th ed. New York: Demos Health.

Leonard H, Thomson M, Glasson E et al. (1999a) Metacarpophalangeal pattern profile and bone age in Rett syndrome. *Am J Med Genet* 83: 88–95.

Leonard H, Thomson MR, Glasson EJ et al. (1999b) A population-based approach to the investigation of osteopenia in Rett syndrome. *Dev Med Child Neurol* 41: 323–328.

Leonard H, Downs J, Jian L et al. (2010) Valproate and risk of fracture in Rett syndrome. *Arch Dis Child* 95: 444–448.

Leonard H, Ravikumara M, Baikie G et al. (2013) Assessment and management of nutrition and growth in Rett syndrome. *J Pediatr Gastroenterol Nutr* 57: 451–460.

Leoncini S, De Felice C, Signorini C et al. (2011) Oxidative stress in Rett syndrome: natural history, genotype, and variants. *Redox Rep* 16: 145–153.

Lotan M, Isakov E, Merrick J (2004) Improving functional skills and physical fitness in children with Rett syndrome. *J Intellect Disabil Res* 48: 730–735.

Maffei S, De Felice C, Cannarile P et al. (2014) Effect of ω-3-PUFAs supplementation on myocardial function and oxidative stress markers in typical Rett syndrome. *Mediators Inflamm* 2014: 983178.

Marchand V, Motil KJ, NASPGHAN Committee on Nutrition (2006) Nutrition support for neurologically impaired children: A clinical report of the North American Society for Pediatric Gastroenterology, Hepatology, and Nutrition. *J Pediatr Gastroenterol Nutr* 43: 123–135.

Meier RP, Perneger TV, Stern R, Rizzoli R, Peter RE (2012) Increasing occurrence of atypical femoral fractures associated with bisphosphonate use. *Arch Intern Med* 172: 930–936.

Morton RE, Bonas R, Minford J, Kerr A, Ellis RE (1997a) Feeding ability in Rett syndrome. *Dev Med Child Neurol* 39: 331–335.

Morton RE, Bonas R, Minford J, Tarrant SC, Ellis RE (1997b) Respiration patterns during feeding in Rett syndrome. *Dev Med Child Neurol* 39: 607–613.

Motil KJ, Schultz RJ, Brown B, Glaze DG, Percy AK (1994) Altered energy balance may account for growth failure in Rett syndrome. *J Child Neurol* 9: 315–319.

Motil KJ, Schultz RJ, Wong WW, Glaze DG (1998) Increased energy expenditure associated with repetitive involuntary movement does not contribute to growth failure in girls with Rett syndrome. *J Pediatr* 132: 228–233.

Motil KJ, Schultz RJ, Browning K, Trautwein L, Glaze DG (1999) Oropharyngeal dysfunction and gastroesophageal dysmotility are present in girls and women with Rett Syndrome. *J Pediatr Gastroenterol Nutr* 29: 31–37.

Motil KJ, Schultz RJ, Abrams S, Ellis KJ, Glaze DG (2006) Fractional calcium absorption is increased in girls with Rett syndrome. *J Pediatr Gastroenterol Nutr* 42: 419–426.

Motil KJ, Ellis KJ, Barrish JO, Caeg E, Glaze DG (2008) Bone mineral content and bone mineral density are lower in older than in younger females with Rett syndrome. *Pediatr Res* 4: 435–439.

Motil KJ, Morrissey M, Caeg E, Barrish JO, Glaze DG (2009) Gastrostomy placement improves height and weight gain in girls with Rett syndrome. *J Pediatr Gastroenterol Nutr* 49: 237–242.

Motil KJ, Barrish JO, Lane J et al. (2011) Vitamin D deficiency is prevalent in girls and women with Rett syndrome. *J Pediatr Gastroenterol Nutr* 53: 569–574.

Motil KJ, Caeg E, Barrish JO et al. (2012) Gastrointestinal and nutritional problems occur frequently throughout life in girls and women with Rett syndrome. *J Pediatr Gastroenterol Nutr* 55: 292–298.

Motil KJ, Barrish JO, Neul JL, Glaze DG (2014) Low bone mineral mass is associated with decreased bone formation and diet in females with Rett syndrome. *J Pediatr Gastroenterol Nutr* 59: 386–392.

Neul JL, Fang P, Barrish J et al. (2008) Specific mutations in methyl-CpG-binding protein 2 confer different severity in Rett syndrome. *Neurology* 70: 1313–1321.

O'Connor RD, Zayzafoon M, Farach-Carson MC, Schanen NC (2009) Mecp2 deficiency decreases bone formation and reduces bone volume in a rodent model of Rett syndrome. *Bone* 45: 346–356.

Oddy WH, Webb KG, Baikie G et al. (2007) Feeding experiences and growth status in a Rett syndrome population. *J Pediatr Gastroenterol Nutr* 45: 582–590.

Platte P, Jaschke H, Herbert C, Korenke GC (2011) Increased resting metabolic rate in girls with Rett syndrome compared to girls with developmental disabilities. *Neuropediatrics* 42: 179–182.

Qvarfordt I, Engerstrom IW, Eliasson AC (2009) Guided eating or feeding: Three girls with Rett syndrome. *Scand J Occup Ther* 16: 33–39.

Rebeiro RA, Romano AR, Birman EG, Mayer MP (1997) Oral manifestations in Rett syndrome: A study of 17 cases. *Pediatr Dent* 19: 349–352.

Reilly S, Cass H (2001) Growth and nutrition in Rett syndrome. *Disabil Rehabil* 23: 118–128.

Roende G, Ravn K, Fuglsang K et al. (2011a) DXA measurements in Rett syndrome reveal small bones with low bone mass. *J Bone Miner Res* 26: 2280–2286.

Roende G, Ravn K, Fuglsang K et al. (2011b) Patients with Rett syndrome sustain low-energy fractures. *Pediatr Res* 69: 359–364.

Roende G, Petersen J, Ravn K et al. (2014) Low bone turnover phenotype in Rett syndrome: results of biochemical bone marker analysis. *Pediatr Res* 75: 551–558.

Schultz RJ, Glaze DG, Motil KJ et al. (1993) The pattern of growth failure in Rett syndrome. *Am J Dis Child* 147: 633–637.

Schwartzman F, Vitolo MR, Schwartzman JS, de Morais MB (2008) Eating practices, nutritional status and constipation in patients with Rett syndrome. *Arq Gastroenterol* 45: 284–289.

Shapiro JR, Bibat G, Hiremath G (2010) Bone mass in Rett syndrome: Association with clinical parameters and *MECP2* mutations. *Pediatr Res* 68: 446–451.

Signorini C, De Felice C, Leoncini S et al. (2014) Altered erythrocyte membrane fatty acid profile in typical Rett syndrome: Effects of omega-3-polyunsaturated fatty acid supplementation. *Prostaglandins Leukot Essent Fatty Acids* 91: 183–193.

Tarquinio DC, Motil KJ, Hou WE et al. (2012) Reference growth standards in Rett syndrome. *Neurology* 79: 1653–1661.

USDA (2012) fnic.nal.usda.gov/dietary-guidance/dietary-reference-intakes (accessed 30 June 2012).

Van den Veyver IB (2002) Genetic effects of methylation diets. *Annu Rev Nutr* 22: 255–282.

Ward BC, Kolodny NH, Nag N, Berger-Sweeney JE (2009) Neurochemical changes in a mouse model of Rett syndrome: Changes over time and in response to perinatal choline nutritional supplementation. *J Neurochem* 108: 361–371.

12
MOLECULAR COMPLEXITIES OF MeCP2 FUNCTION IN RETT SYNDROME

Michael L Gonzales and Janine M LaSalle

Introduction

As a methylated DNA binding protein, MeCP2 serves as a link between epigenetic signals and the gene expression changes they encode. The MeCP2 protein is expressed in tissues throughout the body but the highest levels are found in the brain. MeCP2 protein levels increase over the course of central nervous system (CNS) development and maturation and disruption of MeCP2 expression leads to defects in neuronal maturation. RTT primarily affects girls who are apparently normal at birth, but by 6–18 months of age undergo a transient regression of language and motor milestones, followed by a period where hand sterotypies and autistic features are observed. Mouse models of RTT have recapitulated the major deficits of RTT and restoration of MeCP2 in the mouse is sufficient to ameliorate symptoms (Chen et al. 2001; Guy et al. 2001, 2007). These studies have demonstrated that MeCP2 is required for normal brain development and function. How MeCP2 acts in normal brain development and function will be the topic of this chapter.

MeCP2 domains and isoforms

Proteins are modular molecules that consist of one or more domains, each with a unique function. The overall function of a protein is often defined by the combination of protein domains it contains. The MeCP2 protein can be divided into six distinct domains defined by both functional and structural studies (Fig. 12.1). RTT mutations can be found in the sequences encoding all six of these domains, demonstrating the potential importance of each domain in MeCP2 function relevant to RTT. Two of these domains, the methyl-CpG binding domain (MBD) and transcriptional repression domain (TRD) were initially defined by functional studies. The MBD was identified as the region capable of specific binding to DNA containing symmetrically methylated CpG dinucleotides (Nan et al. 1993). The MBD is also capable of binding to unmethylated DNA, but with a greatly reduced affinity than that for a methylated substrate. RTT mutations in the MBD can disrupt either specific binding to methylated DNA (p.Arg133Cys) or can completely ablate the ability of domain

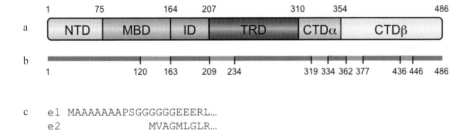

Fig. 12.1. (a) Domain layout of the MeCP2 protein. (b) Regions of disorder (red) and order (green) predicted by Predictor of Naturally Disordered Regions (PONDR). (c) Amino acid sequences of the aminotermini of the MeCP1 e1 and e2 splice variants. NTD, N-terminal domain; MBD, methyl-CpG binding domain; TRD, transcriptional repression domain; CTDα and CTDβ, C-terminal domains. A colour version of this figure can be seen in the plate section between pages 166 and 167.

to interact with DNA (p.Arg106Trp). Interestingly, some MBD mutations have minimal effects on DNA binding, suggesting that the MBD has functions beyond binding to methylated DNA. More than 65% of all pathogenic amino acid substitutions are found in the MBD, a region that comprises less than 20% of the MeCP2 protein. The TRD was identified as the minimal region required to repress transcription in a transient reporter assay (Nan et al. 1997). The TRD also possesses DNA-binding capabilities, although it binds with equal affinity to both methylated and unmethylated DNA (Ghosh et al. 2010). Together, the identification and initial functional characterization of the MBD and TRD led to the classification of MeCP2 as a transcriptional repressor of methylated DNA.

The remaining domains of MeCP2 were identified by limited proteolysis, a biochemical technique that relies on the protective nature of functional units of a protein to prevent degradation by proteolytic enzymes. Application of this technique to MeCP2 resulted in the isolation of six protected domains (Adams et al. 2007). Two of these correspond to the MBD and TRD, confirming their status as functional units of MeCP2. The other four domains constitute most of the remainder of the MeCP2 protein. Since no defining functions could be assigned to these domains at the time, they were named for their position in the molecule (Fig. 12.1). The N-terminal domain (NTD) lies at the extreme N-terminus of the protein, the inter domain lies between the MBD and the TRD, and the C-terminal domains (CTDα and CTDβ) are found after the TRD at the C-terminus of the protein. The NTD is the only region of the protein that differs between the alternatively spliced e1 and e2 isoforms with a 21 amino acid N-terminus in e1 exchanged for nine amino acids in e2 (Fig. 12.1c). Despite the differences in sequence, the structural and functional differences between the two splice variants remains completely unknown. While the NTD does not itself bind to DNA, it does enhance the affinity of the MBD for DNA. The inter domain, like the TRD, contains a DNA binding domain. The inter domain also enhances MBD binding to DNA independent of the inter domain's own DNA binding domain (Ghosh et al. 2010). CTDα also contains a non-specific DNA binding domain, making a total of four DNA binding domains in the MeCP2 protein. CTDβ does not bind directly to DNA but has been proposed to facilitate interactions between MeCP2 and histone proteins (Nikitina et al. 2007a). A majority of the identified RTT frameshift mutations are found in CTDβ, highlighting the importance of MeCP2 functions beyond DNA binding in RTT pathogenesis.

Isoform-specific mutations of *Mecp2* in mouse models have revealed major differences in e1 and e2 isoforms in their functional contributions to RTT phenotypes. Deletion of exon 2 in mouse, creating a specific lack of MeCP2-e2, resulted in no apparent neurological abnormalities, although reproductive effects on placental integrity were observed (Itoh et al. 2012). In striking contrast, a mouse containing a mutation of the translation start site for the e1 isoform in exon 1 of *Mecp2* that modeled a RTT human *MECP2* mutation exhibited a full spectrum of RTT phenotypes, including forelimb stereotypy, hind-limb clasping, excessive grooming, and hypoactivity prior to death between 7 and 31 weeks (Yasui et al. 2014). Although MeCP2-e2 protein levels were elevated in *Mecp2e1* deficient mice compared to wild-type brain, the total MeCP2 levels only reached 50% of control levels. Two additional explanations for the difference in MeCP2 isoform function despite their sharing 96% amino acid sequence was the presence of a unique phosphorylation site in MeCP2-e1 that was associated with distinct subcellular locations, as well as the greater protein stability observed for MeCP2-e1 versus MeCP2-e2 (Yasui et al. 2014). In addition, induced pluripotent stem cells derived from an RTT patient with an *MECP2e1* mutation were differentiated to neurons showing deficits in soma size, dentritic complexity, and excitatory synaptic currents (Djuric et al. 2015). Together, these results imply non-redundant functions of the isoforms of MeCP2 and suggest that investigation of the specific function role of MeCP2-e1 may have the most relevance to RTT.

MeCP2 structure

Classic biochemical thinking suggests that a protein's function is determined by its structure and the ordered folding of its linear amino acid sequence into a defined three-dimensional shape. However, approximately 60% of MeCP2 has been experimentally determined to lack a specific structure (Adams et al. 2007). Because of this, MeCP2 is classified as an intrinsically disordered protein. Intrinsically disordered proteins are a class of proteins in which all or part of the molecule does not adopt a specific three-dimensional structure in the absence of physiological partners. Despite this, intrinsic disorder can be found in a surprisingly large number of proteins that play central roles in important pathways including transcriptional regulation, cellular signaling, and cell cycle control. It is hypothesized that the presence of intrinsically disordered domains allows proteins to undertake multiple roles that would not be possible if the protein was locked into a single rigid structure.

The MBD is the most ordered domain of MeCP2 with approximately 60% of the amino acids adopting a specific structure. The remainder of the MBD and the majority of the rest of the MeCP2 molecule are predicted to lack any defined three-dimensional structure (Fig. 12.1b). Upon interaction with protein partners or substrates (DNA in the case of MeCP2), the disordered domains of intrinsically disordered proteins can adopt defined structures that are unique to each interaction. This feature allows intrinsically disordered domains to interact with a diverse array of partners in a specific manner. DNA binding by the TRD or the inter domain of MeCP2 induces these highly disordered domains to adopt a more ordered structure, which may be important in regulating the function of

MeCP2. Similarly, interactions between MeCP2 and its protein binding partners (see below) may also induce a transition to a more ordered structure. Therefore, the disordered nature of MeCP2 is likely to play an important role in determining and regulating its multiple functions. The importance of intrinsically disordered domains in MeCP2 is apparent by the presence of a number of RTT causing missense mutations in disordered regions of MeCP2.

MeCP2 binding to DNA and chromatin

MeCP2 contains at least four autonomous DNA binding domains that are capable of cooperatively binding to DNA; however, only the MBD is capable of specifically binding to methylated DNA. The remaining DNA binding domains appear to have no specific preference for methylated versus unmethylated DNA. Because of this, MeCP2 only has an approximately three–fold greater affinity for DNA containing a single methylated site than for unmethylated DNA. More recently, MeCP2 has been shown to bind not only to methylated CpG sites but also non-CpG (mCH) sites, as well as hydroxymethylcytosine, although results of different studies have varied based on the composition of the oligonucleotides (Kinde et al. 2015). MeCP2 affinity for methylated DNA appears to increase with methylation density, suggesting that it would have a higher affinity for highly methylated sites. Accordingly, it has been shown that MeCP2 binding throughout the genome is correlated with DNA methylation levels with higher binding at highly methylated regions (Chen et al. 2015). Additionally, the common RTT causing mutation p.Arg133Cys in the MBD specifically disrupts the methylation specific binding of MeCP2 to DNA without disrupting the non-specific binding, indicating that methyl-CpG specific binding is an important component of MeCP2 function. However, the presence of all four DNA binding domains appears to be required for full MeCP2 function. This may be due to the fact that the cooperative binding of MeCP2 to DNA induces significant structural organization of the MeCP2 protein, which may further strengthen MeCP2s interaction with DNA and/or allow for interactions between MeCP2 and specific proteins partners when MeCP2 is bound to DNA.

In the cell, most DNA is packaged into nucleosomes, a DNA and protein complex comprised of DNA wrapped around a core of histone proteins. The MBD, inter domain, TRD, and CTDα of MeCP2 can all bind to DNA packaged into nucleosomes and naked DNA with similar abilities; however, the CTDβ of MeCP2 binds exclusively to nucleosomes (Ghosh et al. 2010), suggesting that this interaction is dependent on more than just DNA binding. Nucleosomes can be further packaged into higher order structures called chromatin. Regulation of the chromatin structure around individual genes is a common mechanism used to regulate their expression. MeCP2 has been shown to promote nucleosome compaction into extremely condensed chromatin, as well as complex looped structures. The ability of MeCP2 to promote chromatin compaction is dependent on both the ability of MeCP2 to bind to DNA and the presence of the CTDs, as compaction is deficient when RTT mutations disrupt either DNA binding by the MBD or cause deletion of the CTDs (Nikitina et al. 2007b).

MeCP2 function

Expression of MeCP2 in both neuronal and glial cells is required for proper neuronal development and maturation (Ballas et al. 2009; Maezawa et al. 2009). These processes require a precise program of transcriptional activation and repression in response to neuronal activity. MeCP2 is required for many of these activity dependent changes in gene expression in the neuronal/glial cell networks involved in the maturation of synapses and synaptic plasticity (Moretti et al. 2006). It is predicted that RTT arises when mutations or truncations of MeCP2 interfere with its ability to properly respond to neuronal activity and modulate gene expression. While the precise mechanisms by which MeCP2 controls this expression are debated, it has become clear that regulation of chromatin states and structure is an important component of MeCP2's control of activity dependent transcription.

The initial characterization of MeCP2 as repressor of methylated DNA stems from observation that highly methylated gene promoters are transcriptionally silenced. This was supported by the report that MeCP2 interacted with the Sin3a/HDAC co-repressor complex and that this interaction was required for MeCP2's ability to silence a reporter construct (Nan et al. 1998). The Sin3a/HDAC complex contains histone deacetylase (HDAC) activity, which removes acetyl groups from histone tails, leading to the establishment of a transcriptionally silent chromatin state. In turn, this leads to a model in which MeCP2 bound to methylated promoter regions to facilitate their silencing by recruiting co-repressors to create a repressive chromatin state. While several genes have since been identified that are regulated by MeCP2 in this fashion, genome-wide expression and binding studies have not supported a role for MeCP2 as a general repressor of gene expression. Only 2% of highly methylated promoters are actually bound by MeCP2, demonstrating that, in general, MeCP2 is not involved in the direct repression of methylated promoters (Yasui et al. 2007). Instead, MeCP2 was more likely to be bound near the promoters of active genes than those of silenced genes. Similarly, expression profiling in the mouse hypothalamus demonstrated that MeCP2 primarily caused activation of gene expression (Chahrour et al. 2008), suggesting that MeCP2 may be playing a role in modulating the expression of active genes rather than silencing inactive genes.

Genome-wide, MeCP2 is actually de-enriched at gene promoters. The mammalian genome is heavily methylated with an average of *c.* 80% methylation of each available CpG site; however, CpG sites and methylation is not evenly distributed throughout the genome. Regions of high CpG density are known as CpG islands. These are frequently found at gene promoters and the majority are unmethylated. Unmethylated CpG island promoters are islands in the genome for both their strikingly different methylation pattern and MeCP2 binding. Almost 60% of MeCP2 binding sites are found between genes, with a majority of this binding occurring at long distances (more than 10 kb) from transcribed regions (Yasui et al. 2007). The presence of MeCP2 binding sites at large distances from any transcribed region indicates that MeCP2 may also be regulating transcription by controlling genome wide changes in chromatin structure. In support of this, MeCP2 was found to be involved in the formation of large scale chromatin loops and that this has dramatic effects on the transcription of genes contained within the loops (Horike et al. 2005). In this way, MeCP2 may affect gene expression across entire chromatin regions without binding directly to gene promoters. Measurements in mature neuronal nuclei have shown that there are nearly as many molecules of MeCP2 as there are nucleosomes (Skene et al. 2010). This raises the possibility that MeCP2 binding may be pervasive throughout chromosomes, a pattern that would be expected of a protein that is regulating global chromatin structure.

Overall, two apparently conflicting models of MeCP2 function have emerged. The first is that of direct regulation whereby MeCP2 binds to distinct genomic sites to directly affect the expression of an associated gene. The second is regulation of gene expression by modulating chromatin structure due to MeCP2 binding throughout the genome. The apparent abundance of MeCP2 in mature neurons is counter to the direct repression model that predicts MeCP2 binding to relatively few, distinct sites within the genome. However, MeCP2 is expressed in CNS cell types other than neurons at much lower levels (Ballas et al. 2009; Maezawa et al. 2009). This suggests that there may be fundamental differences in MeCP2 function in different cell types. It may be that MeCP2 is able to affect gene expression through multiple mechanisms and that both models of MeCP2 function are correct.

MeCP2 interacting partners

How can MeCP2 regulate gene expression through such diverse mechanisms? Often, the individual functions of multifunctional proteins are determined by interactions with specific cofactors. Accordingly, MeCP2 interacts with a wide array of cofactors. The intrinsically disordered nature of MeCP2 permits a large degree of structural flexibility, which allows MeCP2 to interact with many diverse protein partners. This, in turn, allows MeCP2 to utilize a variety of mechanisms to regulate gene expression dependent on the proteins with which it is interacting at any given time.

In addition to the interaction with the co-repressor Sin3a discussed above, MeCP2 has also been shown to interact with the transcription factor YY1 (Forlani et al. 2010). YY1, like MeCP2, is associated with both activation and repression of transcription and the interaction between the two may be important in allowing the regulatory flexibility of MeCP2. Sin3a and YY1 regulate the expression of specific genes by binding to proximal regulatory elements. The association between MeCP2 and these proteins lends support to the direct mechanism of gene regulation by MeCP2. The heterochromatin proteins HP1 α/β/γ also interact with MeCP2 (Agarwal et al. 2007). The HP1 proteins bind to DNA and promote formation of transcriptionally silent heterochromatin. Recently, HP1 isoforms have also been implicated in the activation of gene expression, demonstrating that, like MeCP2, they are multi-functional proteins involved in transcriptional regulation. MeCP2 also interacts with a number of proteins that regulate chromatin structure including ATRX and the cohesin complex (Kernohan et al. 2010). These proteins may work with MeCP2's native ability to induce chromatin compaction to control gene expression both directly and over long distances. It is interesting to note that mutations in ATRX are also associated with neurodevelopmental disorders, highlighting the importance of chromatin structure in brain development. MeCP2 has been shown to interact with a number of other proteins, many of which are involved in the regulation of gene expression, as well as proteins involved in other transcriptionally related processes such as messenger ribonucleic acid (mRNA) splicing, suggesting that MeCP2 may have roles outside of transcriptional regulation.

To date, it is unknown what effect RTT mutations have on the interactions between MeCP2 its cofactors. Many RTT-causing mutations do not affect DNA binding by MeCP2; therefore, other interactions must also be important for MeCP2s ability to modulate transcription. It is likely that the truncation mutations, particularly those that remove large portions of the proteins, would dramatically reduce or destroy the ability of MeCP2 with its interacting partners and thereby impede proper MeCP2 function. Point mutations may also disrupt the interaction between MeCP2 and specific cofactors by altering binding sites, resulting in reduced MeCP2 functionality. The interactions between MeCP2 and its cofactors are likely to be highly regulated and depend on cell or tissue type as well as developmental stages. Within a single cell, individual MeCP2 molecules could be interacting with different proteins allowing MeCP2 to regulate specific genes or groups of genes, each in a unique way, simultaneously.

MeCP2 phosphorylation

As it is involved in the regulation of activity dependent gene expression, MeCP2 requires a mechanism for responding to neuronal activity. MeCP2 achieves this through the use of activity-dependent phosphorylation. Phosphorylation, the addition of a charged phosphate group to specific amino acids of a protein, is frequently used to regulate protein functions, including the formation of protein–protein interactions. Phosphate groups can be quickly added or removed from specific amino acids, allowing for precise control of the timing and location of their placement and, therefore, the functions they regulate.

MeCP2 has been shown to undergo phosphorylation at a number of sites in response to changes in neuronal activity. The two sites of phosphorylation that have been well characterized are serine 421 (S421) and serine 80 (S80). Phosphorylation of S421 occurs in response to neuronal activity and is required for activity dependent expression of brain-derived neurotrophic factor (BDNF) (Zhou et al. 2006). Phosphorylation of S421 is also required for normal dendritic growth and spine maturation, two activity-dependent events. The calcium/calmodulin dependent kinases (CamKs), CamK II and IV, have been implicated in the phosphorylation of MeCP2 on S421 (Tao et al. 2009). These kinases play an important role in neuronal development and synaptic plasticity, processes that also require MeCP2. Alternatively, phosphorylation at S80 is present in resting neurons and is removed in response to neuronal activity (Tao et al. 2009). The homeodomain-interacting protein kinase 2 (HIPK2) has been reported to phosphorylate MeCP2 on serine 80 and this phosphorylation is required for HIPK2-mediated apoptosis (Bracaglia et al. 2009). However, the consequences of this for RTT are unclear as defects in apoptosis do not appear to play a role in the pathogenesis of RTT. Cyclin-dependent kinase like-5 (CDKL5) kinase has also been shown to phosphorylate MeCP2, although the exact site remains to be determined (Mari et al. 2005). Mutations in CKDL5 can be found in the early-onset seizure variant of RTT, demonstrating the two proteins are involved in the same molecular pathway(s).

Intrinsically disordered proteins such as MeCP2 frequently contain multiple phosphorylation sites. The conformationally flexible nature of their disordered regions allows them to interact with many different kinase enzymes, which catalyze the phosphorylation of specific amino acids. Therefore, it is not surprising that MeCP2 has been shown to undergo phosphorylation of several different residues in addition to those discussed above. These phosphorylations allow MeCP2 to dynamically respond to neuronal activity by generating the required changes in activity dependent gene expression.

MeCP2 target genes

As a predicted transcriptional regulator, there has been an ongoing search for downstream gene targets of MeCP2 in order to understand and potentially treat the symptoms of RTT. As discussed above, MeCP2 may directly regulate specific genes at their promoter regions, or control gene expression over long distances by regulating the chromatin structure around genes. Regardless of the mechanism, it is clear that MeCP2 is important for controlling gene expression during neuronal development. While many MeCP2 target genes have been described, this section will focus on the targets that are modulated by MeCP2 in response to neuronal activity and maturation.

Expression of BDNF, a member of the nerve growth factor (NGF) family, is increased in response to neuronal activity and is predicted to promote the maturation of neurons and synapses in the postnatal brain. BNDF has been shown to be dysregulated by MeCP2 deficiency in a number of studies, with the majority showing reduced levels of BDNF in MeCP2-deficient brain. In addition, the retinoic acid responsive proto-oncogene RET, encoding a protein tyrosine kinase implicated in neural crest development, is regulated by MeCP2 binding to a heavily methylated enhancer (Angrisano et al. 2011).

Another activity-dependent gene, early growth response gene 2 (*EGR2*), encodes a Zn finger transcription factor that is important in both early hind-brain development and mature neuronal function. *MECP2* and *EGR2* regulate each other's expression, as MeCP2 binds to an enhancer region within *EGR2* and positively regulates its expression. EGR2 in turn binds to the *MECP2* promoter as a positive regulator of *MECP2* levels (Swanberg et al. 2009). Other developmentally relevant targets of MeCP2 include the four inhibitors of differentiation (ID) genes, *ID1*, *ID2*, *ID3*, and *ID4*, that encode inhibitors of basic-loop helix transcription factors and thereby modulate neuronal differentiation (Peddada et al. 2006). The expression of the differentiation transcription factor myocyte enhancer factor 2C (*MEF2C*), and the transcription factor *CREB1*, are both positively regulated by MeCP2 (Chahrour et al. 2008). Interestingly, microdeletions of the locus containing *MEF2C* show clinical features similar to RTT and reduced levels of both *MECP2* and *CDKL5*, suggesting an additional coregulatory loop (Zweier et al. 2010).

Many of the activity-dependent genes, whose expression is regulated by MeCP2, encode proteins that themselves regulate the expression of genes involved in neuronal maturation. Therefore, MeCP2 is ideally positioned to broadly control the activity-dependent expression patterns required for neuronal development. Consistent with this idea of MeCP2 as a regulator of regulators, MeCP2 targets have now grown to include many noncoding RNAs (ncRNA), particularly microRNAs (miRNAs). miRNAs generally act as negative regulators of transcript and protein levels by specifically targeting transcripts for degradation. MiR-137, a target of MeCP2 regulation (Szulwach et al. 2010), modulates the proliferation and differentiation of adult neural stem cells by targeting the histone methyltrasnferase and polycomb group protein Ezh2. MeCP2 binds to methylated promoters of a number of miRNAs genome-wide, including some targeting *Bdnf* that are upregulated by MeCP2-deficiency (Zweier et al. 2010). The number of noncoding RNAs as targets of MeCP2 in neuronal development are expected to increase with the advent of future high throughput sequencing approaches.

In addition to regulating ncRNAs, MeCP2 itself is subject to regulation by ncRNAs. The long ncRNA, *Evf2*, regulates transcription of *Dlx5* and *Dlx6* by recruitment of MeCP2 to an intergenic enhancer (Bond et al. 2009), while an activation responsive miRNA (miR132), is part of a homeostatic control feedback loop with MeCP2 (Klein et al. 2007). Interestingly, several miRNAs encoded on human chromosome 21 regulate the expression of MeCP2, so that their upregulation from trisomy 21 induces the downregulation of MeCP2 levels in individuals with Down syndrome (Kuhn et al. 2010).

In spite of the strong evidence for dysregulation of specific genes and ncRNAs with MeCP2 deficiency, the abundant nature of MeCP2, coupled with binding to intergenic and repetitive regions, suggests that much of this dysregulation may actually be indirect effects of changes in global chromatin organization. The neuronal nucleus undergoes changes in global chromatin organization, as well as structural changes to heterochromatin and nucleoli during pre- and postnatal brain development. MeCP2 deficient mouse neurons exhibited significant differences in the size and number of heterochromatic clusters (chromocenters) and nucleoli compared to control, and were deficient in the dynamic changes observed in these structures following neuronal activity (Singleton et al. 2011). Coupled with the near histone-octamer levels and the global changes to the level of histone H1 that arise from MeCP2 deficiency, these results suggest that MeCP2 may be primarily a global regulator of neuronal chromatin and the effects of downstream target genes may be a result of both global and local epigenetic changes.

Conclusion

While there is certainly much more to be learned about MeCP2 structure and function and their relevance to RTT, a current picture is emerging of MeCP2 as a 'master regulator' of neuronal differentiation, maturation, and function. Epigenetic mechanisms act at the interface of genetics and environmental influences. MeCP2 can read the epigenetic changes that occur during development in response to activation of neuronal networks and discrete synapses, and translate them into the gene expression patterns they define. MeCP2 seems to be adept at multitasking, acting as a repressor or an activator, depending on the gene, the binding of promoter versus enhancer, or as a long-range chromatin regulator. As a result, MeCP2 is not a single molecule with a single function, but instead appears to posses multiple activities determined by alternative splicing, phosphorylation and interacting proteins, and regulated by neuronal activity. Therefore, understanding the post-translational modifications, isoforms and different interacting partners of MeCP2 is expected to be critical for understanding its functions and their relevance to RTT.

While *MECP2* mutations primarily cause RTT, MeCP2 is also emerging as a key modulator of disease in a number of other neurodevelopmental disorders. Therefore, understanding the basic structural and functional changes that MeCP2 undergoes in its role as a master epigenetic regulator will be critical for designing future therapies that may target not only RTT, but also related neurodevelopmental disorders with a higher prevalence, such as autism, schizophrenia, and epilepsy. In this way, RTT is considered a 'Rosetta's stone' for decoding the complexities of epigenetic pathways in human neurodevelopment in health and disease.

REFERENCES

Adams VH, McBryant SJ, Wade PA, Woodcock CL, Hansen JC (2007) Intrinsic disorder and autonomous domain function in the multifunctional nuclear protein, MeCP2. *J Biol Chem* 282: 15057–15064.

Agarwal N, Hardt T, Brero A et al. (2007) MeCP2 interacts with HP1 and modulates its heterochromatin association during myogenic differentiation. *Nucleic Acids Res* 35: 5402–5408.

Angrisano T, Sacchetti S, Natale, F et al. (2011) Chromatin and DNA methylation dynamics during retinoic acid-induced RET gene transcriptional activation in neuroblastoma cells. *Nucleic Acids Res* 39: 1993–2006.

Ballas N, Lioy DT, Grunseich C, Mandel G (2009) Non-cell autonomous influence of MeCP2-deficient glia on neuronal dendritic morphology. *Nat Neurosci* 12: 311–317.

Bond AM, Vangompel MJ, Sametsky EA et al. (2009) Balanced gene regulation by an embryonic brain ncRNA is critical for adult hippocampal GABA circuitry. *Nat Neurosci* 12: 1020–1027.

Bracaglia G, Conca B, Bergo A et al. (2009) Methyl-CpG-binding protein 2 is phosphorylated by homeodomain-interacting protein kinase 2 and contributes to apoptosis. *EMBO Rep* 10: 1327–1333.

Chahrour M, Jung SY, Shaw C et al. (2008). MeCP2, a key contributor to neurological disease, activates and represses transcription. *Science* 320: 1224–1229.

Chen RZ, Akbarian S, Tudor M, Jaenisch R (2001) Deficiency of methyl-CpG binding protein-2 in CNS neurons results in a Rett-like phenotype in mice. *Nat Genetics* 27: 327–331.

Chen L, Chen K, Lavery LA et al. (2015) MeCP2 binds to non-CG methylated DNA as neurons mature, influencing transcription and the timing of onset for Rett syndrome. *Proc Natl Acad Sci USA* 112: 5509–5514.

Djuric U, Cheung AY, Zhang W et al. (2015) MECP2e1 isoform mutation affects the form and function of neurons derived from Rett syndrome patient iPS cells. *Neurobiol Dis* 76: 37–45.

Forlani G, Giarda E, Ala U et al. (2010) The MeCP2/YY1 interaction regulates ANT1 expression at 4q35: Novel hints for Rett syndrome pathogenesis. *Hum Mol Genet* 19: 3114–3123.

Ghosh RP, Horowitz-Scherer RA, Nikitina T, Shlyakhtenko LS, Woodcock CL (2010) MeCP2 binds cooperatively to its substrate and competes with histone H1 for chromatin binding sites. *Mol Cell Biol* 30: 4656–4670.

Guy J, Hendrich B, Holmes M, Martin JE, Bird A (2001) A mouse Mecp2-null mutation causes neurological symptoms that mimic Rett syndrome. *Nat Genet* 27: 322–326.

Guy J, Gan J, Selfridge J, Cobb S, Bird A (2007) Reversal of neurological defects in a mouse model of Rett syndrome. *Science* 315: 1143–1147.

Horike S, Cai S, Miyano M, Cheng JF, Kohwi-Shigematsu T (2005) Loss of silent-chromatin looping and impaired imprinting of DLX5 in Rett syndrome. *Nat Genet* 37: 31–40.

Itoh M, Tahimic CG, Ide S et al. (2012) Methyl CpG-binding protein isoform MeCP2_e2 is dispensable for Rett syndrome phenotypes but essential for embryo viability and placenta development. *J Biol Chem* 287: 13859–13867.

Kernohan KD, Jiang Y, Tremblay DC et al. (2010) ATRX partners with cohesin and MeCP2 and contributes to developmental silencing of imprinted genes in the brain. *Dev Cell* 18: 191–202.

Kinde B, Gabel HW, Gilbert CS, Griffith EC, Greenberg ME (2015) Reading the unique DNA methylation landscape of the brain: Non-CpG methylation, hydroxymethylation, and MeCP2. *Proc Natl Acad Sci USA* 112: 6800–6806.

Klein ME, Lioy DT, Ma L, Impey S, Mandel G, Goodman RH (2007) Homeostatic regulation of MeCP2 expression by a CREB-induced microRNA. *Nat Neurosci* 10: 1513–1514.

Kuhn DE, Nuovo GJ, Terry AV Jr et al. (2010) Chromosome 21-derived microRNAs provide an etiological basis for aberrant protein expression in human Down syndrome brains. *J Biol Chem* 285: 1529–1543.

Maezawa I, Swanberg S, Harvey D, LaSalle JM, Jin LW (2009) Rett syndrome astrocytes are abnormal and spread MeCP2 deficiency through gap junctions. *J Neurosci* 29: 5051–5061.

Mari F, Azimonti S, Bertani I et al. (2005) CDKL5 belongs to the same molecular pathway of MeCP2 and it is responsible for the early-onset seizure variant of Rett syndrome. *Hum Mol Genet* 14: 1935–1946.

Moretti P, Levenson JM, Battaglia F et al. (2006) Learning and memory and synaptic plasticity are impaired in a mouse model of Rett syndrome. *J Neurosci* 26: 319–327.

Nan X, Meehan RR, Bird A (1993) Dissection of the methyl-CpG binding domain from the chromosomal protein MeCP2. *Nucleic Acids Res* 21: 4886–4892.

Nan X, Campoy FJ, Bird A (1997) MeCP2 is a transcriptional repressor with abundant binding sites in genomic chromatin. *Cell* 88: 471–481.

Nan X, Ng HH, Johnson CA et al. (1998) Transcriptional repression by the methyl-CpG-binding protein MeCP2 involves a histone deacetylase complex. *Nature* 393: 386–389.

Nikitina T, Ghosh RP, Horowitz-Scherer RA, Hansen JC, Grigoryev SA, Woodcock CL (2007a) MeCP2-chromatin interactions include the formation of chromatosome-like structures and are altered in mutations causing Rett syndrome. *J Biol Chem* 282: 28237–28245.

Nikitina T, Shi X, Ghosh RP, Horowitz-Scherer RA, Hansen JC, Woodcock CL (2007b) Multiple modes of interaction between the methylated DNA binding protein MeCP2 and chromatin. *Mol Cell Biol* 27: 864–877.

Peddada S, Yasui DH, LaSalle JM (2006) Inhibitors of differentiation (ID1, ID2, ID3 and ID4) genes are neuronal targets of MeCP2 that are elevated in Rett syndrome. *Hum Mol Genet* 15: 2003–2014.

Singleton MK, Gonzales ML, Leung KN, et al. (2011) MeCP2 is required for global heterochromatic and nucleolar changes during activity-dependent neuronal maturation. *Neurobiol Dis* 43: 190–200.

Skene PJ, Illingworth RS, Webb S et al. (2010) Neuronal MeCP2 is expressed at near histone-octamer levels and globally alters the chromatin state. *Mol Cell* 37: 457–468.

Swanberg SE, Nagarajan RP, Peddada S, Yasui DH, LaSalle JM (2009) Reciprocal co-regulation of EGR2 and MECP2 is disrupted in Rett syndrome and autism. *Hum Mol Genet* 18: 525–534.

Szulwach KE, Li X, Smrt RD et al. (2010) Cross talk between microRNA and epigenetic regulation in adult neurogenesis. *J Cell Biol* 189: 127–141.

Tao J, Hu K, Chang Q et al. (2009) Phosphorylation of MeCP2 at Serine 80 regulates its chromatin association and neurological function. *Proc Natl Acad Sci USA* 106: 4882–4887.

Yasui DH, Peddada S, Bieda MC et al. (2007) Integrated epigenomic analyses of neuronal MeCP2 reveal a role for long-range interaction with active genes. *Proc Natl Acad Sci USA* 104: 19416–19421.

Yasui DH, Gonzales ML, Aflatooni JO et al. (2014) Mice with an isoform-ablating Mecp2 exon 1 mutation recapitulate the neurologic deficits of Rett syndrome. *Hum Mol Genet* 23: 2447–2458.

Zhou Z, Hong EJ, Cohen S et al. (2006) Brain-specific phosphorylation of MeCP2 regulates activity-dependent Bdnf transcription, dendritic growth, and spine maturation. *Neuron* 52: 255–269.

Zweier M, Gregor A, Zweier C et al. (2010) Mutations in MEF2C from the 5q14.3q15 microdeletion syndrome region are a frequent cause of severe mental retardation and diminish MECP2 and CDKL5 expression. *Hum Muta* 31: 722–733.

13
THE NEUROBIOLOGY OF RETT SYNDROME

Walter E Kaufmann, James H Eubanks, Michael V Johnston, and Mary E Blue

Introduction

The study of the neurobiological bases of Rett syndrome (RTT) began shortly after the key 1983 publication by Hagberg and colleagues (1983). Most of the work was based on postmortem brain and other tissue samples from affected individuals, in conjunction with neuroimaging studies of patients with RTT. Experimental paradigms that attempted to model the abnormalities reported in human studies also contributed in this early era of RTT neurobiology. Following the identification of *MECP2* as the main genetic etiology of RTT, a massive body of literature that includes all experimental modalities from whole organism to cell culture models carrying the genetic defect, has been accumulated (Feldman et al. 2016). More recently, the use of new technologies such as induced pluripotent stem cells (iPSC)-derived neurons (Tang et al. 2016) has completed the loop of clinical and experimental samples for the study of the neurobiology and pathophysiology of RTT. Overall, RTT is a developmental disorder that affects virtually all cell types and neurotransmitter and signaling systems in the CNS that results in marked synaptic abnormalities. Taking into consideration the clinical emphasis of this book and the nature of the body of data on the subject, this chapter focuses only on key concepts that would help to understand the genetics, symptomatology, and management of RTT. For details on most of the findings, please refer to the original publications and reviews cited here.

Neurobiological correlates of Rett syndrome

RETT SYNDROME IS A GENERALIZED DISORDER OF NEURONAL DIFFERENTIATION

Two of the earliest neuropathologic findings suggested a global disorder of neuronal differentiation: marked brain volume reduction and increased cell in packing density (associated with reduction in dendritic arborizations) without neuronal loss or overt gliosis (Armstrong 2005; Kaufmann et al. 2005). These findings from the pre-*MECP2* era have been replicated in virtually every cellular and whole organism model of methyl-CpG-binding protein 2 (MeCP2) deficiency (Jung et al. 2003; Kaufmann et al. 2005) and have been expanded by structural neuroimaging (Kaufmann et al. 1998; Carter et al. 2008). The fact that in RTT the brain is typically undersized and underweighted when compared to the brain of an age matched normal child, but without any detectable neuronal loss, supports the notion that RTT is not a neurodegenerative disorder. The lack of neurodegeneration in RTT also implies that interventions in this disorder may be effective throughout the life span of an affected individual.

The relative normal appearance of neurons and other cell populations does not imply that the changes are mild. In fact, their severity is underscored by their widespread nature in both affected patients and animal models. Structural magnetic resonance imaging (MRI) analyses in children with RTT have demonstrated generalized volumetric grey matter reductions (Kaufmann et al. 1998), with mild selective changes affecting the dorsal parietal region and anterior frontal decreases in individuals with greater clinical severity (Carter et al. 2008). Likewise, among other brain regions, smaller than normal neurons displaying increased packing density are observed in the adult Mecp2-deficient mouse hippocampus (Chen et al. 2001), cerebral cortex (Fukuda et al. 2005), locus ceruleus (Zhang et al. 2010; Taneja et al. 2009), substantia nigra (Panayotis et al. 2011), and in the pre-Botzinger complex of the brain stem (Mironov et al. 2009). This decrease in average neuronal soma volume is paralleled by decreases in the average morphological complexity of neurons, as a decrease in dendritic branch structure has been reported for MeCP2-deficient neurons residing within the cortex (Armstrong 2005; Belichenko et al. 2009) and hippocampus (Belichenko et al. 2009; Smrt et al. 2007) in humans and mice.

In addition to displaying attenuated size and diminished morphological complexity, the micro-architecture of MeCP2-deficient neurons is also often altered. Specifically, the density of dendritic spines on MeCP2-deficient excitatory neurons tends to be diminished from normal in several (but not all) regions of the brain. Decreases in dendritic spine densities have been observed along neurons within the Mecp2-deficient mouse cortex, hippocampus, and locus ceruleus (Belichenko et al. 2009; Taneja et al. 2009; Tropea et al. 2009). In cultured hippocampal neurons, silencing Mecp2 with short interference hairpin RNAs caused a decrease in spine density (Chapleau et al. 2009), and spine density of newly born hippocampal dentate granule neurons is also diminished from normal (Smrt et al. 2007). It is important to note, though, that this effect is not ubiquitous: spine density in the Mecp2-null nucleus accumbens (Deng et al. 2010) is preserved at wild-type levels, as is the average density of parallel fiber–Purkinje cell asymmetric synapses in the molecular layer of the cerebellum (Lonetti et al. 2010).

The attenuated morphology and smaller size of neurons in the RTT brain suggest that the loss of MeCP2 function hinders normal neuronal maturation (Johnston et al. 2005; Kaufmann et al. 2005). This model is supported by studies in Mecp2-deficient mice, as neurons displaying hallmarks typically seen in juvenile neurons are over-represented in different regions of their brain. For example, although the overall number of neurons is preserved, the number of mature neurons expressing high levels of tyrosine hydroxylase is diminished in both the locus ceruleus and substantia nigra of *Mecp2*-null mice (Panayotis et al. 2011; Zhang et al. 2010; Taneja et al. 2009). Within these regions, a greater number of smaller neurons with weak or no tyrosine hydroxylase expression are detected, suggestive that their normal progression into mature neurons has been hindered. Similarly, the maturation of newly born hippocampal dentate granule neurons is significantly impaired in *Mecp2*-null mice (Smrt et al. 2007), and the prevalence of mature olfactory receptor neurons is significantly diminished in biopsies of nasal epithelium obtained from RTT patients (Ronnett et al. 2003). Collectively, these observations indicate that MeCP2-deficiency hinders the ability of juvenile neurons to mature into fully differentiated adult neurons. Finally, the developmental profile of MeCP2 expression in humans, beginning prenatally at the brain stem monoaminergic nuclei and progressing throughout childhood into association areas of the cerebral cortex (Shahbazian et al. 2002), underscores the unique role of this transcriptional regulator in brain maturation.

RETT SYNDROME IS A SYNAPTIC DISORDER

A perhaps obvious consequence of the role of MeCP2 in neuronal differentiation and dendritic development is the experimental and human evidence of RTT as a synaptic disorder, a feature shared by most neurodevelopmental disorders. Indeed, both synaptic development and maintenance seem to be influenced by MeCP2 function. However, not all synaptic levels are equally affected. Specifically, the intrinsic properties of Mecp2-null neurons are largely preserved but neuronal communication is abnormal. Given the phenotypic severity of RTT, it was initially expected that the basic neurophysiological properties of MeCP2-deficient neurons would be significantly altered from normal. Surprisingly, this has largely not proven to be the case. In fact, most of the general properties of individual Mecp2-deficient neurons compare favorably with wild-type neurons. For example, in different Mecp2-null mouse models, the resting membrane potential, input resistance, and spike threshold of somato-sensory cortex, motor cortex, hippocampal CA1 and CA3 neurons, inhibitory neurons of the reticular thalamic nucleus, and relay neurons of the nucleus tractus solitarius are comparable to their corresponding wild-type neurons (Dani et al. 2005; Zhang et al. 2008, 2010; Calfa et al. 2015; Kline et al. 2010). Together, these data suggest that the neurophysiological deficiencies that arise in the Mecp2-null brain do not stem from gross alterations in intrinsic neuronal properties. Rather, these deficiencies appear to arise from impairments in synaptic communication.

Despite virtually all neurons and glial cells in the brain expressing MeCP2 (Skene et al. 2010), the absence of MeCP2 does not affect the synaptic properties of all types of neurons within the brain equivalently. For instance, in somatosensory cortical neurons of *Mecp2*-null mice, the average rate and conductance of spontaneously occurring miniature excitatory postsynaptic currents (EPSCs) are diminished from normal, as is the rate of spontaneous action potential firing (Dani et al. 2005). This effect was restricted to excitatory synaptic activity, as the average size of spontaneous miniature inhibitory postsynaptic currents (IPSCs) was not altered (Dani et al. 2005). Another example is a recent study of thalamocortical inputs to the barrel field in 3-week-old *Mecp2*-null mice, which showed normal numbers of both EPSCs and IPSCs but relatively larger inhibitory than excitatory responses due apparently to increased GABA receptor efficacy (Lo et al. 2016). This pattern of diminished excitatory drive has also been observed in the hippocampus of acute brain slices (Zhang et al. 2008), and in cultured Mecp2-null hippocampal neurons in vitro (Nelson et al. 2006). Thus, in forebrain neurons Mecp2 deficiency tends to be associated with diminished excitatory responsiveness. This contrasts dramatically to what has been observed in brain stem regions. In Mecp2-deficient ventral medulla neurons, spontaneous EPSC activity is increased concomitant with decreased spontaneous IPSC activity (Medrihan et al. 2008).

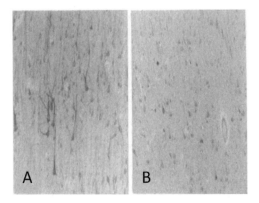

Fig. 13.1. Neuronal abnormalities in RTT. Neuronal somas are typically smaller and associated with less complex dendritic trees (B), when compared to age/sex-matched controls (A). Immunostaining for microtubule-associated protein 2 (MAP-2), a neuronal marker, in motor cortex. Adapted from Kaufmann et al. (1998). A colour version of this figure can be seen in the plate section between pages 166 and 167.

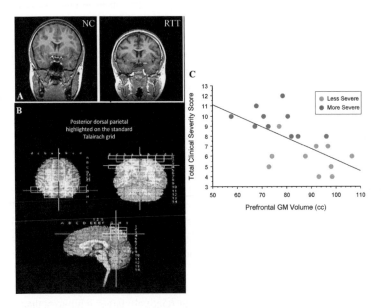

Fig. 13.2. Volumetric brain reductions in RTT. (A) Marked global reductions in brain volume are identified on MRI surveys, when comparing typically developed individuals (NC, normal controls) with affected ones (RTT). (B) MRI quantitative analyses revealed a selective reduction in posterior parietal grey matter volumes, particularly affecting the left hemisphere. The involved region is delineated by the superimposed Talairach 3-dimensional coordinate grid, displayed in the 3 axes. (C) MRI volumetric analyses also revealed that greater overall clinical severity is associated with greater reduction in grey matter volumes affecting the prefrontal cortex, as depicted in the regression plot. Adapted from Kaufmann et al. (1998), and from Carter et al. (2008). A colour version of this figure can be seen in the plate section between pages 166 and 167.

A similar increase in excitatory drive coupled with diminished inhibition has been observed in nucleus tractus solitarius relay neurons (Kline et al. 2010), and this alteration renders the circuitry hyperexcitable. Similarly, neurons within the locus ceruleus also display a hyperexcitable phenotype (Taneja et al. 2009), as do the CA3 hippocampal network (Califa et al. 2015; Zhang et al. 2008). In contrast, there is an increased number of GABAergic synapses in the Mecp2-deficient nucleus accumbens with no evidence of altered glutamate synapse number (Deng et al. 2010).

Changes in synaptic communicative strength are one mechanism that allows neurons to "learn" from experience and tailor their responsiveness appropriately to specific circumstances. Two of the most studied forms of local synapse plasticity are the phenomena of long-term potentiation (LTP) and long-term depression (LTD). Deficits in both LTP and LTD response magnitude have been reported at synapses in cortex and hippocampus in Mecp2-deficient mice when they display overt RTT-like phenotype (Moretti et al. 2006; Lonetti et al. 2010). LTP and LTD impairments appear to be progressive, as these deficits are not evident in younger subjects that display minimal or no overt functional impairments (Moretti et al. 2006; Lonetti et al. 2010), and the magnitude of the LTP deficits increases according to the phenotypic severity of the subject (Weng et al. 2011). These results demonstrate that Mecp2-deficient synapses are not inherently dysfunctional during early perinatal development, and illustrate that the synaptic deficits resulting from the loss of MeCP2 take time to manifest.

While assessments of local synaptic activity provide valuable information on the functional state of small populations of neurons, investigations of local synapses do not address how neural circuits – arguably a better indicator of systemic neural function – are affected by the lack of MeCP2. Neural network investigations in the Mecp2-deficient mouse brain show the presence of network hyperexcitability. In vitro recordings of the Mecp2-deficient hippocampal network revealed only modest alterations in its intrinsic oscillatory activity, illustrating that the lack of Mecp2 did not dramatically alter intrinsic network connectivity (Zhang et al. 2008). However, small excitatory stimuli that had no discernible effect on wild-type hippocampal network activity were sufficient to induce pronounced epileptiform-like discharge activity in the MeCP2-deficient hippocampus (Zhang et al. 2008). Similarly, in vivo assessments using modified electroencephalographic techniques have shown spontaneous epileptiform-like discharges are evident in both the somatosensory cortex and the hippocampus of adult Mecp2-deficient mice (D'Cruz et al. 2010). Despite showing pronounced discharge activity, however, theta wave activity was only modestly altered from normal in Mecp2-deficient when the mice were actively exploring, and a normal delta-like rhythmic pattern was observed in the cortex in the mutant mice during sleep (D'Cruz et al. 2010). Collectively, these results indicate that the neural contacts and intraneuronal communications necessary for network patterning in the MeCP2-deficient brain are largely preserved, but that the networks themselves have a hyperexcitable phenotype. A correlate of these experimental data is the progressive increase in EEG epileptiform activity throughout childhood, even in the absence of clinical seizures, in individuals with RTT (Glaze 2005).

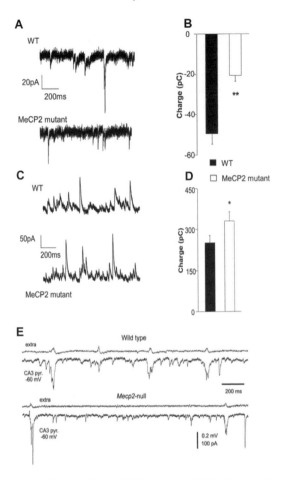

Fig. 13.3. Synaptic abnormalities in Mecp2-deficient mice shift the balance between excitation and inhibition in multiple brain regions. Figures A–D depict L5 pyramidal neurons. Recordings occurred in the presence of ongoing spontaneous activity. Total excitatory and inhibitory synaptic charge was calculated by integrating baseline subtracted spontaneous synaptic current. (A) Representative recordings of spontaneous excitatory postsynaptic currents (EPSCs) (recorded at the chloride-reversal potential) from L5 pyramidal neurons in slices from 4- to 5-week-old wild-type (WT) and mutant mice in modified ACSF. (B) The average excitatory charge was reduced in mutant mice (n = 12 for WT and mutants; P < 0.01, Student's t test). (C) Representative recordings of spontaneous inhibitory postsynaptic currents (IPSCs) (recorded at the reversal potential for spontaneous EPSCs). (D) The average inhibitory charge recorded from the same cells as in C was increased, compared with those from WT mice (n = 12 for WT and mutant, P < 0.05, t test). (E) Basal EPSCs were reduced in CA3 pyramidal neurons. Representative current traces from wild-type (top) and *Mecp2*-null (bottom) mice at −60mV, together with their corresponding local SRFPs detected by extracellular monitoring. Figures A–D reproduced from Dani et al. (2005). Reduced cortical activity due to a shift in the balance between excitation and inhibition in a mouse model of Rett syndrome. *Proc Natl Acad Sci (USA)* 102: 12560–12565 Copyright (2005) National Academy of Sciences, U.S.A. Reproduced with permission. Figure E reproduced from Zhang et al. The *Mecp2*-null mouse hippocampus displays altered basal inhibitory rhythms and is prone to hyperexcitability. Hippocampus 18: 294–309 © 2008 with permission from John Wiley and Sons Ltd.

Human and mouse model anatomical studies have demonstrated variable involvement of virtually every neural pathway (Kaufmann et al. 2005). Likewise, every neurotransmitter system has been implicated in the pathophysiology of RTT. Although in the pre-*MECP2* era the study of CSF and brain postmortem samples mainly revealed abnormalities in mono-amine and opioid levels (Kaufmann et al. 2005), the current view, expanded by mouse models of RTT, is that all major pathways and neurotransmitter systems are involved in the disorder. It is not difficult to understand the complexity of neurochemical abnormal-ities in RTT if one considers the ontogeny of MeCP2 expression in humans mentioned above. Early expression is found in monoaminergic brainstem nuclei, followed by basal forebrain cholinergic nuclei, eventually reaching glutamatergic and GABAergic cortical neurons (Shahbazian et al. 2002). Whether a particular neurotransmitter plays a greater role in RTT pathogenesis and symptomatology appears to be rather time-dependent, although this is still an issue under active discussion. In the next paragraph we provide more details about glutamatergic dysfunction, probably the best-characterized neurotransmitter abnor-mality in RTT, and its potential role in the developmental regression that characterizes RTT (Kaufmann et al. 2016). More recently, MeCP2-related deficits in GABAergic neurons have been linked to a variety of clinical features in RTT (Chao et al. 2010; Abdala et al. 2016). MeCP2 deficiency in GABAergic neurons and abnormalities in GABA receptors may also lead to impairments in a variety of processes, including excitatory-inhibitory balance and other aspects of synaptic plasticity, as well as in epileptogenesis (Calfa et al. 2015; Krishnan et al. 2015). Recent data suggest that the Mecp2 deficiency related network hyperexcitable phenotype is linked to impairments of the GABA system. For example, the postsynaptic responsiveness of GABA receptors in neurons of the thalamus (Zhang et al. 2010) and brain stem (Medrihan et al. 2008) of *Mecp2*-null mice was abnormal, showing directly that GABAergic activity is altered by MeCP2 dysfunction. Further, the selective ablation of Mecp2 from only GABAergic cells in mice is associated with spontaneous hyperexcitable discharges within the cortex and diminished quantal size of GABA release (Chao et al. 2010). These results, therefore, show that proper MeCP2 function in GABAergic cells is required for normal neuronal and brain homeostasis.

In the pre-*MECP2* era, most of the data on CSF and postmortem samples demon-strated abnormalities, primarily decreases in monoamine levels (Kaufmann et al. 2005). A few studies also reported glutamatergic abnormalities, including changes in density or levels of glutamate receptors. Specifically, reductions in AMPA glutamate receptors and increases in NMDA glutamate receptors with relative preservation of GABA receptors in the cerebral cortex were observed (Blue et al. 1999a,b). Interestingly, the glutamate receptor changes, in particular those involving NMDA receptors, were age-dependent with higher levels in younger individuals that decreased below normal levels in late childhood. Some of these abnormalities were also found in other brain regions, such as the basal ganglia, although data were more limited. Extension of this work to mouse models has confirmed the age-dependent change in NMDA receptors and further characterized the regional selectivity of these patterns (i.e. neocortex and striatum but not hippocampus or thalamus [Blue et al. 2011]), as well as delineated an evolution that mimics the regression period in

[³H]CGP binding to NMDA Receptors

A. Human   **B. Mouse**

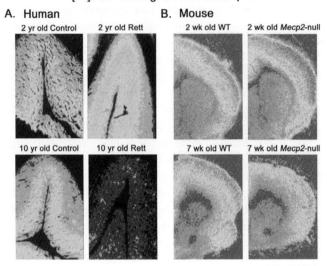

Fig. 13.4. NMDA receptor expression in frontal areas of cortex is altered in RTT and in Mecp2-deficient mice. (A) Receptor autoradiographic labeling of NMDA receptors showed that NMDA binding was enhanced in the prefrontal cortex of patients with RTT compared to controls in the first few years of life but diminished in patients older than 10 years of age. (B) Likewise, in 2-week-old *Mecp2*-null mice, NMDA receptor binding was increased in frontal areas of cortex, but diminished in very symptomatic 7-week-old *Mecp2*-null mice as compared to wild-type (WT) control mice. Adapted from Blue et al. (1999b), and from Blue et al. (2011). A colour version of this figure can be seen in the plate section between pages 166 and 167.

affected patients (Durand et al. 2012). Intriguingly, in the barrel field study mentioned in the preceding section, there was also an increase in extrasynaptic NMDA receptors in the Mecp2-deficient mice (Lo et al. 2016), which could be potentially activated by glutamate spillover from synapses or from release from glial cells. In fact, glutamate levels *per se* also appear to be elevated during early childhood in RTT, as revealed by CSF and magnetic resonance spectroscopy studies (Kaufmann et al. 2005; Horska et al. 2009). This combination of high levels of free glutamate with elevated density of NMDA receptors, particularly during early childhood, supports specific windows and pharmacological agents for intervention in RTT (Kaufmann et al. 2016).

Although little is known about RTT in adulthood, the prevalent parkinsonian features during this period (Humphreys and Barrowman 2016) suggest a prominent dopaminergic or noradrenergic deficit. Indeed, hypopigmentation of the substantia nigra is one of the first neuropathologic abnormalities reported in RTT, and monoamine alterations in CSF have been reported in affected individuals (Kaufmann et al. 2005, 2016). Moreover, selective preservation of MeCP2 function in cathecholaminergic neurons of MeCP2-deficient mice improves many aspects of their RTT-like behavior (Lang et al. 2013). However, little is known about specific dopaminergic abnormalities in early development in RTT or mouse models.

Finally, there are complex patterns of interrelated neurotransmitter abnormalities involving specific brain regions. The best examples are the changes in serotoninergic, glutamatergic, and GABAergic components involving brainstem nuclei that regulate breathing (Ramirez et al. 2013; Abdala et al. 2016).

ASTROCYTES AND MICROGLIA ARE ALSO INVOLVED IN RETT SYNDROME

A major and relatively recent shift in our thinking about RTT neurobiology comes from studies implicating astrocytes and microglia in the neurobiology of the disorder. Although neuronal expression of MeCP2 is relatively higher than in other cells in the CNS, the brain predominant MeCP2E1 isoform is also expressed in astrocytes (Zachariah et al. 2012) and these cells seem to be critical for neuronal and synaptic homeostasis in the context of MeCP2 deficit (Maezawa et al. 2009). Restoration of *Mecp2* expression in astrocytes (Lioy et al. 2011), and even oligodendrocytes (Nguyen et al. 2013), ameliorates RTT-like features in experimental models. Time-dependent increases in myo-inositol, detected by magnetic resonance spectroscopy in patients with RTT (Horska et al. 2009), suggest a process of progressive astrocytic activation in RTT that correlates with earlier postmortem human data (Kaufmann et al. 2005).

Although they are members of the monocyte/macrophage lineage and not true glial cells, microglia interact with astrocytes and there is evidence of an association between *Mecp2* deficiency and abnormal microglia function, most likely through altered phagocytosis or disruption in glutamate homeostasis (Derecki et al. 2012; O'Driscoll et al. 2013). However, additional work is needed in order to determine if microglial-targeted interventions may be useful for treating RTT.

AN EVER MORE COMPLICATED PICTURE

The increasing knowledge of MeCP2 function, indicating that the protein is not only involved in specific gene silencing via recruitment of histone deacetylases (i.e. enzymatic hypothesis) but also in other aspects of transcriptional regulation such as global epigenetic changes (Lombardi et al. 2015) and in cellular homeostatic processes (e.g. mitochondrial function, oxidative stress) (Valenti et al. 2014), raises the possibility that RTT is more than a predominantly neuronal differentiation and synaptic disorder. An example linking novel MeCP2 functions and CNS development is the recent report that the protein modulates cerebral neurogenesis via microRNA (miRNA) regulation (Mellios et al. 2017).

Neurobiological bases of Rett syndrome treatment: genetic and drug rescues

Considering that RTT is associated with a known genetic etiology and the relatively well-characterized neurobiologic mechanisms described above, it is possible to postulate disease-modifying treatments for the disorder. In fact, these interventions have begun to be implemented (Kaufmann et al. 2016). We hope that, eventually, these approaches will lead to prevention and cure of RTT. Meantime, as opposed to generic symptomatic treatments, therapies based on the disorder's neurobiology can result in substantial improvements of a wide range of clinical manifestations with milder side effects. Evidence supporting the latter trends is presented in Chapter 14 on Treatment. In this section,

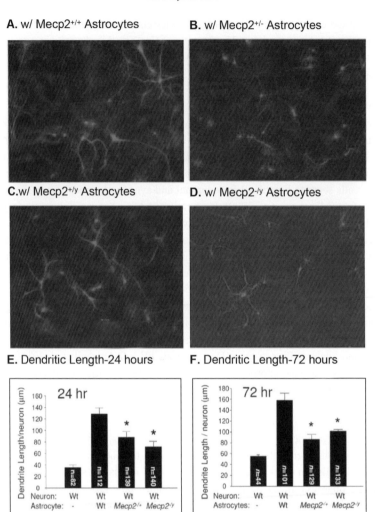

Fig. 13.5. Astrocytic abnormalities in Mecp2-deficient mice. Mecp2-deficient astrocytes support less dendritic growth from wild-type (WT) neurons. E18 WT hippocampal neurons were plated onto confluent monolayers of astrocytes from mice with different genotypes. The dendrites were allowed to grow for 24 h and 72 h. (A–D) Representative photomicrographs of 72 hours co-cultures; dendrites were visualized by immunostaining for the dendritic marker MAP2 (red). Neurolucida and Neuroexplorer software were used to determine the total dendritic length per neuron. Dendrites from the numbers of individual neurons (indicated in the bars) over four independent experiments were imaged and analyzed. Average dendritic length was significantly different among the four groups (p < 0.001) at 24 h (E) and 72 h (F). In post-hoc pairwise comparisons adjusted for multiple comparisons, the mean dendritic length induced by WT-origin astrocytes was significantly higher than by astrocytes from each of the mutant groups (*), but there were no significant differences between astrocytes from heterozygous (Mecp2−/+) and hemizygous (Mecp2−/y) mice. Adapted from Maezawa et al. (2009). Rett syndrome astrocytes are abnormal and spread MeCP2 deficiency through gap Junctions. *J Neurosci* 29: 5051–5061) with permission from *The Journal of Neuroscience*. A colour version of this figure can be seen in the plate section between pages 166 and 167.

we review the foundations of genetic and pharmacological strategies for improving RTT's phenotype.

GENETIC TREATMENTS

Although MeCP2 expression increases significantly within neurons as they transit between immature and mature phenotypes, it is also important to recognize that MeCP2 is expressed in the brain throughout embryonic development (Shahbazian et al. 2002; Jung et al. 2003). Thus, mutations of MeCP2 would be present in neurons of systems during critical periods when synaptic organization and structuring take place. It was initially unclear whether or not the deficits of MeCP2 would prevent proper critical period patterning from being achieved and, therefore, it was also not clear whether certain behavioral deficits were capable of being corrected in mature mice. Studies from Adrian Bird's group has shed insight into this issue, however, and their work suggests that the MeCP2-deficient brain retains the ability to have normal synaptic function restored even in fully adult animals. Using gene reactivation strategies in mice, Guy et al. (2007) showed that restoring Mecp2 function in the adult brain of highly symptomatic *Mecp2*-null mice not only dramatically improved their phenotypic behavior and extended their lifespan, but also corrected their existing synaptic plasticity deficit. The extension of these seminal observations to human trials has not materialized yet, since techniques for activating or introducing *MECP2* have not addressed key issues such as adequate gene dosing and delivery to target organs. Progress has also been reported in vector-mediated delivery of *MECP2* to the brain in Mecp2-deficient mice. Although initial studies employing AAV vectors had showed modest improvements in survival and had relied on intracranial delivery because of systemic toxicity, recently improved safety of intravenous administration (Gadalla et al. 2017) and enhanced survival after intracisternal delivery (Sinnett et al. 2017) have opened the possibility of gene therapy in individuals with RTT. Despite these encouraging data, more work is required to optimize gene therapy systems and delivery protocols.

More promising in the shorter term are approaches targeting *MECP2* nonsense mutations, present in roughly one-third of patients with RTT (Cuddapah et al. 2014). This class of mutation introduces a termination codon into the open reading frame of *MECP2*, and usually occurs at a site normally encoding an arginine amino acid (Nagel-Wolfrum et al. 2016). Although nonsense mutations terminate polypeptide elongation, they generally do not have the normal context of proper termination codons, and in the presence of drugs that alter the ribosomal machinery, certain nonsense mutations can be "read-through" such that a full-length polypeptide is generated. Drugs with the potential to facilitate such read-through include members of the classic aminoglycoside family, synthetic aminoglycoside derivatives, and newer drugs such at PTC124. While there have been no studies to date in Mecp2-deficient mice (only in fibroblasts derived from mice carrying nonsense *MECP2* mutations [Brendel et al. 2011]), work in cultured cells derived from RTT patients, or in cells expressing specific nonsense mutant forms of *MECP2*, have demonstrated that adding these drugs to the culture system allows for some full-length MeCP2 protein to be generated (Brendel et al. 2011; Vecsler et al. 2011). While these studies established "proof-of-principle", issues such as toxicity, blood–brain barrier permeability of specific drugs, whether the MeCP2 generated by the read-through retains function (only rarely is the mutated amino acid appropriately replaced during the read-through process), and whether the amount of full-length MeCP2 generated is at sufficient levels to provide benefit, represent issues that remain to be resolved.

PHARMACOLOGICAL INTERVENTIONS

Drug treatments for RTT could be divided into those targeting multiple neural substrates and pathways and those specific to a cell population or a neural pathway/neurotransmitter system. Among the former are growth factors that modulate synaptic activity that integrates multiple neurotransmitter systems, with brain derived neurotrophic factor (BDNF) being the prime example. Within some regions of the Mecp2-deficient brain, the expression of BDNF is significantly diminished (Li and Pozzo-Miller 2014). However, the effects of BDNF are not only dependent on its level of expression but also by neuronal activity that, under normal conditions strongly influences BDNF signaling, is altered in Mecp2-deficient neurons (Li and Pozzo-Miller 2014). In line with this concept, there are observations that enhancing BDNF levels via transgenesis procedures in Mecp2-deficient mice extends their lifespan, improves their ambulation, and restores the diminished spontaneous excitatory activity in somatosensory cortical neurons to normal levels (Li and Pozzo-Miller 2014). Further, over-expressing BDNF in cultured Mecp2-deficient hippocampal neurons corrected their diminished morphological complexity (Li and Pozzo-Miller 2014), and exogenously applied BDNF corrected synaptic deficiencies within relay neurons of the nucleus tractus solitarius in acute brain stem slices (Kline et al. 2010). The latter study is of particular interest, as the synaptic improvement resulting from BDNF exposure *diminished* the elevated spontaneous excitatory activity that arises within this brain region as a consequence of MeCP2 deficiency. Thus, investigations to date indicate that increasing BDNF levels provides benefit to both neural circuits that display diminished excitatory drive (such as in forebrain structures), and also to circuits that display enhanced excitatory activity (such as in nucleus tractus solitarius of the brain stem) as a consequence of Mecp2 deficiency.

While BDNF administration in order to correct the synaptic consequences of MeCP2 deficiency has a strong rationale, this is not feasible since BDNF does not cross the blood–brain barrier. Among several alternative strategies, for example glatiramer acetate for enhancing BDNF levels (Ben-Zeev et al. 2011), one of the most promising is the administration of another growth factor that modulates synaptic activity: insulin-like growth factor 1 (IGF-1) (Kaufmann et al. 2016). Initial studies have demonstrated that IGF-1 has comparable effects to those of BDNF in terms of correcting dendritic abnormalities in MeCP2-deficient neurons (Li et al. 2013). IGF-1 also stimulates intraneuronal communication and enhances synaptic maturation. Although levels of IGF-1 are not demonstrably diminished in MeCP2-deficient brain, there is evidence that insulin growth factor binding protein 3 (IGFBP3), a factor that binds IGF-1 and inhibits its signaling, is significantly induced in the Mecp2-deficient mouse brain and in the brains of RTT patients (Itoh et al. 2007). Using this rationale, Tropea and colleagues (2009) tested whether behavioral rescue and synaptic communication improvements could be achieved by long-term treatment of

Mecp2-deficient mice with IGF-1's active peptide. Their results showed that a 2-week treatment with the IGF-1 tripeptide significantly improved excitatory transmission in the Mecp2-deficient somatosensory cortex, increased the levels of postsynaptic density protein 95 (PSD95) in motor cortex, increased the density of dendritic spines along neurons of the motor cortex, and restored ocular dominance plasticity in the Mecp2-deficient visual cortex (Tropea et al. 2009). A more recent study administering full-length IGF-1 confirmed the overall findings of the IGF-1 tripeptide report (Kaufmann et al. 2016). These results show generalized synaptic deficits associated with Mecp2 deficiency in mice can be, at least partially, overcome by pharmacological intervention, and support the hypothesis that attenuated excitatory activity contributes to RTT pathophysiology.

SPECIFIC NEUROTRANSMITTER SYSTEMS

The multiple disruptions in neurotransmitter systems secondary to MeCP2 deficit reviewed above suggest that there is a wide range of pharmacological options for RTT. Nevertheless, the complexity of neurotransmitter balances, such as those involving glutamate and GABA, encourage a cautious approach since drug treatments may lead to worsening of symptoms or significant side effects. Unless targeting the period in which the specific neurotransmitter abnormality plays the greatest role, the effects of treatment may be limited in range and duration. Pharmacological studies of the centers underlying the respiratory phenotype in Mecp2-deficient mice illustrate the possibilities and challenges of targeting specific neurotransmitter systems in RTT (Ramirez et al. 2013; Abdala et al. 2016). Therefore, this section will focus on this body of literature as a model for preclinical testing of drug interventions.

There is a clear link between excitatory activity and pulsatile BDNF expression and signaling. The diminished level of spontaneous forebrain excitatory activity observed in Mecp2-deficient mice, together with the impaired activity-dependent BDNF responsiveness of MeCP2-deficient neurons in culture, suggests stimulating excitatory activity could facilitate enhanced BDNF responsiveness in MeCP2-deficient systems. Ampakines are a type of drug that enhances the activity of glutamatergic AMPA receptors. Ogier et al.'s (2007) administration of the ampakine CX546 for 3 days to Mecp2-deficient mice resulted in elevated levels of BDNF in nodose cranial sensory ganglia, and significantly improved the respiratory deficit of Mecp2-deficient mice.

As discussed above, however, the deficits in synaptic responsiveness in the MeCP2-deficient brain are not equivalent between regions. While attenuated excitatory drive has been seen at forebrain synapses, attenuated inhibitory activity and hyperexcitability has been observed in other MeCP2-deficient brain regions. In addition to genetic reactivation and reintroduction investigations, recent pharmacological studies indicate that enhancing GABA receptor conductance with benzodiazepine treatment in Mecp2-deficient mice rescues the hyperexcitability of breathing center networks, and improves their respiratory deficit (Ramirez et al. 2013). Emphasizing the complexity of the synaptic abnormalities associated with Mecp2 deficit, Banerjee and colleagues (2016) have recently reported that visually-driven excitatory and inhibitory conductances are both reduced in cortical pyramidal neurons.

Several other neurotransmitter receptors influence respiratory and other phenotypes in Mecp2-deficient brains: NMDA receptor antagonists decrease the severity of apneas, as well as of other phenotypes (Kaufmann et al. 2016); and monoaminergic modulators such as serotonin 1a agonists, alone (Abdala et al. 2014) or in combination with GABA agonists (Abdala et al. 2016), also have a powerful corrective effect on respiratory abnormalities in preclinical models. The postulated dopaminergic abnormalities underlying the parkinsonian features in late stages of RTT are also an area that deserves investigation in mouse and other experimental models. Recently, abnormalities in neuronal cation chloride cotransporters NKCC1 and KCC2, specifically reduced levels of KCC2 and KCC2/NKCC1 (Duarte et al. 2013), represent a new potential therapeutic target in RTT (Tang et al. 2016).

In addition to modulators of neuronal function, drugs that regulate astrocytic or microglial function have the potential to ameliorate brain abnormalities secondary to MeCP2 deficit. Treatment with NF-κβ inhibitors (O'Driscoll et al. 2013) or the mitochondrial peptide antioxidant Szeto-Schiller 31 (Kaufmann et al. 2016), which target glutaminase levels and the effects of glutamine transporter SNAT1 over-activity, respectively, lead to decreased glutamate release from microglia and the possibility of developing glia-based therapies for RTT.

Finally, new knowledge on MeCP2's role in homeostasis and metabolism, including mitochondrial function and oxidative stress, expands the target options for RTT. Additional information on neurobiologically based treatments can be found in recent reviews by Katz et al. (2016) and Kaufmann et al. (2016).

Conclusion

The explosion of neurobiology knowledge in RTT, in particular after the identification of *MECP2* mutations as the main genetic defect, has led to a better understanding of the symptoms and the intricate evolution of the disorder. It has also opened the possibility of treatments specific to the CNS abnormalities secondary to MeCP2 deficiency throughout life. However, our current perspective of the neurobiology of RTT highlights the complexity of the cellular and circuit abnormalities of the disorder and the fact that achieving an adequate functional balance would be difficult. Delivering the right treatment at the right place and the right time is a challenge. This humbling realization suggests that, while aiming for cure during the next 50 years, our realistic goal should be neurobiologically based amelioration of symptoms in the near future.

REFERENCES

Abdala AP, Bissonnette JM, Newman-Tancredi A (2014) Pinpointing brainstem mechanisms responsible for autonomic dysfunction in Rett syndrome: therapeutic perspectives for 5-HT1A agonists. *Front Physiol* 5: 205.

Abdala AP, Toward MA, Dutschmann M, Bissonnette JM, Paton JF (2016) Deficiency of GABAergic synaptic inhibition in the Kolliker-Fuse area underlies respiratory dysrhythmia in a mouse model of Rett syndrome. *J Physiol* 594(1): 223–237.

Armstrong DD (2005) Neuropathology of Rett syndrome. *J Child Neurol* 20(9): 747–753.

Banerjee A, Rikhye RV, Breton-Provencher V, Tang X, Li C, Li K et al. (2016) Jointly reduced inhibition and excitation underlies circuit-wide changes in cortical processing in Rett syndrome. *Proc Natl Acad Sci USA* 113(46): E7287–E7296.

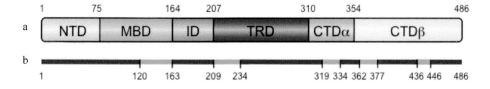

a
| NTD | MBD | ID | TRD | CTDα | CTDβ |

1   75   164   207   310   354   486

b

1   120   163   209 234   319 334 362 377   436 446   486

c   e1 MAAAAAAAPSGGGGGGGEEERL...
     e2   MVAGMLGLR...

Fig. 12.1. (p 143) (a) Domain layout of the MeCP2 protein. (b) Regions of disorder (red) and order (green) predicted by Predictor of Naturally Disordered Regions (PONDR). (c) Amino acid sequences of the aminotermini of the MeCP1 e1 and e2 splice variants. NTD, N-terminal domain; MBD, methyl-CpG binding domain; TRD, transcriptional repression domain; CTDα and CTDβ, C-terminal domains.

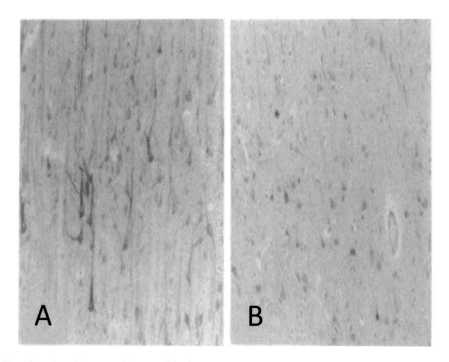

Fig. 13.1. (p 156) Neuronal abnormalities in RTT. Neuronal somas are typically smaller and associated with less complex dendritic trees (B), when compared to age/sex-matched controls (A). Immunostaining for microtubule-associated protein 2 (MAP-2), a neuronal marker, in motor cortex. Adapted from Kaufmann et al. (1998).

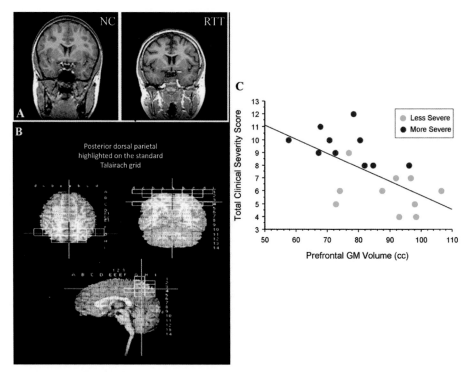

Fig. 13.2. (p 156) Volumetric brain reductions in RTT. (A) Marked global reductions in brain volume are identified on MRI surveys, when comparing typically developed individuals (NC, normal controls) with affected ones (RTT). (B) MRI quantitative analyses revealed a selective reduction in posterior parietal grey matter volumes, particularly affecting the left hemisphere. The involved region is delineated by the superimposed Talairach 3-dimensional coordinate grid, displayed in the 3 axes. (C) MRI volumetric analyses also revealed that greater overall clinical severity is associated with greater reduction in grey matter volumes affecting the prefrontal cortex, as depicted in the regression plot. Adapted from Kaufmann et al. (1998), and from Carter et al. (2008).

[³H]CGP binding to NMDA Receptors

A. Human

B. Mouse

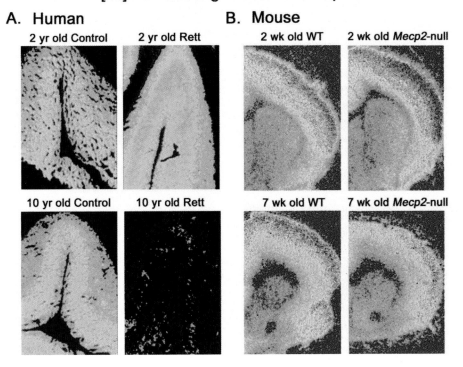

Fig. 13.4. (p 160) NMDA receptor expression in frontal areas of cortex is altered in RTT and in Mecp2-deficient mice. (A) Receptor autoradiographic labeling of NMDA receptors showed that NMDA binding was enhanced in the prefrontal cortex of patients with RTT compared to controls in the first few years of life but diminished in patients older than 10 years of age. (B) Likewise, in 2-week-old *Mecp2*-null mice, NMDA receptor binding was increased in frontal areas of cortex, but diminished in very symptomatic 7-week-old *Mecp2*-null mice as compared to wild-type (WT) control mice. Adapted from Blue et al. (1999b), and from Blue et al. (2011).

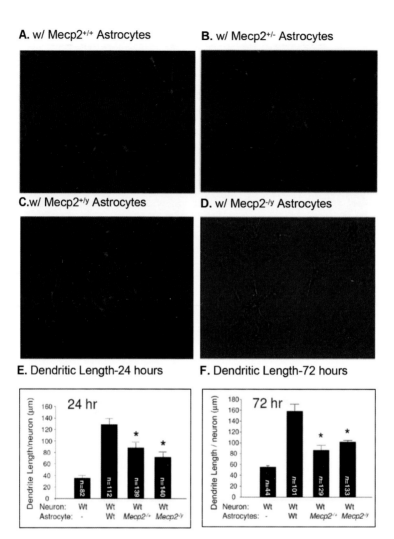

A. w/ Mecp2$^{+/+}$ Astrocytes

B. w/ Mecp2$^{+/-}$ Astrocytes

C. w/ Mecp2$^{+/y}$ Astrocytes

D. w/ Mecp2$^{-/y}$ Astrocytes

E. Dendritic Length-24 hours

F. Dendritic Length-72 hours

Fig. 13.5. (p 162) Astrocytic abnormalities in Mecp2-deficient mice. Mecp2-deficient astrocytes support less dendritic growth from wild-type (WT) neurons. E18 WT hippocampal neurons were plated onto confluent monolayers of astrocytes from mice with different genotypes. The dendrites were allowed to grow for 24 h and 72 h. (A–D) Representative photomicrographs of 72 hours co-cultures; dendrites were visualized by immunostaining for the dendritic marker MAP2 (red). Neurolucida and Neuroexplorer software were used to determine the total dendritic length per neuron. Dendrites from the numbers of individual neurons (indicated in the bars) over four independent experiments were imaged and analyzed. Average dendritic length was significantly different among the four groups (p < 0.001) at 24 h (E) and 72 h (F). In post-hoc pairwise comparisons adjusted for multiple comparisons, the mean dendritic length induced by WT-origin astrocytes was significantly higher than by astrocytes from each of the mutant groups (*), but there were no significant differences between astrocytes from heterozygous (Mecp2−/+) and hemizygous (Mecp2−/y) mice. Adapted from Maezawa et al. (2009). Rett syndrome astrocytes are abnormal and spread MeCP2 deficiency through gap Junctions. *J Neurosci* 29: 5051–5061) with permission from *The Journal of Neuroscience.*

Belichenko PV, Wright EE, Belichenko NP, Masliah E, Li HH, Mobley WC, Francke U (2009) Widespread changes in dendritic and axonal morphology in Mecp2-mutant mouse models of Rett syndrome: evidence for disruption of neuronal networks. *J Comp Neurol* 514(3): 240–258.

Ben-Zeev B, Aharoni R, Nissenkorn A, Arnon R (2011) Glatiramer acetate (GA, Copolymer-1) an hypothetical treatment option for Rett syndrome. *Med Hypotheses* 76(2): 190–193.

Blue ME, Kaufmann WE, Bressler J, Eyring C, O'Driscoll C, Naidu S, Johnston MV (2011) Temporal and regional alterations in NMDA receptor expression in *Mecp2*-null mice. *Anat Rec (Hoboken)* 294(10): 1624–1634.

Blue ME, Naidu S, Johnston MV (1999a) Altered development of glutamate and GABA receptors in the basal ganglia of girls with Rett syndrome. *Exp Neurol* 156(2): 345–352.

Blue ME, Naidu S, Johnston MV (1999b) Development of amino acid receptors in frontal cortex from girls with Rett syndrome. *Ann Neurol* 45(4): 541–545.

Brendel C, Belakhov V, Werner H, Wegener E, Gartner J, Nudelman I et al. (2011) Readthrough of nonsense mutations in Rett syndrome: evaluation of novel aminoglycosides and generation of a new mouse model. *J Mol Med (Berl)* 89(4): 389–398.

Calfa G, Li W, Rutherford JM, Pozzo-Miller L (2015) Excitation/inhibition imbalance and impaired synaptic inhibition in hippocampal area CA3 of Mecp2 knockout mice. *Hippocampus* 25(2): 159–168.

Carter JC, Lanham DC, Pham D, Bibat G, Naidu S, Kaufmann WE (2008) Selective cerebral volume reduction in Rett syndrome: a multiple-approach MR imaging study. *AJNR Am J Neuroradiol* 29(3): 436–441.

Chao HT, Chen H, Samaco RC, Xue M, Chahrour M, Yoo J et al. (2010) Dysfunction in GABA signalling mediates autism-like stereotypies and Rett syndrome phenotypes. *Nature* 468(7321): 263–269.

Chapleau CA, Calfa GD, Lane MC, Albertson AJ, Larimore JL, Kudo S et al. (2009) Dendritic spine pathologies in hippocampal pyramidal neurons from Rett syndrome brain and after expression of Rett-associated *MECP2* mutations. *Neurobiol Dis* 35(2): 219–233.

Cuddapah VA, Pillai RB, Shekar KV, Lane JB, Motil KJ, Skinner SA et al. (2014) Methyl-CpG-binding protein 2 (*MECP2*) mutation type is associated with disease severity in Rett syndrome. *J Med Genet* 51(3): 152–158.

Dani VS, Chang Q, Maffei A, Turrigiano GG, Jaenisch R, Nelson SB (2005) Reduced cortical activity due to a shift in the balance between excitation and inhibition in a mouse model of Rett syndrome. *Proc Natl Acad Sci USA* 102(35): 12560–12565.

D'Cruz JA, Wu C, Zahid T, El-Hayek Y, Zhang L, Eubanks JH (2010) Alterations of cortical and hippocampal EEG activity in MeCP2-deficient mice. *Neurobiol Dis* 38(1): 8–16.

Deng JV, Rodriguiz RM, Hutchinson AN, Kim IH, Wetsel WC, West AE (2010) MeCP2 in the nucleus accumbens contributes to neural and behavioral responses to psychostimulants. *Nat Neurosci* 13(9): 1128–1136.

Derecki NC, Cronk JC, Lu Z, Xu E, Abbott SB, Guyenet PG, Kipnis J (2012) Wild-type microglia arrest pathology in a mouse model of Rett syndrome. *Nature* 484(7392): 105–109.

Duarte ST, Armstrong J, Roche A, Ortez C, Perez A, del Mar O'Callaghan M (2013) Abnormal expression of cerebrospinal fluid cation chloride cotransporters in patients with Rett syndrome. *PLoS One* 8(7): e68851.

Durand S, Patrizi A, Quast KB, Hachigian L, Pavlyuk R, Saxena A et al. (2012) NMDA receptor regulation prevents regression of visual cortical function in the absence of Mecp2. *Neuron* 76(6): 1078–1090.

Feldman D, Banerjee A, Sur M (2016) Developmental dynamics of Rett syndrome. *Neural Plast* 2016: 6154080.

Gadalla KKE, Vudhironarit T, Hector RD, Sinnett S, Bahey NG, Bailey MES (2017) Development of a novel AAV gene therapy cassette with improved safety features and efficacy in a mouse model of Rett syndrome. *Mol Ther Methods Clin Dev* 5: 180–190.

Glaze DG (2005) Neurophysiology of Rett syndrome. *J Child Neurol* 20(9): 740–746.

Guy J, Gan J, Selfridge J, Cobb S, Bird A (2007) Reversal of neurological defects in a mouse model of Rett syndrome. *Science* 315(5815): 1143–1147.

Hagberg B, Aicardi J, Dias K, Ramos O (1983) A progressive syndrome of autism, dementia, ataxia, and loss of purposeful hand use in girls: Rett's syndrome: report of 35 cases. *Ann Neurol* 14(4): 471–479.

Horska A, Farage L, Bibat G, Nagae LM, Kaufmann WE, Barker PB, Naidu S (2009) Brain metabolism in Rett syndrome: age, clinical, and genotype correlations. *Ann Neurol* 65(1): 90–97,

Humphreys P, Barrowman N (2016) The incidence and evolution of parkinsonian rigidity in Rett syndrome: a pilot study. *Can J Neurol Sci* 43(4): 567–573.

Itoh M, Ide S, Takashima S, Kudo S, Nomura Y, Segawa M et al. (2007) Methyl CpG-binding protein 2 (a mutation of which causes Rett syndrome) directly regulates insulin-like growth factor binding protein 3 in mouse and human brains. *J Neuropathol Exp Neurol* 66(2): 117–123.

Johnston MV, Blue ME, Naidu S (2005) Rett syndrome and neuronal development. *J Child Neurol* 20(9): 759–763.

Jung BP, Jugloff DG, Zhang G, Logan R, Brown S, Eubanks JH (2003) The expression of methyl CpG binding factor MeCP2 correlates with cellular differentiation in the developing rat brain and in cultured cells. *J Neurobiol* 55(1): 86–96.

Katz DM, Bird A, Coenraads M, Gray SJ, Menon DU, Philpot BD, Tarquinio DC (2016) Rett syndrome: crossing the threshold to clinical translation. *Trends Neurosci* 39(2): 100–113.

Kaufmann WE, Johnston MV, Blue ME (2005) MeCP2 expression and function during brain development: implications for Rett syndrome's pathogenesis and clinical evolution. *Brain Dev* 27 *Suppl* 1, S77–S87.

Kaufmann WE, Pearlson GD, Naidu S (1998) The neuroanatomy of Rett syndrome: neuropathological and neuroimaging studies. *Rivista Medica* 4: 189–202.

Kaufmann WE, Stallworth JL, Everman DB, Skinner SA (2016) Neurobiologically-based treatments in Rett syndrome: opportunities and challenges. *Expert Opin Orphan Drugs* 4(10): 1043–1055.

Kline DD, Ogier M, Kunze DL, Katz DM (2010) Exogenous brain-derived neurotrophic factor rescues synaptic dysfunction in *Mecp2*-null mice. *J Neurosci* 30(15): 5303–5310.

Krishnan K, Wang BS, Lu J, Wang L, Maffei A, Cang J, Huang ZJ (2015) MeCP2 regulates the timing of critical period plasticity that shapes functional connectivity in primary visual cortex. *Proc Natl Acad Sci USA* 112(34): E4782–E4791.

Lang M, Wither RG, Brotchie JM, Wu C, Zhang L, Eubanks JH (2013) Selective preservation of MeCP2 in catecholaminergic cells is sufficient to improve the behavioral phenotype of male and female Mecp2-deficient mice. *Hum Mol Genet* 22(2): 358–371.

Li W, Pozzo-Miller L (2014) BDNF deregulation in Rett syndrome. *Neuropharmacology* 76 *Pt C*, 737–746.

Li Y, Wang H, Muffat J, Cheng AW, Orlando DA, Lovén J et al. (2013) Global transcriptional and translational repression in human-embryonic-stem-cell-derived Rett syndrome neurons. *Cell Stem Cell* 13(4): 446–58.

Lioy DT, Garg SK, Monaghan CE, Raber J, Foust KD, Kaspar BK et al. (2011) A role for glia in the progression of Rett's syndrome. *Nature* 475(7357): 497–500.

Lo FS, Blue ME, Erzurumlu RS (2016) Enhancement of postsynaptic GABAA and extrasynaptic NMDA receptor-mediated responses in the barrel cortex of *Mecp2*-null mice. *J Neurophysiol* 115(3): 1298–1306.

Lonetti G, Angelucci A, Morando L, Boggio EM, Giustetto M, Pizzorusso T (2010) Early environmental enrichment moderates the behavioral and synaptic phenotype of MeCP2 null mice. *Biol Psychiatry* 67(7): 657–665.

Maezawa I, Swanberg S, Harvey D, LaSalle JM, Jin LW (2009) Rett syndrome astrocytes are abnormal and spread MeCP2 deficiency through gap junctions. *J Neurosci* 29(16): 5051–5061.

Medrihan L, Tantalaki E, Aramuni G, Sargsyan V, Dudanova I, Missler M, Zhang W (2008) Early defects of GABAergic synapses in the brain stem of a MeCP2 mouse model of Rett syndrome. *J Neurophysiol* 99(1): 112–121.

Mellios N, Feldman DA, Sheridan SD, Ip JPK, Kwok S, Amoah SK et al. (2017) MeCP2-regulated miRNAs control early human neurogenesis through differential effects on ERK and AKT signaling. *Mol Psychiatry* doi: 10.1038/mp.2017.86.

Mironov SL, Skorova E, Hartelt N, Mironova LA, Hasan MT, Kugler S (2009) Remodelling of the respiratory network in a mouse model of Rett syndrome depends on brain-derived neurotrophic factor regulated slow calcium buffering. *J Physiol* 587(Pt 11): 2473–2485.

Moretti P, Levenson JM, Battaglia F, Atkinson R, Teague R, Antalffy B et al. (2006) Learning and memory and synaptic plasticity are impaired in a mouse model of Rett syndrome. *J Neurosci* 26(1): 319–327.

Nagel-Wolfrum K, Moller F, Penner I, Baasov T, Wolfrum U (2016) Targeting nonsense mutations in diseases with Translational Read-Through-Inducing Drugs (TRIDs). *BioDrugs* 30(2): 49–74.

Nelson ED, Kavalali ET, Monteggia LM (2006) MeCP2-dependent transcriptional repression regulates excitatory neurotransmission. *Curr Biol* 16(7): 710–716.

Nguyen MV, Felice CA, Du F, Covey MV, Robinson JK, Mandel G, Ballas N (2013) Oligodendrocyte lineage cells contribute unique features to Rett syndrome neuropathology. *J Neurosci* 33(48): 18764–18774.

O'Driscoll CM, Kaufmann WE, Bressler JP (2013) MeCP2 deficiency enhances glutamate release through NF-kappaβ signaling in myeloid derived cells. *J Neuroimmunol* 265(1–2): 61–67.

Ogier M, Wang H, Hong E, Wang Q, Greenberg ME, Katz DM (2007) Brain-derived neurotrophic factor expression and respiratory function improve after ampakine treatment in a mouse model of Rett syndrome. *J Neurosci* 27(40): 10912–10917.

Panayotis N, Pratte M, Borges-Correia A, Ghata A, Villard L, Roux JC (2011) Morphological and functional alterations in the substantia nigra pars compacta of the Mecp2-null mouse. *Neurobiol Dis* 41(2): 385–397.

Ramirez JM, Ward CS, Neul JL (2013) Breathing challenges in Rett syndrome: lessons learned from humans and animal models. *Respir Physiol Neurobiol* 189(2): 280–287.

Ronnett GV, Leopold D, Cai X, Hoffbuhr KC, Moses L, Hoffman EP, Naidu S (2003) Olfactory biopsies demonstrate a defect in neuronal development in Rett's syndrome. *Ann Neurol* 54(2): 206–218.

Shahbazian MD, Antalffy B, Armstrong DL, Zoghbi HY (2002) Insight into Rett syndrome: MeCP2 levels display tissue- and cell-specific differences and correlate with neuronal maturation. *Hum Mol Genet* 11(2): 115–124.

Sinnett SE, Hector RD, Gadalla KKE, Heindel C, Chen D, Zaric V et al. (2017) Improved *MECP2* Gene Therapy Extends the Survival of *MeCP2*-Null Mice without Apparent Toxicity after Intracisternal Delivery. *Mol Ther Methods Clin Dev* 5: 106–115.

Skene PJ, Illingworth RS, Webb S, Kerr AR, James KD, Turner DJ et al. (2010) Neuronal MeCP2 is expressed at near histone-octamer levels and globally alters the chromatin state. *Mol Cell* 37(4): 457–468.

Smrt RD, Eaves-Egenes J, Barkho BZ, Santistevan NJ, Zhao C, Aimone JB et al. (2007) Mecp2 deficiency leads to delayed maturation and altered gene expression in hippocampal neurons. *Neurobiol Dis* 27(1): 77–89.

Taneja P, Ogier M, Brooks-Harris G, Schmid DA, Katz DM, Nelson SB (2009) Pathophysiology of locus ceruleus neurons in a mouse model of Rett syndrome. *J Neurosci* 29(39): 12187–12195.

Tang X, Kim J, Zhou L, Wengert E, Zhang L, Wu Z et al. (2016) KCC2 rescues functional deficits in human neurons derived from patients with Rett syndrome. *Proc Natl Acad Sci USA* 113(3): 751–756.

Tropea D, Giacometti E, Wilson NR, Beard C, McCurry C, Fu DD et al. (2009) Partial reversal of Rett Syndrome-like symptoms in MeCP2 mutant mice. *Proc Natl Acad Sci USA* 106(6): 2029–2034.

Valenti D, de Bari L, De Filippis B, Henrion-Caude A, Vacca RA (2014) Mitochondrial dysfunction as a central actor in intellectual disability-related diseases: an overview of Down syndrome, autism, Fragile X and Rett syndrome. *Neurosci Biobehav Rev* 46(Pt 2) 202–217.

Vecsler M, Ben Zeev B, Nudelman I, Anikster Y, Simon AJ, Amariglio N et al. (2011) Ex vivo treatment with a novel synthetic aminoglycoside NB54 in primary fibroblasts from Rett syndrome patients suppresses *MECP2* nonsense mutations. *PLoS One* 6(6): e20733.

Weng SM, McLeod F, Bailey ME, Cobb SR (2011) Synaptic plasticity deficits in an experimental model of rett syndrome: long-term potentiation saturation and its pharmacological reversal. *Neuroscience* 180: 314–321.

Zachariah RM, Olson CO, Ezeonwuka C, Rastegar M (2012) Novel MeCP2 isoform-specific antibody reveals the endogenous MeCP2E1 expression in murine brain, primary neurons and astrocytes. *PLoS One* 7(11): e49763.

Zhang L, He J, Jugloff DG, Eubanks JH (2008) The MeCP2-null mouse hippocampus displays altered basal inhibitory rhythms and is prone to hyperexcitability. *Hippocampus* 18(3): 294–309.

Zhang X, Cui N, Wu Z, Su J, Tadepalli JS, Sekizar S, Jiang C (2010) Intrinsic membrane properties of locus coeruleus neurons in *Mecp2*-null mice. *Am J Physiol Cell Physiol* 298(3): C635–C646.

14
TREATMENTS FOR RETT SYNDROME: PROSPECTS FOR TARGETED THERAPIES

Wendy A Gold, SakkuBai Naidu, and John Christodoulou

Introduction

Rett syndrome (RTT, OMIM #312750) is an X-linked neurodevelopmental disorder that predominantly affects females. The RTT clinical phenotype is very broad, encompassing classical, as well as a number of phenotypically heterogeneous variants or atypical forms of the disorder, with clinical features overlapping into the autism spectrum of disorders.

Since the first reports of RTT by the Austrian pediatrician, Andreas Rett in 1966, intensive research efforts have been undertaken to unravel the enigmas associated with the disorder, with a primary objective being to develop targeted therapies. Subsequent to the initial suggestions that RTT may be a mitochondrial disorder, mutations in the methyl-CpG-binding protein 2 (*MECP2*) gene were identified in patients with RTT in 1999, which opened the scope of research into the function and targets of MeCP2. The search for a cure however, has been impeded by the multiple mutations in *MECP2*, as well as the imperfect genotype-phenotype associations, and most importantly, the pleiotropic functions of MeCP2 itself. Although we have gained many insights into the disorder and the functions of associated genes in the half century since the first clinical diagnosis of RTT, we have not, as yet, been able to find therapeutic agents that have the capacity to cure or even substantially ameliorate the disease in humans. Recent trials using mouse models, however, show that it is possible to reverse aspects of the RTT phenotype, as well as therapies aimed at downstream targets of MeCP2, which has greatly increased optimism that human therapeutic trials now being implemented raise the prospect that RTT could be a curable childhood neurological disorder.

Clinical trials

This information corresponds to the status of clinical trials in RTT as of August 2016.

A number of clinical trials for RTT have been conducted over the years, targeting the consequences of MeCP2 deficiency on neuronal dysfunction and behavior of patients with RTT. To date, however, no therapeutic strategy has been translated into the clinic. This is not necessarily due to the lack of efficacy of these treatments, but rather to the confounding and complex nature of the disorder. RTT is a rare clinically and genetically heterogeneous disorder, in which patients display a broad range of phenotypic symptoms, each manifesting at varying time points throughout development. Thus, small sample groups and appropriate primary outcome measure selection, along with funding resources, have in the past greatly impinged on the capacity to execute clinical trials successfully.

PREVIOUS CLINICAL TRIALS

To date, a number of completed clinical trials testing potentially therapeutic agents have been reported for RTT (Table 14.1). These include the ketogenic diet, bromocriptine, the opiate antagonist naltrexone, L-carnitine dietary supplementation, cerebrolysin, folate-betaine supplementation, folic acid, the dietary supplement creatine, ω-3 polyunsaturated fatty acids (PUFAs), IGF-1, NNZ-2566, the novel redox therapeutic EPI-743 and dextromethorphan. The outcomes of these studies were variable, with some showing no beneficial effects and some at best modest effects; however, potentially encouragingly, most studies showed improvements in at least one outcome measure. It is important to note that these trials were not necessarily unsuccessful and that factors such as study design, lack of patient phenotype homogeneity, and end-point selection were confounding factors in some of these studies. It is pleasing to note that follow-up studies to re-examine some of these compounds and their derivatives are still under investigation.

CURRENT CLINICAL TRIALS

Currently, a number of promising clinical trials are being conducted in patients with RTT, including both observational and interventional designs, with the latter involving drug and dietary supplementation. Table 14.2 lists the current and recently completed interventional studies being conducted in patients with RTT, which include insulin-like growth factor (IGF-1), sarizotan, trofinetide, glatiramer acetate, dextromethorphan, desipramine, fingolimond, triheptanoin, ketamine and lovastatin.

The full-length form of insulin-like growth factor, recombinant human IGF-1 (hrIGF-1, Mecasermin or INCRELEX), has been tested in two clinical trials. The first trial consisted of a phase 1 trial to test the safety and efficacy of IGF-1 in 12 patients. The results from this trial have been published, and showed not only safety and tolerability, but promising improvements in a number of neurobehavioral parameters, specifically measures of anxiety and depression and a reduction in the incidence of apnea (Khwaja et al. 2014). This trial has led to a second phase 2 double-blind, placebo-controlled, crossover clinical trial and has influenced the design and goals of the current trofinetide and sarizotan trials.

Sarizotan, a selective serotonin (5-HT1A) receptor agonist and domapine 2 (D2) receptor antagonist, is currently being used in a randomized, double-blind, placebo-controlled study to evaluate its capacity to reduce respiratory deficits such as apnea in patients with RTT. The trial is not yet at the recruiting phase. Trofinetide (previously known as NZ-2566), a synthetic analog derived from the tri-peptide of IGF-1, has previously been tested in a phase 2 randomized, double-blind, placebo-controlled, parallel-group, dose-escalation study in patients between the ages of 16 and 45 years old and is in the process of being set up for another phase 2 trial for pediatric (5–15 year old) patients. Both trials have the same primary outcomes measures to determine incidence of adverse events.

TABLE 14.1

Completed interventional clinical trials in RTT

Name	Date	Target	Outcome	Status	Intervention	Phase
Ketogenic diet	1986	Carbohydrate metabolism	Improvement in seizures in some patients with other minor changes	Completed	Dietary supplementation of medium chain triglyceride oil	NA
Bromocriptine	1990	Dopamine receptor	Improvements in communication and relaxation and decreased hand movements	Completed	Treatment with drug	NA
Naltrexone	1994	B-endorphins	Some beneficial effects on respiratory parameters	Completed	Treatment with drug	NA
L-Carnitine	1999	Mitochondrial fatty acid metabolism and dysfunction	Modest improvement in respiratory features and Patient Well-being Index	Completed	Oral dose of L-carnitine	NA
Cerebrolysin	2001	Synaptic maturation	Improvements in motor function and behavior, reduced seizure frequency, improved EEG	Completed	Daily intramuscular doses	NA
Folate-betaine	2009	DNA methylation	No improvements were observed in motor function, breathing, and growth parameters. Subjective improvement based on a parent questionnaire was observed in patients <5 y	Completed	Oral dose of betaine and folate	NA
Creatine monohydrate (CMH)	2010	Global DNA methylation	Statistical increase in global DNA methylation. Improvement in total and sub-scores of Rett Syndrome Motor-Behavior Assessment Scale but without statistical significance	Completed	Dietary supplementation of creatine monohydrate	NA

Continued

TABLE 14.1
Continued

Name	Date	Target	Outcome	Status	Intervention	Phase
ω-3 PUFAs		Oxidative stress	Moderately reduces clinical severity, significantly reduces oxidative stress biomarker levels, and improved biventricular myocardial systolic function	Completed	Dietary supplementation of ω-3 PUFAs	NA
rhIGF1/Mecasermin [rDNA] injection]/ INCRELEX	2011	Synaptic maturation	Confirmed safety and tolerability. Observed improvements in mood and anxiety scores and reduced apnea incidence	Completed	Treatment with drug	1
NNZ-2566	2012	General	No study results posted	Completed	Treatment with drug vs placebo	2
EPI-743	2013	Oxidative stress	No study results posted	Completed	Treatment with drug vs placebo	NA
Dextromethorphan and donepezil hydrochloride	2003	Glutamate NMDA receptors	Not available	Recruitment status is unknown	Treatment with drug	2
Dextromethorphan with topiramate and donepezil	2000	Glutamate NMDA receptors	No study results posted	Completed	Treatment with drug	NA
Dextromethorphan	2008	Glutamate NMDA receptors	Terminated with results	Terminated	Treatment with drug	2

NA, not applicable; ω-3 PUFAs, ω-3 polyunsaturated fatty acids; NMDA, N-methyl-D-aspartate.

TABLE 14.2
Recently completed and current interventional clinical trials in RTT

Name	Date	Target	Outcome	Status	Intervention	Phase
rhIGF1/ Mecasermin/ INCRELEX	2013	Synaptic maturation	In progress	Recruiting	Treatment with drug vs placebo	2
Glatiramer acetate	2013	BDNF	In progress	Recruiting (phase 1) Not recruiting (phase 2)	Open label treatment	1 and 2
Dextromethorphan	2012	Glutamate NMDA receptors	In progress	Recruiting	Treatment with drug vs placebo	2
Desipramine	2009	Respiratory disturbances	In progress	Recruiting	Treatment with high and low doses of drug	2
Fingolimond (FTY720)	2013	BNDF	In progress	Recruiting	Treatment with drug vs placebo	1 and 2
Ketamine	2015	General	In progress	Active, not recruiting	Treatment with drug vs placebo	1
Lovastatin	2015	Cholesterol	In progress	Recruiting	Treatment with drug	2
Trofinetide (NZ-2566)	2016	General	In progress	Recruiting	Treatment with drug vs placebo	2
Sarizotan	2016	Serotonin and dopamine receptors	In progress	Not yet open for participant recruitment	Treatment with drug vs placebo	2 and 3
Triheptanoin	2016	Mitochondrial function	In progress	Recruiting	Treatment with drug	2

BDNF, brain derived neurotrophic factor; NMDA, N-methyl-D-aspartate.

Two clinical trials of glatiramer acetate are being conducted, one in Israel (led by principle investigator Professor Bruria Ben Zeev, at the Sheba Medical Center) and one in the USA (led by principle investigator Aleksandra Djukic) and conducted at the Montefiore Medical Center, New York, United States). Both are open label with a number of outcome measures including EEG, seizure frequency, respiratory regulation, and quality of life measures. The recruitment status of the study in Israel is unknown; however, the US study is still active and ongoing, and have published some results. The authors reported on the efficacy of glatiramer acetate in improving gait velocity in female patients 10 years or older. They also highlighted that although the trial provides valuable preliminary information a larger scale, controlled trial is much needed (Djukic et al. 2016) in RTT.

The efficacy of the N-methyl-D-aspartate (NMDA) receptor antagonist dextromethorphan is currently being assessed in a randomized, double-blind placebo-controlled study that is still recruiting patients. This study, led by the principal investigator Dr. Sakkubai Naidu and conducted at the Pediatric Clinical Research Unit (PCRU) of the Johns Hopkins Hospital/Kennedy Krieger Institute, has the highest number of patients in any RTT study ($n = 60$) with primary outcome measures assessing the cognitive status of patients using the neuropsychologist Mullen Scales of Early Learning test. Dextromethorphan has also being tested in other studies to evaluate the independent effects of the drugs dextromethorphan, topiramate, and donepezil. Although these studies have been completed, no study results have been posted to date.

The desipramine trial has recently been completed (in 2015 sponsored by Assistance Publique Hopitaux De Marseille) and consisted of an unbalanced, double-blind placebo-controlled parallel study. Desipramine is a tricyclic antidepressant that inhibits norepinephrine reuptake. The primary outcome measures of the trial were to assess the efficacy of desipramine on respiratory disturbances in patients with RTT. Although this study has been completed, no study results have been posted.

Fingolimod, a compound known to increase brain derived neurotrophic factor (BDNF) is in a phase 1 open label study, led by the principal investigator Professor Ludwig Kappos, Department of Neurology - University Hospital Basel – Switzerland, and is still recruiting patients. Oral fingolimod (FTY720) modulates sphingosine-1 phosphate (S1P) receptors by acting as a 'super agonist' on the S1P receptor on thymocytes and lymphocytes, inducing uncoupling and internalization of the receptor. The outcome measures are based on serum and cerebrospinal fluid (CSF) BDNF level measurements.

Triheptanoin, a triglyceride shown to improve mitochondrial function and preserve cellular energy, is currently being tested in a non-randomized open label triglyceride trial led by the principal investigator Daniel Tarquinio at the Children's Healthcare of Atlanta, Georgia, United States. The trial is currently recruiting patients (maximum of 10) with primary aims to evaluate the safety and tolerability as well as to determine whether triheptanoin can improve overall seizure frequency and dystonia in RTT.

The use of ketamine is being investigated in a randomized, crossover, double blinded phase 1 clinical trial led by the principal investigator Daniel Sessler at the Cleveland Clinic, Cleveland, Ohio, United States. Ketamine is a sedative, most commonly used as an anesthetic; however, animal studies and case reports in humans suggest that ketamine may improve some clinical abnormalities in RTT. The purpose of this study is to determine the safety and efficacy of ketamine for treating breathing and behavioral abnormalities of patients with RTT. Primary outcome measures include measuring behavioral parameters, apnea/breath-hold index, hyperventilation and cardiorespiratory coupling indices, as well as EEG before, during, and after each treatment. Auditory evoked potentials (AEP) will be recorded on the day after each treatment. This trial is active, but not yet recruiting patients.

Lovastatin, a statin drug, used for lowering cholesterol, is being tested in an open label phase 2 clinical trial, and currently participants are being recruited into the study. The study is led by the principal investigator Aleksandra Djukic and conducted at the Montefiore Medical center, New York, United States. Patients with RTT have increased levels of neuronal cholesterol, which may be inhibited by lovastatin and lead to the improvement in RTT-related symptoms. The primary outcome measure of this trial is gait velocity with secondary measures including visual attention and memory, respiratory function, EEG, quality of life measures, and visual pursuit.

Conducting clinical trials in rare disorders such as RTT has many challenges; however, lessons from past clinical trials together with new information from preclinical studies will enable clinical trials research to move forward to achieve a therapeutic strategy for RTT.

Current therapies

At present, treatment of RTT is largely symptomatic, and with integrated multidisciplinary health care and symptomatic drug treatment, patients with RTT have a better quality of life and a considerably longer lifespan. Anticonvulsant medications often help to reduce seizure activity. Dopamine agonists may be used to help to alleviate spasticity in patients with late motor impairment. Opiate antagonists such as naltrexone have been tried for their potential ability to alleviate breathing irregularities, however clinical trials have been inconclusive. Where certain anticonvulsant drug therapy is used (e.g. sodium valproate), patients may suffer from secondary carnitine deficiency, which can be managed with replacement L-carnitine. An L-carnitine clinical trial was undertaken in 1999 which revealed that L-carnitine was associated with an improvement in two of the measured outcomes; the behavioral/social and orofacial/respiratory scales of the Rett Syndrome Motor Behavioural Assessment and the Patient Well-Being Index (Ellaway et al. 1999).These effects, however, were not as substantial as those reported earlier (Plioplys and Kasnicka, 1993; Plochl et al. 1996), and to date no long-term studies have been reported using L-carnitine. Some patients with RTT may have a prolonged QT interval on ECG, and so certain drugs, including antipsychotics, anti-arrhythmics, certain antibiotics, anesthetic agents, and cisapride, need to be avoided as these may cause potentially life-threatening arrhythmias. Supportive medical management includes physical, occupational, speech therapy, special academic, social, vocational, and supportive services. Early intervention is often required to reduce the possibility of inadequate weight gain resulting in growth failure, and may require nasogastric or gastrostomy feeding.

Potential future therapies under investigation

In order to develop relevant targeted therapies for patients with RTT, a deeper understanding of the underlying biology leading to dysfunction is needed. Translational research requires the synergistic approaches between clinical, behavioral and genotype-phenotype studies in humans, functional studies in cellular models, and phenotype studies in animal models. Over the years there have been many studies that have revealed functional abnormalities in patients with RTT and mouse models, as well as aberrant function or expression of MeCP2 and associated molecules. The possibility that phenotypic rescue is possible has inspired the search for therapeutic agents that have the potential to restore the functional abnormalities found in patients with RTT. These therapeutic approaches are largely focused on ameliorating or reversing the existing symptoms. There are a number of pathogenic pathways that are prime targets for therapies, and for the purposes of this chapter we have classified them into five areas of potential therapeutic approaches. The most obvious candidate is the *MECP2* gene, with RTT-causing mutations leading to loss of function of the protein. Other likely targets

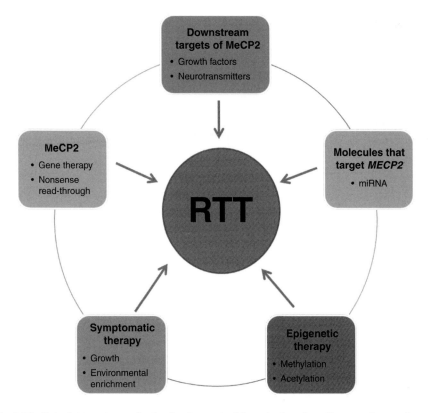

Fig. 14.1. Potential target areas for the development of therapies based on disease pathogenesis.

are downstream processes that are direct targets of MeCP2, molecules that either enhance or repress *MECP2*, symptomatic therapy, and finally epigenetic therapy (Figure 14.1). Additional information on potential treatments can be found in Chapter 13.

TARGETING *MECP2*

Targeting *MECP2* and other primary causative genes is one of the most obvious areas to focus in terms of developing therapeutic opportunities.

Over 300 pathogenic *MECP2* mutations have been identified in classic and variant patients with RTT (RettBASE(http://mecp2.chw.edu.au/) Christodoulou et al. 2003) with many of the mutations involving a C > T transition resulting in missense or nonsense mutations. In addition, small (<100 bp) to large deletions, some encompassing whole exons and even the whole gene have been identified, resulting in truncated, unstable proteins that render MeCP2 non-functional. Thus, mutations involving *MECP2* can result in complete loss of MeCP2 function or in hypomorphic alleles, with some residual function or in the overproduction of MeCP2 due to gene duplication, the latter of which causes a phenotype very distinct from RTT (Van Esch et al. 2005).

MECP2 is located on the X chromosome and is subject to X-chromosome inactivation (XCI) in females, where one X chromosome in each cell is usually randomly inactivated. This produces a mosaic of MeCP2 expression, whereby some cells express the mutant allele and others express the wild type (normal) allele. Pharmacological approaches aimed at augmenting the expression of *MECP2* hold great potential for patients with RTT. One such approach is an epigenetic approach that targets the existing wild type allele and either leads to a compensatory increase in the expression of the active wild type allele, or re-activates the inactive wild type allele in cells where the mutant allele is being expressed. Other approaches include the use of gene therapy, where a functional copy of *MECP2* can be delivered to deficient cells, or read-through agents that can circumvent mutated nonsense sequences thus producing full-length functional protein transcripts.

Read-through

Read-through, using small molecules based on the aminoglycoside structure is a potential emerging pharmacological approach for patients with RTT harboring nonsense mutations. The ability of the these molecules to allow for partial read through of nonsense codons, allows the transcription machinery to bypass the premature stop codon and produce full length transcripts that are able to encode partially functional proteins. Encouraging studies using gentamicin show a 10–22% *MECP2* read-through efficiency in constructs containing the most common RTT nonsense mutations p.Arg168X, p.Arg255X, p.Arg270X, and p.Arg294X (Brendel et al. 2009). However, gentamicin cannot easily traverse the blood–brain barrier and is associated with toxicity after long-term use, thus rendering it inappropriate as a therapeutic agent. Novel and less toxic synthetic aminogylcosides have been recently shown to be more promising with NB54 and NB84, derivatives of the antibiotic paromomycin, showing a high efficiency in their ability to suppress nonsense mutations than gentamicin (Vecsler et al. 2011; Brendel et al. 2011). NB54 is also able to increase the expression of one of the most well-known targets of MeCP2 and *BDNF* (Vecsler et al. 2011).

Gene therapy

Another potentially useful therapeutic approach is the use of gene therapy where an exogenous copy of the working gene in question can be delivered to the patient to compensate for endogenous loss. Gene therapy has been shown to be of some value in neurodegenerative disorders such as Parkinson disease, which is currently in phase 2 of clinical trials using NLX-P101 therapy. For patients with RTT with loss of function mutations in *MECP2*, this approach would be theoretically useful, as working copies of the complete transcript of *MECP2* could be administered to patients to compensate for the deficient gene. Practically, however, this approach has major hurdles, which include the risk of overexpression of MeCP2, as well as targeting the correct cells. As the target cells are post-mitotic neurons, which have become senescent and no longer have the capacity to divide, in vivo viral gene therapy delivery is the most feasible option. However, if a suitable vector can be sourced, the vector has to have the capacity to avoid transgene repression and be delivered in the correct dosage in order to transduce enough cells without causing overexpression of *MECP2*.

Several strategies using mouse models have been reported where working copies of the *MECP2* gene have been introduced using lentiviral, retroviral, or adenoviral vector transduction. Earlier work using adenoviral delivery of *MECP2* into the striatum of *Mecp2*-null mice showed promising results of phenotypic recovery, where decreased motor deterioration and restoration of voluntary motor activity was reported (Kosai, 2005); however, this work has not been repeated, nor has any follow-up work been reported. Adenoviral vector strategies for gene therapy are being implemented in clinical trials in a number of disorders including neurodegenerative lipid storage disorders and Parkinson disease. Adenoviral vectors are an appealing viral source for gene therapy in RTT, and in particular the serotype AAV9, as it is able to transduce neuronal cells with a high efficiency and maintain the long-term expression of the transduced gene, as well as being able to traverse the blood–brain barrier.

Regardless of the viral vector employed, however, one of the major hurdles that needs to be overcome is the effect of dosage of MeCP2 in patients with RTT. Introduction of wild type MeCP2 into neuronal and glial cells already expressing the wild type endogenous allele could result in a doubling in expression of MeCP2, which is likely to be toxic given the phenotypic abnormalities seen in transgenic mice overexpressing Mecp2 and based on the observed phenotype in patients with the MeCP2 duplication phenotype (Van Esch et al. 2005). An attractive solution to this would be to repress all endogenous MeCP2 expression and just allow the expression of the exogenous MeCP2 to take place. This strategy was employed by Zhou et al. in 2006 whereby a bicistronic cassette was designed containing a short hairpin RNA (shRNA) element with the capacity to suppress translation of Mecp2 from endogenous message RNA (mRNA) (both mutated and wild type), leaving only the exogenous Mecp2 expression to exert its effects (Zhou et al. 2006). The lentivirus-mediated protein-replacement assay (LEMPRA) constructs were able to replace MeCP2 in neuronal cells with about 90% efficiency. Recently, a proof-of-principle targeted gene-re-introduction strategy was employed, whereby modest levels of introduced MeCP2 were able to rescue some behavior and motor deficits in heterozygous females of an RTT mouse model. Heterozygous Mecp2-overexpressing mice were generated expressing a Mecp2 transgene in forebrain neurons, resulting in a 1.6-fold increase in MeCP2 expression. Although gene therapy was not used directly, these authors showed that crossing the Mecp2 overexpressing mice with heterozygous Mecp2 null mice confirmed that compensation of expression of MeCP2, within a specific developmental time window, can be therapeutically advantageous (Jugloff et al. 2008). These proof-of-principle studies, in which the mobility and locomotive activity were restored in heterozygous female mice with return of Mecp2 expression to wild type levels, indicate that the phenotype may indeed be rescued.

Avoiding transgene expression is another major concern when implementing gene therapy strategies. Self-inactivating lentiviral vectors containing genes encoding the E1 and E2 *MECP2* isoforms have been used to transduce neurons derived from neuronal stem cells (NSCs) of *Mecp2*-null mice (Mnatzakanian et al. 2004; Rastegar et al. 2009). These vectors were created such that the expression of each isoform was either under the control of the ubiquitous *EF1α* promoter, to circumnavigate any silencing elements, or the endogenous *Mecp2* promoter to allow for archetypal cellular gene expression. Transduced neurons with the *MECP2* isoforms under the *EF1α* promoter successfully evaded silencing elements, maintained long-term expression and displayed improved dendritic growth and branching. Transduced glia and neurons with the isoform vectors under the control of the endogenous *Mecp2* promoter were also successfully generated, with expression patterns identical to that of endogenous *Mecp2* being achieved. As it is critically important to deliver the correct dosage of *MECP2*, an endogenous promoter is more preferable, and thus this study provides a potentially suitable system for RTT therapy (Rastegar et al. 2009).

Recently, *Mecp2*-null make mice treated neonatally by intracranial delivery of a single-stranded AAV9/CBA-*MECP2* vector showed improved survival and locomotor function and exploratory activity, as well as normal neuronal nuclear volume in transduced cells. As the wild type mice that received the same vector did not show any significant abnormalities, it appears that modest levels of MeCP2 overexpression can be tolerated. Furthermore, the intravenous delivery (more appropriate for human use) of a self-complementary AAV vector designed to drive MeCP2 expression from a fragment of the *Mecp2* promoter, still showed modest improvements in survival. Although the brain transduction efficiency in juvenile mice was low, these results support the notion of *MECP2* gene therapy for RTT (Gadalla et al. 2013).

Gene therapy holds great promise as a therapeutic tool, and once the hurdles of targeted delivery that avoid transgene expression and delivery of *Mecp2* at nontoxic doses have been overcome, gene therapy could be a viable strategy for restoration of the RTT phenotype.

DOWNSTREAM TARGETS OF MeCP2 OR CONSEQUENCES OF MeCP2 DEFICIENCY
Downstream targets of MeCP2 are other obvious avenues to explore for the development of novel therapies for RTT. Targeting downstream genes that are misregulated as a consequence of a lack of MeCP2, may be a solution to restoring at least some aspects of the RTT phenotype back toward normal. Several putative targets of MeCP2 have been identified, including molecules involved in neuronal repression [xHairy2α], neuronal development [BDNF], cell proliferation [IGF2], proteolysis [UBE3A], gamma-amino butyric acid (GABA) signaling [GABRB3], as well as the transcription factors [DLX5/Dlx5, DLX6/Dlx6].

MeCP2 has been shown to be capable of responding to neuronal activation signals and once activated, has the capability to decipher epigenetic markers and regulate the transcription of genes distal as well as proximal MeCP2 binding sites. The activation and subsequent phosphorylation of MeCP2, leads to many of its target genes, such as *BDNF*, to undergo rapid changes in expression (Zhou et al. 2006). It is feasible, therefore, that the identification of all the physiologically important targets of MeCP2 has been hindered by the heterogeneous nature of the activity-dependent activation and epigenetic status of neurons in the maturing brain.

Targeting growth factors
Alterations in the neurotrophic factors NGF (nerve growth factor) and BDNF and the growth factor IGF-1 have been reported in RTT. These molecules are integral in early development and in the mature brain, as they as they are widely expressed in the central nervous system (CNS), and support activity-dependent neuronal plasticity, which plays a role in cognitive

processes such as learning and memory, and have consequently gained attention in RTT as possible therapeutic targets.

NGF, a trophic factor with nerve growth stimulating activity, is primarily involved in the regulation of growth and the differentiation of basal forebrain cholinergic neurons. Studies have shown deficits in NGF levels in brain and CSF of girls with RTT, in the plasma of patients with RTT with corrected QT (QTc) interval prolongation compared with those with a normal QTc interval, and more recently in the hippocampus of *Mecp2* null mice.

Postnatal dietary choline supplementation has been shown to increase cortical and hippocampal NGF as well as BDNF expression. Furthermore, it has also been demonstrated to have some therapeutic benefits in *Mecp2* null mice, with mice showing improvements in motor, behavioral, and neurobiological deficits. However, further studies are needed to determine whether dietary choline has any adverse side effects that could preclude it from consideration for clinical trials.

BDNF falls under the neurotrophin growth factor subclass, which plays a pivotal role in postnatal survival and neuronal outgrowth. Studies have shown that reduced neurotrophin levels are associated with reduced neuronal complexity and impaired learning, which can be rescued upon neurotrophin administration. Demonstration that BDNF is a direct target of MeCP2 (Chen et al. 2003; Martinowich et al. 2003), that it has a crucial role in neuronal survival, differentiation and maturation during early development, as well as more dynamic functions that are a consequence of neuronal plasticity, learning, memory, and synaptic function, have led to the suggestion that BDNF could be a therapeutic target in patients with RTT. Various studies have confirmed the functional interaction between BDNF and MeCP2 and that BDNF is a target of MeCP2 (Chen et al. 2003; Chahrour et al. 2008; Chang et al. 2006; Martinowich et al. 2003), whereby MeCP2 exerts promoter selective and phosphorylation dependent transcriptional control over BDNF (Chen et al. 2003). The levels of MeCP2 and BDNF in the brain have been shown to be closely correlated (Chang et al. 2006). Overexpression of MeCP2 in cultured mouse cortical neurons increases BDNF expression (Klein et al. 2007), whereas Mecp2-deficient mice show reduced levels of BDNF and earlier onset of RTT-like symptoms (Chang et al. 2006). Furthermore, restoring BDNF in the brains of Mecp2-deficient mice ameliorates many of their RTT-like physiological and behavioral deficits (Larimore et al. 2009; Kondo et al. 2008). Studies like these infer that dysregulation of BDNF could be contributing to the neurological phenotype and pathophysiology of RTT; however, no clinical study has demonstrated abnormal BDNF protein levels in blood or CSF of patients with RTT, and the underlying functional dynamics between BDNF and MeCP2 still remain unclear.

A possible therapeutic option would be to administer recombinant BDNF, working on the supposition that increased BDNF will have a beneficial effect on a patient's clinical progress. However, as attractive as BDNF is as a target for therapy, it cannot traverse the blood–brain barrier. To circumvent this problem, compounds such as glatiramer acetate (also known as Copolymer-1 or Copazone) and Fingolimod (FTY720) that are capable of enhancing BDNF expression are being investigated. These two compounds are currently being tested in phase 1 and 2 open label clinical trials, and are both U S Food and Drug Administration (FDA)-approved drugs for the treatment of multiple sclerosis. Fingolimod is a modulator of the sphingosine-1 phosphate receptor, which leads to an increase in BDNF expression and activation of TrkB downstream signalling pathways. Glatiramer acetate is a cocktail of synthetic polypeptides with immunomodulation properties, and is capable of augmenting BDNF expression in neurons in an autoimmune encephalomyelitis (EAE) mouse model, where it exhibits neuroprotective properties. In a preclinical study, glatiramer acetate was found to increase the levels of BDNF expression in the cortex of the *Mecp2*-deficient mouse model (*Mecp2^{tm1Hzo/J}*) compared to the wild type mice, although no phenotypic changes were observed after treatment, and the levels of *Mecp2*/Mecp2 were not reported (Ben-Zeev et al. 2011).

Studies using exogenous BDNF have been undertaken with certain success. *Mecp2*-deficient mice (*Mecp2^{tm1-1Jae}*) demonstrated dysregulation of primary afferent synaptic transmission in the brainstem nucleus tractus solitarius (nTS), the principal target of peripheral sensory neurons, and a crucial site for reflex modulation of autonomic and respiratory function (Kline et al. 2010; Balkowiec and Katz, 2000; Balkowiec et al. 2000). This was accompanied by significantly increased amplitude of spontaneous miniature and evoked excitatory postsynaptic currents (EPSCs) in nucleus tractus solitarius (nTS) neurons, which are prone to fire action potentials in response to primary afferent stimulation compared to wild type cells. Furthermore, these cells showed significantly reduced levels of BDNF. The synaptic phenotype was shown to be rescued when brain slices of Mecp2-deficient mice were treated with exogenous BDNF. Bath application of BDNF restored the amplitude of EPSCs to wild type levels, and significantly reduced the number of action potentials elicited by tractus solitarius stimulation (Kline et al. 2010). Given that BDNF can modulate glutamatergic excitation of second-order nTS neurons , and that BDNF regulates the synaptic function in the brainstem, it is therefore likely that the abnormal sensory gating in the nTS may be underpinning the cardiorespiratory phenotype observed in RTT, which can be rescued by exogenous BDNF administration.

IGF-1 is gaining attention because of its promising results in clinical trials. IGF-1 is primarily secreted by the liver and regulates cell growth and development. Unlike BDNF, IGF-1 is able to cross the blood–brain barrier, making it a more viable therapeutic candidate. IGF-1 is also widely expressed in the brain during normal development, and plays an essential role both developmentally and during adulthood by supporting neuronal integrity and activity-dependent neuronal plasticity. Of its six potential protein-binding partners, IGF-1 predominantly binds to IGFBP3. Interestingly, IGFBP3 also has a binding site for MeCP2 (Chang et al. 2004), and exhibits unusually high levels of expression in patients with RTT and Mecp2-deficient mice, which may result in defective IGF-1 signaling. The tri-peptide derivative (1-3)-IGF-1 has been tested in Mecp2-deficient mice to investigate its potential to stimulate synaptic maturation and alleviate key motor and behavioral abnormalities associated with the RTT phenotype (Tropea et al. 2009). IGF-1 was able to reverse some locomotor and respiratory deficits in the null mice as well as extending their lifespan. Furthermore, treated mice showed an increase in brain weight, partial restoration of spine density, and amelioration of synaptic strength and plasticity deficits, as well as an increase in synaptic amplitude. Clinical trials testing the efficacy of rhIGF-1 have shown promising results with improvements in neurobehavioral parameters, specifically measures of anxiety and depression and a reduction in apnea frequency have been reported (Khwaja et al. 2014). These studies have led to a phase 2 double-blind, placebo-controlled, crossover study and have greatly shaped the design and initiation of the current trofinetide and sarizotan trials.

Treatment using a cocktail of neuropeptides has been investigated using the neuroprotective and neurotrophic drug, cerebrolysin, in a RTT Mecp2-deficient mouse model. Cerebrolysin, a peptide-based drug consisting of a combination of several neurotrophic factors such as BDNF, glial cell-derived neurotrophic factor (GDNF), NGF, and ciliary neurotrophic factor (CNTF), have nerve growth factor like activity, particularly on cholinergic neurons, and has been shown to promote neurogenesis in rat models. Clinical trials of cerebrolysin have shown a reduction in memory deficits in dementia patients. Importantly, cerebrolysin was trialled on a small cohort of patients with RTT. Following treatment with cerebrolysin, these patients showed a promising improvement in their motor and behavioral function, their EEG parameters were normalized, and they had a decrease in seizure frequency (Gorbachevskaya et al. 2001).

One of the neuropathological hallmarks of RTT is reduced brain size, with decreased dendritic branching and synaptic formation. The $Mecp2^{308/y}$ RTT mouse model closely mimics the behavioral features of patients with RTT (Shahbazian et al. 2002) with male mice over 4 months of age showing behavioral alterations and a reduction in dendritic complexity (Doppler et al. 2008). These mice were treated with cerebrolysin at 4 months of age for 3 months, which resulted in ameliloration of dendritic damage in the basal ganglia, hippocampus and neocortex of these mice. Furthermore, cerebrolysin-treated mice showed an improvement in their motor performance using open field test and pole tests (Doppler et al. 2008). Interestingly, the younger mice, which were treated at 1 month of age for 6 months, did not respond as positively to cerebrolysin, and although a trend was observed, they showed no significant changes in their behavioral performance. At 1 month, $Mecp2^{308/y}$ mice show no dendritic differences to those of their wild type counterparts, suggesting that the manifestations of the RTT phenotype had not yet been initiated. It would appear that cerebrolysin acts in a specific window of disease development and is able to act in a trophic manner, whereby it has the capacity to restore normal neuronal function as seen in the 4 month old mice, rather than a preventative one, where the 1 month old mice could not be protected from disease progression.

Targeting neurotransmitters

Despite the severe neurological and associated behavioral abnormalities observed in RTT, no overt differences in the gross anatomy of the brains of patients with RTT, apart from a reduced volume and weight, is evident (Chahrour and Zoghbi, 2007). At the cellular level, however, decreased neuronal cell body size and reduced dendritic arborisation are seen, suggesting that the neurological features arise from more subtle changes in neuronal morphology and function rather than gross anatomical abnormalities. Furthermore, there is no evidence to support neuronal and glial cell death, atrophy, or degeneration that are typically associated with neurodegenerative disorders, which fosters the notion that RTT is a disorder of neuronal development and plasticity rather than one of neuronal degeneration.

In addition to cellular morphological abnormalities, synaptic alterations are also observed in RTT. Synaptic plasticity is the ability of neurons to alter their morphology and synapse strength in response to environmental changes. Synaptic plasticity is most prevalent during 'critical periods' of early postnatal life which are vital for the normal development of neuronal circuits (Hensch, 2004). These periods coincide with the emergence of RTT features, and together with the growing body of evidence revealing potentially reversible defects of long-term and short-term potentiation in MeCP2 mutant mouse models (Asaka et al. 2006; Lonetti et al. 2010; Moretti et al. 2006; Guy et al. 2007), suggest that neuronal synaptic plasticity is impaired in patients with RTT and may play a role in the pathogenesis of the disorder.

As stated earlier, neurotrophic factors play a pivotal role in establishing neuronal networks during development and activity-dependent plasticity in adulthood, and also on neurotransmitter systems such as the inhibitory GABAergic circuits and excitatory glutamate receptor system.

Biogenic amines and neuropeptides: Biogenic amines are a group of neurotransmitters, which include serotonin, acetylcholine, dopamine, and norepinephrine. Although these molecules are implicated in a wide range of behavioral, cognitive and homeostatic functions in adults, these neuromodulators are produced during early embryogenesis, well before the onset of synaptogenesis, suggesting their possible importance in early brain development.

Reports focused on neurochemical studies in patients with RTT are limited and show some inconsistencies. While some studies have shown no differences in CSF metabolites of dopamine (homovanillic acid, HVA), noradrenaline (3-methoxy-4-hydroxy-phenylglycol, MHPG), and serotonin (5-hydroxyindoleacetic acid, 5HIAA) in patients with typical RTT (Lekman et al. 1990), other studies of post-mortem brains and CSF in patients with RTT, as well as RTT mouse models, have shown abnormalities in biogenic amines. These include dopamine, serotonin, norepinephrine, and their respective metabolites HVA, 5HIAA and MHPG, the neuromodulator acetylcholine, as well as the neuropeptide substance P, the endogenous opioid peptide neurotransmitter β-endorphin, and melatonin. In addition, dysfunction of the primary excitatory neurotransmitter, glutamate and its receptors, and abnormalities of the potential primary inhibitory neurotransmitter, GABA, and its receptors, have also been reported.

These neuromodulators are primary targets for pharmacological action based on their involvement in the regulation and activation of the neuronal circuitry. Recent approaches have focused on ameliorating the deficits observed in these modulators associated with an absence of MeCP2 expression.

Patients with RTT exhibit breathing deficits with an erratic respiratory rhythm and life-threatening apneas, with 26% of deaths in female patients with RTT being attributed to sudden cardiorespiratory arrhythmia (Kerr et al. 1997). No treatments are presently available for these neurological abnormalities. Early reports revealing reduced levels of norepinephrine as well as its metabolites in patients with RTT suggested that bio-aminergic deficits could account for the breathing irregularities observed (Brucke et al. 1987; Lekman et al. 1989). Norepinephrine plays a key role in the maturation and modulation of the respiratory network, and studies of norepinephrine modulation have increased our awareness of the relevance of norepinephrine in the breathing irregularities in these patients (Hilaire et al. 2004; Viemari et al. 2005; Viemari et al. 2004; Zoghbi et al. 1989; Zoghbi et al. 1985).

Male *Mecp2^{tm1-Bird}* also show breathing abnormalities, which increase with age until their demise. These abnormalities manifest as mild variability in the duration of the respiratory cycle/rhythm when they are young, and progress onto severe apneas and highly variable cycle periods, finally culminating in fatal respiratory arrest at around 2 months. These breathing disturbances resonate closely with the clinical features reported in a number of patients with RTT (Weese-Mayer et al. 2006), and developmentally correlate with bio-aminergic deficits. These mice showed a reduction in medullary norepinephrine and serotonin levels, suggesting that the respiratory disturbances are partially due to a deficiency in noradrenergic and serotonergic modulation of the medullary respiratory network (Viemari et al. 2005). An important observation from this study was that the norepinephrine deficits preceded any apparent respiratory deficits, suggesting that they may contribute to their development. Furthermore, in vitro studies have shown that exogenous norepinephrine is able to stabilize the firing pattern of the respiratory pacemaker neurons in Mecp2-deficient brainstem slices (Viemari et al. 2005). This, together with the reduction in the catecholamine biogenic amine levels, leads to the hypothesis that breathing disturbances in Mecp2-deficient mice may be due to a medullary bio-aminergic defect. Reduced CO_2 chemosensitivity may also contribute to breathing abnormalities because of the importance of serotonin in CO_2 chemosensitivity, and so restoring the levels of serotonin in these mice may be of clinical value. Indeed, male Mecp2-deficient mice treated with citalopram, a selective serotonin reuptake inhibitor, showed restored levels of serotonin which rescued the aberrant levels of CO_2 chemosensitivity (Toward et al. 2013). The recent work on restoring Mecp2 exclusively into astrocytes in globally Mecp2-deficient mice was associated with a recovery of respiratory abnormalities to normal patterns (Lioy et al. 2011), suggests that first the reinstatement of Mecp2 is able to reverse the respiratory abnormalities, and second, that this is effective in cells that normally express only minute levels of MeCP2 compared to their neighbouring neurons. This opens up a therapeutic opportunity where the breathing irregularities could be restored by treatment with regulators of norepinephrine metabolism.

The tricyclic antidepressant desipramine is therefore a likely therapeutic agent in this context, as it inhibits norepinephrine uptake in nerve terminals by blocking the norepineph-rine-selective transporter proteins, thereby increasing the availability of norepinephrine. In recent studies, desipramine treated Mecp2-deficient mice showed a significant improvement in their respiratory rhythm as well as an extended lifespan (Roux et al. 2007; Zanella et al. 2008). Furthermore, the number of tyrosine hydroxylase-producing medullary neurons was restored to wild-type levels, suggesting that in a MeCP2-deficient environment tyrosine hydroxylase-expressing neurons lose their ability to synthesize tyrosine hydroxylase during development, and that by pharmacological stimulation using the noradrenergic stimulant desipramine, these breathing irregularities can be restored. Although desipramine is able to relieve breathing difficulties of these mice, it does not correct them completely. It is tempting to speculate that concomitant therapy with other catecholamines such as serotonin could potentially have a synergistic effect on the respiratory phenotype.

Glutamate: Glutamate binds with high specificity to two primary receptors α-amino-3-hydroxyl-5-methyl-4-isoxazole-propionate (AMPA) and NMDA. The ampakine drug CX546, a positive AMPA receptor modulator and cognitive enhancer, which also has the capacity to increase BDNF levels, has been shown to restore normal breathing frequency and minute volume in *Mecp2*-null mice, suggesting that BDNF expression can be induced in these mice and that CX546 may be a possible therapeutic candidate (Ogier et al. 2007).

Electrophysiological defects in RTT have been shown to correlate with disease severity (Glaze et al. 1998). Approximately 80% of patients with RTT develop seizures with the risk of epilepsy being primarily dependent on the severity of the developmental tribulations, mutation type, and age (Glaze et al. 2010; Jian et al. 2007). It has been shown that brain glutamate and NMDA receptors are increased in the brains of younger patients with RTT, resulting in toxic damage to neurons and contributing to EEG spikes. Dextromethorphan exerts its effect through its major metabolite dextrorphan and acts as an NMDA receptor antagonist, by blocking NMDA/glutamate receptors. Dextromethorphan is currently in a placebo-controlled phase 2 clinical trial to determine its efficacy on cognition, behavior, and seizures in patients with RTT. If dextromethorphan can improve cognition and behavior deficits, as well as reduce seizures, this would be a major advance in ameliorating some of the age-associated symptoms in RTT. Memantine, a drug used in Alzheimer disease for its ability to block NMDA receptors and reduce neuronal excitotoxicity, has been tried in ex vitro hippocampal slices from *Mecp2*-null mice as well as in vivo. Although some deficits in synaptic plasticity were reversed, these positive effects of memantine did not translate into improving the RTT phenotype or survival time of treated animals (Weng et al. 2011).

GABA: Therapeutic options to alleviate aberrant GABA signaling in RTT have also been investigated. Midazolam, a benzodiazepine, used for its ability to enhance GABA activity on GABA receptors to treat acute seizures, has recently been shown to reduce apneas and other associated breathing abnormalities in *Mecp2*-null mice (Voituron et al. 2009, 2010a, b; Voituron and Hilaire 2011). Other compounds that act as GABA enhancers, such as GABA-reuptake blockers, have shown a promising ability to improve the respiratory phenotype in *Mecp2*-null mice (Abdala et al. 2010). Furthermore, a serotonin 1a receptor agonist, which depresses expiratory neuronal activity, was shown to reduce apneas, correct irregular breathing patterns, and increase survival in *Mecp2*-null male mice (Abdala et al. 2010). Interestingly, the synergistic approach of both chemicals completely corrected the respiratory defects in the *Mecp2*-null female mice. These results suggest that GABA enhancing drugs are likely candidates for the treatment of the respiratory disorders in RTT (Abdala et al. 2010).

Drugs aimed at the downstream consequences of MeCP2 deficiency (ω-3 PUFA)
Depriving a cell of the functions of the MeCP2 protein has many potential detrimental cellular ramifications. Among those already mentioned, is the increase in oxidative stress and the production of reactive oxygen species (ROS) that target primarily phospholipids

resulting in lipid peroxidation. ω-3 Polyunsaturated fatty acids (ω-3 PUFA) are known pleiotropic antioxidants, and have been shown to have multiple therapeutic beneficial effects including in cardiac disease (Kris-Etherton et al. 2002), in experimental brain hypoxia in rats, and recently in patients with RTT (De Felice et al. 2012).

Mitochondria are major producers of cellular ROS, and consequently dysfunctional mitochondrial respiratory chain activity observed in patients with RTT has the potential to trigger oxidative stress. One of the primary targets of ROS attack is phospholipids containing polyunsaturated fatty acids, which are predominantly susceptible to peroxidation resulting in the production of a class of compounds known as isoprostanes (IsoPs). F_2-isoprostanes (F_2-IsoPs) and non-protein-bound iron (NPBI) are considered to be the most reliable markers of oxidative stress.

Enhanced oxidative stress, lipid peroxidation, and abnormal mitochondrial metabolism have been demonstrated in patients with RTT (De Felice et al. 2009; Ruch et al. 1989; Sierra et al. 2001), and specifically show significantly elevated levels of F_2-IsoPs and NPBI compared to normal controls, with levels in classic patients with RTT being even higher than in atypical patients with RTT (De Felice et al. 2009; Leoncini et al. 2011).

Two pilot studies of typical female patients with RTT have shown that ω-3 PUFA oil treatment significantly reduced the levels of the oxidative stress markers, F_2-isoPs, and NPBI, and resulted in improved clinical severity scores (De Felice et al. 2009; Leoncini et al. 2011), suggesting that oral supplementation of the safe, FDA approved ω-3 PUFA oil could potentially be of therapeutic value in patients with RTT patients. Another study, treating female patients with RTT with oral supplementation of ω-3 PUFAs-containing fish oil for 12 months in a randomized controlled study, has also shown positive outcomes. Patients treated with the ω-3 PUFAs showed an improved ω-6/ω-3 ratio and serum plasma lipid profile (total cholesterol and triglycerides) and decreased PUFAs peroxidation end products compared to the untreated RTT group. In addition, the abnormal fatty acid composition observed in erythrocytes of these patients was partially restored after treatment. These data indicate that cell membrane lipid composition may be a potential therapeutic target for patients with RTT (Signorini et al. 2014). A fourth study testing the effects of ω-3 PUFAs on echocardiographic parameters and systemic oxidative stress markers in 66 typical patients with RTT has been conducted whereby patients were treated for 12 months with high doses of dietary supplementation of ω-3 PUFAs. ω-3 PUFAs were able to improve the biventricular myocardial systolic function along with a decrease in the oxidative stress markers levels in the treated patients (Maffei et al. 2014).

MOLECULES THAT TARGET MECP2

Another therapeutic option is an indirect form of therapy that involves targeting those molecules that modulate *MECP2* expression. Although the regulation of *MECP2* expression is poorly understood, it has recently been shown that microRNAs (miRNAs) contribute to the regulation of *MECP2* translation by binding to recognition elements in the *MECP2* three prime untranslated region (3'UTR). The *MECP2* 3'UTR is one of the longest known in the human genome, and, produces four transcripts of different length. The expression of each transcript is tissue-specific and temporally regulated, with the longest transcript being most highly expressed in the brain (Reichwald et al. 2000; Pelka et al. 2005). Multiple microRNA recognition elements (MRE) are present in the long 3'UTR of the *MECP2_e1* transcript that are not present in the shorter *MECP2_e2* isoform. Among these are binding sites for miR132 and miR212, which have been shown to repress MeCP2 translation. MiR132 is enriched in the brain and known to be involved in neurite outgrowth. Together with the observed decreased levels in a RTT mouse model, this suggests a role for miR132 in the regulation of *MECP2* expression during brain development. Interestingly, it has recently been shown that the interaction between miR212 and MeCP2 is important in regulating BDNF (Im et al. 2010). Given that *MECP2_e1* levels are ten times higher in the human adult brain and cerebellum than the *e2* isoform (Kriaucionis and Bird, 2004; Mnatzakanian et al. 2004), the manipulation of these regulators, in particular miR132, could potentially serve as a therapeutic strategy to either restore MeCP2 deficiency in patients with mutations or reduce *MECP2* expression in patients with a *MECP2* duplication.

Antisense oligonucleotides (ASOs) and their derivatives are currently being used to inhibit specific miRNAs and thereby prevent the degradation of the latter's target mRNA transcripts, some of which are in preclinical and clinical trials. However, delivering therapeutic RNA to its target tissue necessitates that these molecules exit the circulatory system, cross the cell membrane and evade the degradative machinery of the endosomes. Advances in miRNA therapies such as lipid-based delivery systems, are providing promising potential solutions.

SYMPTOMATIC THERAPY: TARGETING GROWTH AND ENVIRONMENTAL ENRICHMENT

Although neuronal plasticity and survival are rescued in Mecp2-deficient mice when Mecp2 levels are restored, a closer assessment of the more subtle RTT features, such as social behavior deficits and anxiety, also need to be addressed. Impaired MeCP2 function in mice results in synaptic deficits associated with motor, cognitive, and emotional alterations (Young et al. 2005). The use of the rearing condition and environmental enrichment has been shown to enhance synapse formation and plasticity as well as restore BDNF expression back toward normal in heterozygous Mecp2-deficient mice, but not in hemizygous male Mecp2-deficient mice (Kondo et al. 2008; Nag et al. 2009, Nithianantharajah and Hannan, 2006). However, work on environmental enrichment reared pre-weaned (P10) Mecp2-deficient male mice has shown that environmental enrichment is able to induce long term potentiation (LTP) as well as the expression of BDNF, thereby promoting synaptic plasticity at this early stage of development. Both male and female mice showed an improvement in the behavioral studies, with males showing improvement of motor coordination and motor learning deficits, and females showing reduced anxiety levels, as well as recovery of memory deficits (Lonetti et al. 2010). In another study, male mice (aged 3–5 weeks) exposed to environmental enrichment, showed an attenuated neuromotor phenotype, with improved motor skills and anxiety levels equivalent to those of wild type mice (Kerr et al. 2010). The effect of an enriched environment on Mecp2-deficient mice, particularly during early development, has vindicated the therapeutic importance of introducing an early rehabilitation intervention strategy in patients with RTT. More recently, environmental enrichment has been shown to reverse affective dysfunction and anxiety in female Mecp2-deficient mice exposed to environmental enrichment from 4 weeks of age (Kondo et al. 2015). In addition, this study showed that environmental enrichment also rescued basal serum corticosterone and hippocampal BDNF protein levels suggesting that environmental enrichment regulates downstream pathways of MeCP2 targets and thus the synergistic use of environmental enrichment together with pharmacological intervention is a possible therapeutic option (Kondo et al. 2015).

Other growth factors, such as ghrelin, an acetylated peptide hormone which is predominantly produced in gastrointestinal tissue, has therapeutic potential for patients with RTT. Ghrelin has the ability to stimulate growth hormone secretion and gastrointestinal motility, as well as promoting caloric intake by enhancing the sensation of hunger, both important management issues in patients with RTT. A recent study revealed that patients with RTT have lower plasma ghrelin levels than controls, and this significantly correlated with plasma IGF-1 levels. Patients with eating and digestive difficulties displayed lower ghrelin levels, which could contribute to the growth failure (which is difficult to reconcile with the observation that girls with RTT eat without satiety), and the autonomic dysfunction that these patients display.

EPIGENETIC THERAPIES

The regulation of epigenetic marking, which plays an integral part in determining whether a gene is expressed or not, is mediated by methylation (the addition of methyl groups to DNA and histones), acetylation (the addition of acetyl groups to histones), and by small interfering RNA (siRNA). Epigenetic dysregulation is a common theme in disorders of synaptic plasticity and cognition, including neurodegenerative disorders such as Huntington disease, and neurodevelopmental disorders such as RTT. MeCP2 has traditionally been thought to be a transcriptional repressor by virtue of its capacity to bind to methylated CpG islands via its methyl binding domain (MBD) and repress transcription via its transcriptional repressor domain (TRD). The interactions between the TRD of MeCP2 and transcriptional corepressors, such as mSin3A and histone deacetylases (HDACs), provide evidence that there is a link between DNA methylation and chromatin remodelling. As new evidence emerges, our understanding of the function of MeCP2 is being challenged. It has been recently shown that MeCP2 is one of the most abundant nuclear proteins (as abundant as histone H1) found in mature neurons, and globally binds chromatin and tracks with the density of methyl CpG sites (Skene et al. 2010). Furthermore, neuronal nuclei, deficient of MeCP2, show a two-fold increase in expression of histone H1, which implies that MeCP2 may have a similar function to that of histone H1 in neuronal cells, and thus may be involved in chromatin remodelling and epigenetic changes.

Methylation

In vitro DNA methylation is carried out by DNA methyltransfereases (DNMTs), which catalyse the transfer of a methyl group from an S-adenosyl-L-methionine to the nucleotide cytosine. Altering the methylation levels of DNA, resulting in epigenetic changes and thereby altering regulation of gene expression, may be possible through dietary means. Methyl-group rich compounds such as choline (mentioned in the section 'Targeting growth factors'), methionine, and betaine, and methyl-group donors such as folate, can alter DNA and histone methylation during critical periods in development, and are available as dietary supplements for therapeutic treatment. Transmethylation metabolic pathways closely link the metabolism of choline, methionine, and folate. These pathways intersect at the formation of methionine from homocysteine. Thus, the effects of these nutrients on epigenetic marking are interrelated.

Cerebral folate deficiency (CFD), characterized by low cerebrospinal fluid (CSF) concentrations of 5MTHF, has been reported in RTT (Ormazabal et al. 2006), although subsequent studies have not been able to reproduce this. A clinical trial involving the use of folate-betaine supplementation in 68 patients with RTT (Glaze et al. 2009) has been conducted, with no objective evidence of improvement being observed. Moreover, a recent study, using folinic acid supplementation, was shown to increase cerebrospinal fluid 5-MTHF levels in patients with RTT, but this did not translate into clinical improvement (Hagebeuk et al. 2011).

Creatine is a potent methyl group donor and currently used as a therapeutic agent for improving muscle strength. The dietary supplement creatine monohydrate (CMH), has the capacity to increase methylation and has been used for clinical trials in patients with RTT (Freilinger et al. 2011). In this trial, a statistically significant increase in global DNA methylation was observed, as well as a general tendency for motor and behavioral assessment scores to increase, however the latter did not reach statistical significance (Freilinger et al. 2011).

Acetylation

Epigenetic remodeling resulting in alterations in gene expression via changes in acetylation may be the consequence of the action of the epigenetic modifiers histone acetyltransferases (HATs), histone deacetylases (HDACs), and HDAC inhibitors. Transcriptional control is tightly regulated and is in constant flux between an open chromatin structure mediated through histone acetylation by HATs facilitating gene transcription, and a closed unavailable chromatin structure mediated through histone deacetylation by HDACs, which dampen transcription, resulting in the down-regulation of gene transcription. Current developments in the field of DNA remodeling and epigenetic gene regulation have greatly altered our understanding of gene regulation, and this knowledge, coupled with the increase in the development of new HDAC inhibitors, holds promise for the identification of new compounds that may have therapeutic effects on CNS disorders such as RTT. HDAC inhibitors display neuroprotective and neuroregenerative properties and are emerging as an exciting new class of therapeutic agents. These small drug molecules are proving to have beneficial effects in a number of diseases including cancer, inflammatory disorders, and as well as neurological disorders including Parkinson disease, Rubinstein-Taybi syndrome, Friedreich ataxia, Huntington disease, Alzheimer disease, Fragile X syndrome, and RTT, and have already been tested in a number of disease models. Treating CNS disorders by drug delivery is challenging because of the blood–brain barrier. Another obstacle is the unique metabolic properties of the brain, which can alter the kinetics and dynamics as well as the ADMET (adsorption, distribution, metabolism, excretion, toxicity) properties of a drug, rendering it unsafe, non-specific, or ineffective. HDAC inhibitors are currently being explored in CNS disorders for their ability to remain stable, to penetrate the blood–brain barrier to reach specific areas of the brain, and to be potent and selective for specific intracellular molecular targets, as well as be isoform specific to reduce any nonspecific side effects.

The HDAC super-family of proteins are well known for their ability to deacetylate histones, as well as microtubules, and thus investigations are warranted into isoform-specific HDAC inhibitors. Promising results in a mouse model of Huntington disease following treatment with the HDAC inhibitors sodium butyrate and phenylbutyrate showed attenuation of neuronal loss, as well as increased motor function and survival. These results led to clinical trials in patients with Huntington disease, for which a phase 2 trial has been completed. Microtubule instability and the need to stabilize the microtubule network in neuronal cells of neurological disorders is becoming increasingly evident. Specifically to RTT, recent reports have shown RTT cells to have an unstable microtubule network and through the utility of pharmacological HDAC6 inhibition, stability can be restored (Delepine et al. 2013; Nectoux et al. 2012; Gold et al. 2015; Xu et al. 2014). Small molecule HDAC6-specific inhibitors are thus emerging as promising therapeutic options in a growing number of neurological disorders, including Alzheimer disease, Huntington disease, Charcot-Marie-Tooth disease, Parkinson disease, as well as in RTT (Gold et al. 2015; Xu et al. 2014).

RTT is a very good candidate for HDAC inhibitor therapy by virtue of the fact that it is one of the first disorders to link neurobiology and epigenetics in human diseases. The potential success of HDAC inhibitor therapy in RTT is based on a number of factors. First, there is the requirement for histone acetylation and concomitant increased transcription, based on the transcriptional repression/chromatin remodeling mode of action of MeCP2. Second, based on emerging reports of microtubule instability in RTT, there is a need to stabilize the microtubule network of neuronal cells. Third, RTT being a neurodevelopmental CNS disorder makes it a suitable disorder for the use of small drug molecules that can traverse the blood–brain barrier. Despite the number of years that have been invested into translational and clinical research, drug delivery to specific areas of the brain still remains a major hurdle in designing therapies for RTT. HDAC inhibitors provide tremendous therapeutic potential for RTT and other CNS disorders, and as the biology of these small molecules and their efficacy as novel therapeutic compounds are better understood, there is every possibility that they could become a successful approach for treating RTT.

Reversibility of Rett syndrome in mouse models

The recent innovative studies demonstrating that neurological deficits resulting from loss of MeCP2 function can be reversed upon restoration of gene function are very promising (Giacometti et al. 2007; Guy et al. 2007). The very idea that MeCP2-deficient neurons, deprived of the consequences of the protein's expression, are able to regain functionality when MeCP2 is reinstated, challenges the paradigm that RTT is a neurodevelopmental disorder but rather that it is a disorder of neuronal plasticity, providing credence to the possibility that potentially corrective therapy for RTT could be a feasible option. With the development of a number of Mecp2-deficient mouse models that recapitulate many of the phenotypic hallmarks of RTT, we are now in a position to investigate whether this reversibility can be achieved using targeted therapies.

Simple reinstatement of MeCP2 levels is not without problems though, as excess MeCP2 is as deleterious as too little (Van Esch et al. 2005; Luikenhuis et al. 2004; Collins et al. 2004). Also, potentially contributing to the disease phenotype may be non-cell autonomous toxic effects from neighboring MeCP2-deficient glial cells (Ballas et al. 2009; Lioy et al. 2011), and the inefficient phagocytic function of microglial cells (Derecki et al. 2012).

Recent evidence has highlighted the importance of glial cells and their non-cell autonomous effects on neuronal cells in RTT (Lioy et al. 2011). This work is an extension of the previous discovery that *Mecp2*-null non-neuronal cells such as astrocytes, oligodendrocyte progenitor cells (OPCs), and oligondendrocytes exert a negative and detrimental non-cell autonomous effect on surrounding wild type neurons (Ballas et al. 2009). Using the cleverly engineered globally Mecp2-deficient *Mecp2^stop^-hGFAPcreT2* mice, harboring an allele with a tamoxifen-inducible Cre recombinase transgene driven by the astrocyte-specific promoter (hGFAP), and an allele with a Cre-excisable transcriptional Stop sequence in the *Mecp2* gene, the exclusive expression of *Mecp2* in astrocytes of these mice was achieved by the administration of tamoxifen. This study showed that the astrocyte-specific re-expression of *Mecp2* is able to correct, or partially correct, a number of key clinical features found in RTT mice, including anxiety levels, locomotion, respiratory abnormalities, and lifespan. Furthermore, through positive non-cell autonomic effects, these authors were able to show that the reintroduction of *Mecp2* in astrocytes restored normal dendritic morphology as well as increasing the levels of an important excitatory neurotransmitter, VGLUTI (vesicular glutamate transporter).

Traditionally, glial cells have been thought not to express *MECP2* and so were not considered to be a major contributor to the pathogenesis of RTT. This study opens up a potentially new therapeutic avenue for RTT, whereby glial cells, rather than neuronal cells, could be targeted. An increase in expression of the wild type *Mecp2* allele in glial cells (either by gene therapy, read-through drugs, or small drug molecules), and the reliance on the non-cell autonomous effects of these cells on their neighboring Mecp2-deficient neurons, may be enough to ameliorate the RTT phenotype.

Even more recently, it has been shown that microglial cells may also contribute to the pathogenesis of RTT, although the precise mode of action is currently undetermined. Derecki et al. (2012) have shown that transplanting bone marrow cells containing a wild-type *Mecp2* copy of the gene into P28 irradiated *Mecp2*-null mice, leads to the engraftment of microglial-like cells in the brain, attenuation of disease progression, and an increased lifespan. Microglial cells are a subpopulation of immune cells that originate from bone marrow and populate the brain, where they primarily function as debris-removing phagocytes. Microglial cells of the *Mecp2*-null mouse models used in these experiments had defective phagocytic and immunological response capabilities, suggesting that impaired phagocytosis with less efficient removal of debris in the brain, may be contributing to the underlying pathology of RTT. Although certain phenotypic aspects were corrected in the (P28) mice, restoration of phenotype could not be accomplished in older mice (P40 or

P45) that received the same transplantation treatment, or in very young mice (P2) that did not receive cranial irradiation prior to the transplantation (Derecki et al. 2012). Given the small time window in which the transplantation is successful, this study suggests that bone marrow transplant is able to exert its effects in the young maturing brain at a relatively early stage of the disease.

Despite these promising results, others have not been able to replicate these studies. Four independent groups, some utilizing the same mice, same bone marrow transplantation methods, and same outcome measures as the original study, have pooled their data and demonstrated that, in all cases, RTT mice showed no benefit to bone marrow transplant as far as alleviating symptoms or extending lifespan were concerned. Furthermore, they showed that even early, targeted rescue of *MECP2* expression in microglia cells did not rescue the mice from the disease (Wang et al. 2015). These subsequent studies challenge the original study and raise significant doubts as to the potential efficacy of bone marrow transplantation therapy for RTT.

Given the sensitivity of MeCP2 dosage and the diversity of cells implicated, we are faced with the challenge of finding therapeutic strategies that deliver MeCP2 in a correct spatial and temporal manner to only those neuronal and non-neuronal cells that are MeCP2-deficient. Identification of causative underlying molecular mechanisms of RTT, including the crucial factors that function downstream of *MECP2*, will produce a feasible approach to finding pharmacological options for RTT.

Conclusion

The paradigm shift that RTT is more a disorder of neuronal plasticity, and that it is possible to reverse symptoms toward normality, makes the notion of RTT being a treatable disorder a very viable one.

Recent research advances, coupled with knowledge already gained, are propelling RTT research into a new realm of therapeutic possibilities. The diversity of animal models expressing *Mecp2* mutations, together with our improved understanding of the biology of MeCP2, has the potential to lead to the development of innovative therapies for RTT. Pursuit of all possible therapeutic options is warranted, and based on recent research advances, there is every reason to believe that at least some of these will be successfully translated into the clinic in the near future.

REFERENCES

Abdala AP, Dutschmann M, Bissonnette JM and Paton JF (2010). Correction of respiratory disorders in a mouse model of Rett syndrome. *Proc Natl Acad Sci U S A* 107: 18208–18213.
Asaka Y, Jugloff DG, Zhang L, Eubanks JH and Fitzsimonds RM (2006). Hippocampal synaptic plasticity is impaired in the Mecp2-null mouse model of Rett syndrome. *Neurobiol Dis* 21: 217–227.
Balkowiec A and Katz DM (2000). Activity-dependent release of endogenous brain-derived neurotrophic factor from primary sensory neurons detected by ELISA in situ. *J Neurosci* 20: 7417–7423.
Balkowiec A, Kunze DL and Katz DM (2000). Brain-derived neurotrophic factor acutely inhibits AMPA-mediated currents in developing sensory relay neurons. *J Neurosci* 20: 1904–1911.
Ballas N, Lioy DT, Grunseich C and Mandel G (2009). Non-cell autonomous influence of MeCP2-deficient glia on neuronal dendritic morphology. *Nat Neurosci* 12: 311–317.

Ben-Zeev B, Aharoni R, Nissenkorn A and Arnon R (2011). Glatiramer acetate (GA, Copolymer-1) an hypothetical treatment option for Rett syndrome. *Med Hypotheses* 76: 190–193.

Brendel C, Belakhov V, Werner H, Wegener E, Gartner J, Nudelman I, Baasov T and Huppke P (2011). Readthrough of nonsense mutations in Rett syndrome: evaluation of novel aminoglycosides and generation of a new mouse model. *J Mol Med (Berl)* 89: 389–398.

Brendel C, Klahold E, Gartner J and Huppke P (2009). Suppression of nonsense mutations in Rett syndrome by aminoglycoside antibiotics. *Pediatr Res* 65: 520–523.

Brucke T, Sofic E, Killian W, Rett A and Riederer P (1987). Reduced concentrations and increased metabolism of biogenic amines in a single case of Rett-syndrome: a postmortem brain study. *J Neural Transm* 68: 315–324.

Chahrour M, Jung SY, Shaw C, Zhou X, Wong ST, Qin J and Zoghbi HY (2008). MeCP2, a key contributor to neurological disease, activates and represses transcription. *Science* 320: 1224–1229.

Chahrour M and Zoghbi HY (2007). The story of Rett syndrome: from clinic to neurobiology. *Neuron* 56: 422–437.

Chang Q, Khare G, Dani V, Nelson S and Jaenisch R (2006). The disease progression of Mecp2 mutant mice is affected by the level of BDNF expression. *Neuron* 49: 341–348.

Chang YS, Wang L, Suh YA, Mao L, Karpen SJ, Khuri FR, Hong WK and Lee HY (2004). Mechanisms underlying lack of insulin-like growth factor-binding protein-3 expression in non-small-cell lung cancer. *Oncogene* 23: 6569–6580.

Chen WG, Chang Q, Lin Y, Meissner A, West AE, Griffith EC, Jaenisch R and Greenberg ME (2003). Derepression of BDNF transcription involves calcium-dependent phosphorylation of MeCP2. *Science* 302: 885–889.

Christodoulou J, Grimm A, Maher T, Bennetts B (2003) RettBASE: The IRSA MECP2 variation database-a new mutation database in evolution. *Hum Mutat* 21(5): 466–472.

Collins AL, Levenson JM, Vilaythong AP, Richman R, Armstrong DL, Noebels JL, David Sweatt J and Zoghbi HY (2004). Mild overexpression of MeCP2 causes a progressive neurological disorder in mice. *Hum Mol Genet* 13: 2679–2689.

De Felice C, Ciccoli L, Leoncini S, Signorini C, Rossi M, Vannuccini L, Guazzi G, Latini G, Comporti M, Valacchi G and Hayek J (2009). Systemic oxidative stress in classic Rett syndrome. *Free Radic Biol Med* 47: 440–448.

De Felice C, Signorini C, Durand T, Ciccoli L, Leoncini S, D'esposito M, Filosa S, Oger C, Guy A, Bultel-Ponce V, Galano JM, Pecorelli A, De Felice L, Valacchi G and Hayek J (2012). Partial rescue of Rett syndrome by omega-3 polyunsaturated fatty acids (PUFAs) oil. *Genes Nutr* 7: 447–458.

Delepine C, Nectoux J, Bahi-Buisson N, Chelly J and Bienvenu T (2013). MeCP2 deficiency is associated with impaired microtubule stability. *FEBS Lett* 587: 245–253.

Derecki NC, Cronk JC, Lu Z, Xu E, Abbott SB, Guyenet PG and Kipnis J (2012). Wild-type microglia arrest pathology in a mouse model of Rett syndrome. *Nature* 484: 105–109.

Doppler E, Rockenstein E, Ubhi K, Inglis C, Mante M, Adame A, Crews L, Hitzl M, Moessler H and Masliah E (2008). Neurotrophic effects of Cerebrolysin in the Mecp2(308/Y) transgenic model of Rett syndrome. *Acta Neuropathol* 116: 425–437.

Ellaway C, Williams K, Leonard H, Higgins G, Wilcken B and Christodoulou J (1999). Rett syndrome: randomized controlled trial of L-carnitine. *J Child Neurol* 14: 162–167.

Freilinger M, Dunkler D, Lanator I, Item CB, Muhl A, Fowler B and Bodamer OA (2011). Effects of creatine supplementation in Rett syndrome: a randomized, placebo-controlled trial. *J Dev Behav Pediatr* 32: 454–460.

Gadalla KK, Bailey ME, Spike RC, Ross PD, Woodard KT, Kalburgi SN, Bachaboina L, Deng JV, West AE, Samulski RJ, Gray SJ and Cobb SR (2013). Improved survival and reduced phenotypic severity following AAV9/MECP2 gene transfer to neonatal and juvenile male Mecp2 knockout mice. *Mol Ther* 21: 18–30.

Giacometti E, Luikenhuis S, Beard C and Jaenisch R (2007). Partial rescue of MeCP2 deficiency by postnatal activation of MeCP2. *Proc Natl Acad Sci U S A* 104: 1931–1936.

Glaze DG, Percy AK, Motil KJ, Lane JB, Isaacs JS, Schultz RJ, Barrish JO, Neul JL, O'brien WE and Smith EO (2009). A study of the treatment of Rett syndrome with folate and betaine. *J Child Neurol* 24: 551–556.

Glaze DG, Percy AK, Skinner S, Motil KJ, Neul JL, Barrish JO, Lane JB, Geerts SP, Annese F, Graham J, Mcnair L and Lee HS (2010). Epilepsy and the natural history of Rett syndrome. *Neurology* 74: 909–912.

Glaze DG, Schultz RJ and Frost JD (1998). Rett syndrome: characterization of seizures versus non-seizures. *Electroencephalogr Clin Neurophysiol* 106: 79–83.

Gold WA, Lacina TA, Cantrill LC and Christodoulou J (2015). MeCP2 deficiency is associated with reduced levels of tubulin acetylation and can be restored using HDAC6 inhibitors. *J Mol Med (Berl)* 93: 63–72.

Gorbachevskaya N, Bashina V, Gratchev V and Iznak A (2001). Cerebrolysin therapy in Rett syndrome: clinical and EEG mapping study. *Brain Dev* 23 Suppl 1: S90–3.

Guy J, Gan J, Selfridge J, Cobb S and Bird A (2007). Reversal of neurological defects in a mouse model of Rett syndrome. *Science* 315: 1143–1147.

Hagebeuk EE, Duran M, Koelman JH, Abeling NG, Vyth A and Poll-The BT (2011). Folinic Acid Supplementation in Rett Syndrome Patients Does Not Influence the Course of the Disease: A Randomized Study. *J Child Neurol* 27: 304–309.

Hensch TK (2004). Critical period regulation. *Annu Rev Neurosci* 27: 549–579.

Hilaire G, Viemari JC, Coulon P, Simonneau M and Bevengut M (2004). Modulation of the respiratory rhythm generator by the pontine noradrenergic A5 and A6 groups in rodents. *Respir Physiol Neurobiol* 143: 187–197.

Im HI, Hollander JA, Bali P and Kenny PJ (2010). MeCP2 controls BDNF expression and cocaine intake through homeostatic interactions with microRNA-212. *Nat Neurosci* 13: 1120–1127.

Jian L, Nagarajan L, De Klerk N, Ravine D, Christodoulou J and Leonard H (2007). Seizures in Rett syndrome: an overview from a one-year calendar study. *Eur J Paediatr Neurol* 11: 310–317.

Jugloff DG, Vandamme K, Logan R, Visanji NP, Brotchie JM and Eubanks JH (2008). Targeted delivery of an Mecp2 transgene to forebrain neurons improves the behavior of female Mecp2-deficient mice. *Hum Mol Genet* 17: 1386–1396.

Kerr AM, Armstrong DD, Prescott RJ, Doyle D and Kearney DL (1997). Rett syndrome: analysis of deaths in the British survey. *Eur Child Adolesc Psychiatry* 6 Suppl 1: 71–74.

Kerr B, Silva PA, Walz K and Young JI (2010). Unconventional transcriptional response to environmental enrichment in a mouse model of Rett syndrome. *PLoS One* 5: e11534.

Khwaja OS, Ho E, Barnes KV, O'leary HM, Pereira LM, Finkelstein Y, Nelson CA, 3Rd, Vogel-Farley V, Degregorio G, Holm IA, Khatwa U, Kapur K, Alexander ME, Finnegan DM, Cantwell NG, Walco AC, Rappaport L, Gregas M, Fichorova RN, Shannon MW, Sur M and Kaufmann WE (2014). Safety, pharmacokinetics, and preliminary assessment of efficacy of mecasermin (re-combinant human IGF-1) for the treatment of Rett syndrome. *Proc Natl Acad Sci U S A* 111: 4596–4601.

Klein ME, Lioy DT, Ma L, Impey S, Mandel G and Goodman RH (2007). Homeostatic regulation of MeCP2 expression by a CREB-induced microRNA. *Nat Neurosci* 10: 1513–1514.

Kline DD, Ogier M, Kunze DL and Katz DM (2010). Exogenous brain-derived neurotrophic factor rescues synaptic dysfunction in Mecp2-null mice. *J Neurosci* 30: 5303–5310.

Kondo M, Gray LJ, Pelka GJ, Christodoulou J, Tam PP and Hannan AJ (2008). Environmental enrichment ameliorates a motor coordination deficit in a mouse model of Rett syndrome--Mecp2 gene dosage effects and BDNF expression. *Eur J Neurosci* 27: 3342–3350.

Kondo MA, Gray LJ, Pelka GJ, Leang SK, Christodoulou J, Tam PP and Hannan AJ (2015). Affective dysfunction in a mouse model of Rett syndrome: Therapeutic effects of environmental stimulation and physical activity. *Dev Neurobiol* 76: 209–224.

Kosai K, et al. (2005). Rett Syndrome Is Reversible and Treatable by MeCP2 Gene Therapy into the Striatum in Mice. *Mol Ther* 11(Suppl 1): S24.

Kriaucionis S and Bird A (2004). The major form of MeCP2 has a novel N-terminus generated by alternative splicing. *Nucleic Acids Res* 32: 1818–1823.

Larimore JL, Chapleau CA, Kudo S, Theibert A, Percy AK and Pozzo-Miller L (2009). Bdnf overexpression in hippocampal neurons prevents dendritic atrophy caused by Rett-associated MECP2 mutations. *Neurobiol Dis* 34: 199–211.

Lekman A, Witt-Engerstrom I, Gottfries J, Hagberg BA, Percy AK and Svennerholm L (1989). Rett syndrome: biogenic amines and metabolites in postmortem brain. *Pediatr Neurol* 5: 357–362.

Lekman A, Witt-Engerstrom I, Holmberg B, Percy A, Svennerholm L and Hagberg B (1990). CSF and urine biogenic amine metabolites in Rett syndrome. *Clin Genet* 37: 173–178.

Leoncini S, De Felice C, Signorini C, Pecorelli A, Durand T, Valacchi G, Ciccoli L and Hayek J (2011). Oxidative stress in Rett syndrome: natural history, genotype, and variants. *Redox Rep* 16: 145–153.

Lioy DT, Garg SK, Monaghan CE, Raber J, Foust KD, Kaspar BK, Hirrlinger PG, Kirchhoff F, Bissonnette JM, Ballas N and Mandel G (2011). A role for glia in the progression of Rett's syndrome. *Nature* 475: 497–500.

Lonetti G, Angelucci A, Morando L, Boggio EM, Giustetto M and Pizzorusso T (2010). Early environmental enrichment moderates the behavioral and synaptic phenotype of MeCP2 null mice. *Biol Psychiatry* 67: 657–665.

Luikenhuis S, Giacometti E, Beard CF and Jaenisch R (2004). Expression of MeCP2 in postmitotic neurons rescues Rett syndrome in mice. *Proc Natl Acad Sci U S A* 101: 6033–6038.

Maffei S, De Felice C, Cannarile P, Leoncini S, Signorini C, Pecorelli A, Montomoli B, Lunghetti S, Ciccoli L, Durand T, Favilli R and Hayek J (2014). Effects of omega-3 PUFAs supplementation on myocardial function and oxidative stress markers in typical Rett syndrome. *Mediators Inflamm* 2014: 983178.

Martinowich K, Hattori D, Wu H, Fouse S, He F, Hu Y, Fan G and Sun YE (2003). DNA methylation-related chromatin remodeling in activity-dependent BDNF gene regulation. *Science* 302: 890–893.

Mnatzakanian GN, Lohi H, Munteanu I, Alfred SE, Yamada T, Macleod PJ, Jones JR, Scherer SW, Schanen NC, Friez MJ, Vincent JB and Minassian BA (2004). A previously unidentified MECP2 open reading frame defines a new protein isoform relevant to Rett syndrome. *Nat Genet* 36: 339–341.

Moretti P, Levenson JM, Battaglia F, Atkinson R, Teague R, Antalffy B, Armstrong D, Arancio O, Sweatt JD and Zoghbi HY (2006). Learning and memory and synaptic plasticity are impaired in a mouse model of Rett syndrome. *J Neurosci* 26: 319–327.

Nag N, Moriuchi JM, Peitzman CG, Ward BC, Kolodny NH and Berger-Sweeney JE (2009). Environmental enrichment alters locomotor behaviour and ventricular volume in Mecp2 1lox mice. *Behav Brain Res* 196: 44–48.

Nectoux J, Florian C, Delepine C, Bahi-Buisson N, Khelfaoui M, Reibel S, Chelly J and Bienvenu T (2012). Altered microtubule dynamics in Mecp2-deficient astrocytes. *J Neurosci Res* 90: 990–998.

Nithianantharajah J and Hannan AJ (2006). Enriched environments, experience-dependent plasticity and disorders of the nervous system. *Nat Rev Neurosci* 7: 697–709.

Ogier M, Wang H, Hong E, Wang Q, Greenberg ME and Katz DM (2007). Brain-derived neurotrophic factor expression and respiratory function improve after ampakine treatment in a mouse model of Rett syndrome. *J Neurosci* 27: 10912–10917.

Ormazabal A, Garcia-Cazorla A, Perez-Duenas B, Gonzalez V, Fernandez-Alvarez E, Pineda M, Campistol J and Artuch R (2006). Determination of 5-methyltetrahydrofolate in cerebrospinal fluid of paediatric patients: reference values for a paediatric population. *Clin Chim Acta* 371: 159–162.

Pelka GJ, Watson CM, Christodoulou J and Tam PP (2005). Distinct expression profiles of Mecp2 transcripts with different lengths of 3'UTR in the brain and visceral organs during mouse development. *Genomics* 85: 441–452.

Plioplys AV and Kasnicka I (1993). L-carnitine as a treatment for Rett syndrome. *South Med J* 86: 1411–1412.

Plochl E, Sperl W, Wermuth B and Colombo JP (1996). [Carnitine deficiency and carnitine therapy in a patient with Rett syndrome]. *Klin Padiatr* 208: 129–134.

Rastegar M, Hotta A, Pasceri P, Makarem M, Cheung AY, Elliott S, Park KJ, Adachi M, Jones FS, Clarke ID, Dirks P and Ellis J (2009). MECP2 isoform-specific vectors with regulated expression for Rett syndrome gene therapy. *PLoS One* 4: e6810.

Reichwald K, Thiesen J, Wiehe T, Weitzel J, Poustka WA, Rosenthal A, Platzer M, Stratling WH and Kioschis P (2000). Comparative sequence analysis of the MECP2-locus in human and mouse reveals new transcribed regions. *Mamm Genome* 11: 182–190.

Roux JC, Dura E, Moncla A, Mancini J and Villard L (2007). Treatment with desipramine improves breathing and survival in a mouse model for Rett syndrome. *Eur J Neurosci* 25: 1915–1922.

Ruch A, Kurczynski TW and Velasco ME (1989). Mitochondrial alterations in Rett syndrome. *Pediatr Neurol* 5: 320–323.

Shahbazian M, Young J, Yuva-Paylor L, Spencer C, Antalffy B, Noebels J, Armstrong D, Paylor R and Zoghbi H (2002). Mice with truncated MeCP2 recapitulate many Rett syndrome features and display hyperacetylation of histone H3. *Neuron* 35: 243–254.

Sierra C, Vilaseca MA, Brandi N, Artuch R, Mira A, Nieto M and Pineda M (2001). Oxidative stress in Rett syndrome. *Brain Dev* 23 Suppl 1: S236–239.

Signorini C, De Felice C, Leoncini S, Durand T, Galano JM, Cortelazzo A, Zollo G, Guerranti R, Gonnelli S, Caffarelli C, Rossi M, Pecorelli A, Valacchi G, Ciccoli L and Hayek J (2014). Altered erythrocyte membrane fatty acid profile in typical Rett syndrome: effects of omega-3 polyunsaturated fatty acid supplementation. *Prostaglandins Leukot Essent Fatty Acids* 91: 183–193.

Skene PJ, Illingworth RS, Webb S, Kerr AR, James KD, Turner DJ, Andrews R and Bird AP (2010). Neuronal MeCP2 is expressed at near histone-octamer levels and globally alters the chromatin state. *Mol Cell* 37: 457–468.

Toward MA, Abdala AP, Knopp SJ, Paton JF and Bissonnette JM (2013). Increasing brain serotonin corrects CO2 chemosensitivity in methyl-CpG-binding protein 2 (Mecp2)-deficient mice. *Exp Physiol* 98: 842–849.

Tropea D, Giacometti E, Wilson NR, Beard C, Mccurry C, Fu DD, Flannery R, Jaenisch R and Sur M (2009). Partial reversal of Rett Syndrome-like symptoms in MeCP2 mutant mice. *Proc Natl Acad Sci U S A* 106: 2029–2034.

Van Esch H, Bauters M, Ignatius J, Jansen M, Raynaud M, Hollanders K, Lugtenberg D, Bienvenu T, Jensen LR, Gecz J, Moraine C, Marynen P, Fryns JP and Froyen G (2005). Duplication of the MECP2 region is a frequent cause of severe mental retardation and progressive neurological symptoms in males. *Am J Hum Genet* 77: 442–453.

Vecsler M, Ben Zeev B, Nudelman I, Anikster Y, Simon AJ, Amariglio N, Rechavi G, Baasov T and Gak E (2011). Ex vivo treatment with a novel synthetic aminoglycoside NB54 in primary fibroblasts from Rett syndrome patients suppresses MECP2 nonsense mutations. *PLoS One* 6: e20733.

Viemari JC, Bevengut M, Burnet H, Coulon P, Pequignot JM, Tiveron MC and Hilaire G (2004). Phox2a gene, A6 neurons, and noradrenaline are essential for development of normal respiratory rhythm in mice. *J Neurosci* 24: 928–937.

Viemari JC, Roux JC, Tryba AK, Saywell V, Burnet H, Pena F, Zanella S, Bevengut M, Barthelemy-Requin M, Herzing LB, Moncla A, Mancini J, Ramirez JM, Villard L and Hilaire G (2005). Mecp2 deficiency disrupts norepinephrine and respiratory systems in mice. *J Neurosci* 25: 11521–11530.

Wang J, Wegener JE, Huang TW, Sripathy S, De Jesus-Cortes H, Xu P, Tran S, Knobbe W, Leko V, Britt J, Starwalt R, Mcdaniel L, Ward CS, Parra D, Newcomb B, Lao U, Nourigat C, Flowers DA, Cullen S, Jorstad NL, Yang Y, Glaskova L, Vigneau S, Kozlitina J, Yetman MJ, Jankowsky JL, Reichardt SD, Reichardt HM, Gartner J, Bartolomei MS, Fang M, Loeb K, Keene CD, Bernstein I, Goodell M, Brat D J, Huppke P, Neul JL, Bedalov A and Pieper AA (2015). Wild-type microglia do not reverse pathology in mouse models of Rett syndrome. *Nature* 521: E1–4.

Weese-Mayer DE, Lieske SP, Boothby CM, Kenny AS, Bennett HL, Silvestri JM and Ramirez JM (2006). Autonomic nervous system dysregulation: breathing and heart rate perturbation during wakefulness in young girls with Rett syndrome. *Pediatr Res* 60: 443–449.

Weng SM, Mcleod F, Bailey ME and Cobb SR (2011). Synaptic plasticity deficits in an experimental model of rett syndrome: long-term potentiation saturation and its pharmacological reversal. *Neuroscience* 180: 314–321.

Xu X, Kozikowski AP and Pozzo-Miller L (2014). A selective histone deacetylase-6 inhibitor improves BDNF trafficking in hippocampal neurons from Mecp2 knockout mice: implications for Rett syndrome. *Front Cell Neurosci* 8: 68.

Young JI, Hong EP, Castle JC, Crespo-Barreto J, Bowman AB, Rose MF, Kang D, Richman R, Johnson JM, Berget S and Zoghbi HY (2005). Regulation of RNA splicing by the methylation-dependent transcriptional repressor methyl-CpG binding protein 2. *Proc Natl Acad Sci U S A* 102: 17551–17558.

Zanella S, Mebarek S, Lajard AM, Picard N, Dutschmann M and Hilaire G (2008). Oral treatment with desipramine improves breathing and life span in Rett syndrome mouse model. *Respir Physiol Neurobiol* 160: 116–121.

Zhou Z, Hong EJ, Cohen S, Zhao WN, Ho HY, Schmidt L, Chen WG, Lin Y, Savner E, Griffith EC, Hu L, Steen JA, Weitz CJ. and Greenberg ME (2006). Brain-specific phosphorylation of MeCP2 regulates activity-dependent Bdnf transcription, dendritic growth, and spine maturation. *Neuron* 52: 255–269.

Zoghbi HY, Milstien S, Butler IJ, Smith EO, Kaufman S, Glaze DG and Percy AK (1989). Cerebrospinal fluid biogenic amines and biopterin in Rett syndrome. *Ann Neurol* 25: 56–60.

Zoghbi HY, Percy AK, Glaze DG, Butler IJ and Riccardi VM (1985). Reduction of biogenic amine levels in the Rett syndrome. *N Engl J Med* 313: 921–924.

15
REHABILITATION IN RETT SYNDROME

Sarojini Budden

Introduction

Rett syndrome (RTT) is not a degenerative condition and, therefore, the potential for functional development is difficult to measure since the expression of *MECP2* mutations on neurobiological mechanisms change with age. Brain immaturity in RTT Armstrong 1992; Armstrong et al. 1995 provides opportunities to encourage development of new skills and maintain current function. Studies on knock out mice placed in challenging learning environments show learning and development of neural pathways (Kondo et al. 2005). This evidence provides opportunities for intervention in enriched environments to maximize abilities and facilitate emerging skills. Females with RTT typically survive into adulthood (Kirby et al. 2010; Anderson et al. 2014), which requires their physicians to provide long-term care and treatment.

Partnerships in care

Against this background, a physician caring for individuals with RTT is challenged in providing continuity of coordinated care with primary physicians, subspecialists, therapists, social services, educational systems, and above all, the parents or caregivers, who are important members of this team. By creating partnerships there are opportunities to share current understanding of the biological mechanisms that may impact on individuals with RTT. Partnerships should be child and family-centered, community-based, accessible, comprehensive, continuous, collaborative, compassionate, communicative, and culturally competent. There is increasing evidence to support this view and studies have shown improved learning and maintenance of motor function (Lotan et al. 2004). Management draws heavily on clinical experience and general principles applied to other neurodevelopmental disorders. The overarching principle in rehabilitation is maintaining medical stability and providing continuity of therapy.

Assessments should identify seizures, sleep disorders, respiratory problems, dysphagia, reflux, gall stones, constipation, scoliosis, and osteoporosis, as well as other precipitating causes for agitation and behavioral dysfunctions. Careful documentation of growth, dental status, vision, hearing, and EEGs for long QTc and peripheral autonomic disturbances is essential. Radiological studies are carried out when indicated, including dual-energy X-ray absorptiometry (DEXA) scans.

Emotion and behavior

The biological underpinnings of emotional and behavioral disturbances probably result from dysfunctions in mono-aminergic systems secondary to genetic mutations and are age related (Banerjee et al. 2012). Neuropathological studies have shown high binding of serotonin type 1 and 2 receptors in the brainstem, reflecting the immaturity of the neurons. Neurochemical changes in the synapses of cortical and subcortical regions of the brain and alterations in synaptic function (Blue et al. 1999) further support possible mechanisms for behavioral disturbances. Hypofunction of noradrenaline and serotonin are present as early as 36 weeks of gestational age (Nomura et al. 1984; Nomura and Segawa 1990, 2001) and may explain the placidity noted in infants and toddlers. Early behavioral changes are replaced by sleep disturbances, crying, irritability, followed by social withdrawal and loss of language and hand use. Subsequently, disruptive behaviors such as screaming, hair pulling, biting, hitting, pacing, anxiety, inattentiveness, and hyperactivity are reported in 5–10-year-old girls. This behavior may also result from increased glutamate levels in early childhood (Lappalainen and Riikonen 1996; Naidu et al. 2001). It is well recognized that cortisol levels are elevated in anxiety and stress and elevated corticotrophin release factor has also been documented in an RTT mouse model (McGill et al. 2006).

Other neurotransmitter abnormalities, such as elevated levels of B-endorphins (Budden et al. 1990a) and decreasing levels of biogenic amines with age (Zoghbi et al. 1985; Budden et al. 1990a) further support the biological basis for behavior disorders in RTT. The range of behavioral abnormalities in RTT includes the following:

1. Behaviors that may result from an impaired autonomic nervous system include respiratory disturbances, agitation, panic-like attacks, disordered arousal and sleep, mood changes, intermittent strabismus, tremors, myoclonic jerks, abnormal motor activity, gastrointestinal dysfunction, vasomotor changes, cardiac irregularities, and fluctuating blood pressure.
2. Undesired behaviors may result from unrecognized medical conditions such as seizures, dental problems, ear infections, reflux, constipation, gall stones, renal stones, fractures, dystonic spasms at night, menstrual discomfort, sleep apnea, and day-time sleepiness. Clinicians must remain alert in making a correct diagnosis before treating.
3. In maturing girls, depression is suspected based on history of sleeplessness, poor appetite, weight loss, and lack of interest in activities they previously enjoyed. Although other reasons for unexplained crying, sadness, and loneliness can result from changes in school, in caregivers, loss of social contacts, and school peers, sometimes agitation and negative reaction can result from changes in daily routine and unrecognized abuse.

Some individuals using augmentative communication programs can assist providers in understanding their feelings and emotions. A knowledgeable team can assist in addressing these issues in the most effective way with the family, care provider, and staff at activity centers and make a major difference in the individual's life. Management is based on a clear understanding of causes of particular behaviors and providing appropriate treatment.

Various medications are available for use, such as neuroleptics for injurious behavior, mood stabilizers, antidepressants, and anxiolytics such as selective serotonin reuptake inhibitors (SSRIs) and serotonin and norepinephrine reuptake inhibitors (SNRIs) for obsessive behaviors. Responses are variable among individuals with RTT.

Motor Function
FACTORS AFFECTING MOBILITY

Changing tone

Hypotonia is well documented in the majority of infants, toddlers, and preschoolers with RTT. Children who have not sat up by the age of 2 years seldom acquire ambulation and generally are more affected medically and developmentally. Rigidity is noted between 5 and 9 years of age. The first sign is rigidity in heel cords with increased ankle reflexes and is frequently asymmetrical. Radiological studies of spine and hips have not revealed any localized abnormalities, and neither have brain and spinal cord MRIs shown any asymmetries. This problem probably originates in the cerebral cortex.

Extrapyramidal motor dysfunction and onset of rigidity are a result of decreasing dopamine levels with age (Budden et al. 1990). Bruxism, oculogyric crises, bradykinesia, and proximal myoclonus are also noted. Leg length discrepancy is being recognized as being frequently associated with asymmetric posture. Thorough evaluation of the spine, hip, and leg measurements are necessary. If the discrepancy is over 19 mm then shoe lifts should be considered.

Medical management of dystonia/rigidity is a challenge as it impairs motor function. It is often noted in the extremities and in the neck, and may result in intermittent painful spasms and discomfort; it also may be one of the causes for frequent night awakenings. Medical treatment includes diazepam at bedtime. Trihexylphenidyl and other anti-Parkinson drugs such as carbidopa/levodopa have been used with variable results. Oral baclofen is minimally effective since large doses result in undesirable sedative effects. Baclofen pumps are successful in controlling dystonia in older females, but the drawbacks are a need for team management and monitoring, and it is an expensive proposition for many families.

Dronabinol (2.5 mg/day) was shown to be very effective in one patient with acute dystonia that was unresponsive to other commonly used medications. She was monitored as an in-patient and a trial of weaning her off it was unsuccessful in maintaining lower tone and comfort. She remains on 2.5 mg once a day without any side effects. Other options include warm baths, massages, and aquatic therapy.

Deformities

Older women often have deformities of ankles and feet, asymmetrical hip positions with obliquity, scoliosis with or without kyphosis, restricted flexion extension of the elbows, difficulty with supination/pronation of the forearm, hand and finger deformities, and abnormal postures of the jaw with malalignment. Protracted and retracted shoulders impact on swallowing and should be considered if the individual presents with swallowing difficulties. Unfortunately, physical therapy interventions and monitoring can become infrequent with age and should be addressed, and efforts made to continue therapy.

Fractures

Osteoporosis has been recognized with increasing frequency (Hass et al. 1997; Leonard et al. 1999) and supported by bone histomorphometric studies (Budden and Gunness 2003; Shapiro et al. 2010). Individuals are treated preventively with vitamin D and sufficient intake of calcium, folic acid, and vitamin C. If an ambulatory child suddenly stops weight bearing and walking, she must be assessed for a fracture and treated appropriately. Loss of motor function in RTT is never a sudden event and minimal injury can result in fractures of small and long bones. Another reason for avoiding weight bearing is swollen, painful feet as a result of regional sympathetic dystrophy. Management requires long-term multidisciplinary treatment including physical therapy, and pain-relieving measures including medications, sympathetic/somatic blockade, and spinal analgesia. Elevating feet during sitting and sleeping is useful, along with padded shoes.

Scoliosis

Scoliosis occurs in 85% of individuals with RTT and probably has a neurogenic basis. Girls with severe hypotonia are prone to developing it early. Onset is usually between 8 and 11 years and progresses with age. About 64% of girls below 6 years of age show spinal curvature and in 17% it remains unchanged. Individuals with significant hypotonia show scoliosis as early as 2 years of age and it progresses rapidly, resulting in serious secondary respiratory, gastrointestinal, and orthopedic problems. It is best treated with a soft neoprene brace to stabilize the trunk. Seating posture is extremely important and slouching on the couch watching television is to be avoided.

Sitting on a firm surface while wearing the brace and with feet supported resting at a 90 degree angle is optimal. Standing for short periods of time such as 10 to 15 minutes in a stander at home or school is very beneficial. Those individuals with better balance should use a treadmill with support.

Early weight bearing and improving postural alignment is essential (Hanks 1990; Lotan and Hanks 2006). Scoliosis is influenced by loss of equilibrium responses, poor spatial perception, loss of transitional motor skills due to dyspraxia, onset of rigidity, and pelvic asymmetry with leg length discrepancy. Encouraging balance and spatial perception using a therapy ball, weighted vests, or neoprene suits makes a notable difference.

When young children with RTT start to lean to one side or another and compulsively wring their hands then postural changes occur in the trunk and spine. Using bilateral soft neoprene elbow braces or weighted wrist bands assist in keeping hands down and away from compulsive wringing. Guidelines for management of scoliosis (Downs et al. 2009) provide a comprehensive approach to management.

MEDICAL AND THERAPEUTIC MANAGEMENT FOR MOBILITY

Anemia may exaggerate underlying hypotonia and needs treatment. Hypotonia responds to oral L-carnitine in a dose of 75 mg/kg/day in three separate doses; it also has been found to be very effective in improving tone, strength, general health, and appetite. It can also help alleviate constipation. It is important to coordinate use of carnitine with the physical therapist monitoring improvement. L-Carnitine may have a preventative role in improving cardiac dysautonomia (Guideri et al. 1999, 2005; Byard 2006) and general health (Ellaway et al. 2001).

Hip support shorts are used in young children to promote stability at the hip joints and bring them into adduction to facilitate movement, improve sitting, and assist in standing. Another option is to use neoprene vests to stabilize a hypotonic trunk.

It is crucial that all young children bear weight to promote adequate skeletal integrity and aid proper development of the acetabulum to prevent subluxation or dislocation of the hip. Standing also improves spatial perception. The focus is on getting children upright for future transfers if ambulation is restricted.

Prone or supine standers can also be used. Treadmills and walkers are introduced based on the individual's age, abilities, space at home, transportation, and use in school (Lotan and Hanks 2006).

Ankle foot orthoses (AFOs) are commonly used to maintain the foot in a neutral position and prevent deformities. Girls with marked hypotonia and hyperextended knees benefit from using higher AFOs. These are worn inside the shoes comfortably. Botulinum neurotoxin type A (BoNT-A) injections, along with use of AFOs, are very useful in maintaining the foot position correctly. In some individuals, serial casting may be necessary, along with BoNT-A, to maintain adequate stretch on the heel cords. Night splints are used for positioning.

Aquatic therapy is introduced as early as 2 years of age to help children weight bear and use their limbs in a reciprocal fashion. The buoyancy they experience helps maintain an upright posture. Girls have achieved ambulation as late as 8, 12, and 16 years (in the author's personal experience) refuting the early theories that RTT was degenerative (Bumin et al. 2003).

Hippotherapy, or horseback riding, could effectively maintain an upright posture, improves balance, delays onset of scoliosis, prevents hip problems, alleviates constipation, and provides added benefits in socialization with other people of all ages, giving a sense of independence (Whalen and Case-Smith 2012; O'Haire 2013).

Individuals with RTT who suddenly refuse to weight bear should be evaluated for fractures in the lower extremities. Other causes are peripheral neuropathy causing pain on weight bearing. Raising an individual's legs and providing stockings and padded shoes to aid weight bearing can be helpful. Painful feet respond well to gabapentin.

Surgical interventions become necessary in individuals who present with fractures, dislocated hips, marked untreated equinus deformity, or who are unresponsive to therapy and medical management. Surgery becomes necessary with increasing scoliosis of 40 degree angle or more.

UPPER EXTREMITY FUNCTION AND EVALUATION

Changing pattern of hand involvement

Girls with RTT may develop typical hand use and a pincer grasp, which can persist in a few girls, but the majority revert to a palmar grasp or raking movements. Ability to maintain sustained grasp is affected, causing them to drop objects or leaving them unable to complete a grasping movement (Nomura et al. 1984). Girls with RTT may show intention, but dyspraxia or apraxia affects function. Abnormal hand movements might be very subtle in infants, becoming more evident as development progresses when further hand use is expected. Philippart (1992) observed that the hand postures are a typical developmental pattern in infants who persist having minimal functional improvement.

Characteristics of hand movements

Abnormal hand movements, or stereotypies, are one of the classic signs of RTT. Initially, they are non-specific hand waving, hand mouthing, or clapping. Others have noted movements such as peculiar rubbing movements of the hands on either side, hand washing movements in the midline with wringing or squeezing, or rubbing the backs of the hands. Others frequently tap their chest or pull at their hair or clothes, put their hands in their mouths, bite their fingers, or poke at their eyes. Hand movements are often repetitive, distinctive in their pattern, and asymmetrical, with the dominant hand showing stereotyped movements while the other hand may remain more or less inactive (Hagberg et al. 1983).

Factors affecting hand movements

Hand movements often vary with changes in respiration and emotions (Elian and Rudolf 1996). Anxiety, anger, happiness, or excitement may increase frequency and intensity of movements and are often accompanied by bruxism, hyperventilation, squeezing of the eyes, and occasionally tremors. Interestingly, these movements subside during sleep and change with age and maturation. The frequency of hand movements decreases with onset of rigidity, presence of flexion contractures, or marked adduction of the thumb. Hands may be held folded in front with tapping or strumming movements, with little function in adults.

Elastic wrist weights are the least restrictive option for low intensity hand patterning. Soft neoprene elbow sleeves give a tactile cue, emphasizing elbow extension, and break up hand patterning for younger girls. A neoprene sleeve with a rigid thermoplastic insert is helpful for a school-aged child who is a more 'driven' to engage in hand patterning (Naganuma and Bellingsley 1998). An orthotic rigid elbow extension may be the best option for an older girl who engages in self-harming behaviors, such as hitting her face or eyes and thus causing injuries. Hand splints include thumb abduction splints or protective gloves to reduce skin breakdown. The possibility of increased agitation as a result of wearing splints should be noted.

Splints are only rarely used during sleep. It is frequently observed that elbow splints may only be worn during purposeful play and while using hand-activated communication devices. Individuals who are mobile and bring their hands up to their chest may develop lateral flexion, which exacerbates scoliosis. Often, the use of wrist weights or soft elbow splints facilitates a more typical gait pattern, since girls with RTT wring their hands in front or to the side, and over time, it can affect their posture resulting in scoliosis (McClure et al. 1998).

Evaluation for activities of daily living

An essential part of activities of daily living management requires a clear understanding of the person's developmental stage for feeding, communication, hand use, mobility, and neurological stability, and a holistic solution should be provided.

FEEDING

Common parental concerns are chewing, swallowing, choking, gagging, spitting up, drooling, and the time it takes to feed an individual with RTT. Clearly there are differences based on age, motor skills, tone, associated medical problems, the caregiver's experience, and oral motor development.

Feeding specialist/speech therapist

A feeding specialist or speech therapist assesses oral motor function, tongue and jaw placement, sensory issues that interfere with accepting certain textures, consistencies and flavors of foods, swallowing of liquids, soft solids, and regular foods. Abnormal tone affects oral-motor function, neck posture, and position. The therapist can also provide insights into communication, making food choices, accepting or refusing foods, and can assess risk factors for aspiration.

Nutritionist/dietician

A nutritionist or dietician is an essential member of the team who will assess whether girls with RTT are receiving adequate caloric and nutritional intake and they will assist parents, other therapists and the individual's physician with recommendations regarding varieties of foods, caloric boosters, daily requirements, and amounts. In conjunction with the physician, laboratory assessments are performed to rule out anemia, assess nutritional risk for osteoporosis, and give advice on adequate caloric intake using a variety of foods best tolerated by the person.

Occupational therapist

An occupational therapist will evaluate proper seating, head and neck positioning, tone, and the person's ability to self-feed using hands and/or utensils. Assistive devices such as a universal cuff allow using a spoon or fork with greater ease, or an elbow splint to prevent interference with the opposite hand (Sharpe and Ottenbacher 1990).

The decision to use gastrostomy tube to feed an individual is based on several factors, for example, significant growth failure and weight loss, chronic dehydration, low body mass index, dysphagia, severe and frequent vomiting, recurrent aspiration pneumonias, fatigue during feeding, increased feeding time, and associated serious medical problems (Motil et al. 2009).

COMMUNICATION

Morphological studies of the cytoarchitecture of the speech areas of the brain (Belichenko et al. 1994), indicate the existence of an interhemispheric difference that forms part of the infrastructure for speech processing and support clinical observations that girls with RTT have better receptive language skills than expressive language skills. Late speech onset has been noted and reported in individuals with RTT (Kerr et al. 2001).

Girls with RTT use intense eye gaze to communicate and fixate on food or toys they want, but are restricted because of dyspraxia and hand tremors that are often observed while reaching. They also have response latency, probably as a result of delayed ipsi-contralateral auditory responses (Pelson and Budden 1987), and/or low hearing thresholds.

Girls with RTT may display frustration, including agitation and self-injurious behavior, due to lack of communicative abilities. Clinical observations consistently identify that restricting stereotypic activity of the less dominant hand will facilitate functional use of the dominant hand. Gently blocking the arm or applying deep pressure decreases the intense need to bring hands together and provides relaxation, improves focus, and facilitates intentional hand use (Aaron 1990).

The majority of individuals with RTT do not have expressive verbal language and should be introduced to a variety of assisted augmentative communication AAC programs.

Therapists providing treatment should take into consideration the level of cognitive function, delayed response latency, delayed auditory processing, oral-motor dyspraxia, and dysarthria. The majority of girls with RTT develop 'cause and effect', a basic underpinning for learning and it has been documented that girls with RTT have this basic ability to learn and comprehend (Budden et al. 1990b) and are able to participate in AAC, which has become an accepted option for therapies in school and at home.

AUGMENTATIVE COMMUNICATION

When assessing individuals for augmentative communication, the following prerequisites should be assessed: communicative intent, object permanence, cause and effect, the ability to follow directions, the ability to make choices, a receptive function of at least 18 months, and effective eye gaze. All individuals with RTT have a communicative intent. It is important for the therapist to believe in the person's ability to respond and to be able to understand her emotions, facial expressions, eye gaze, body language, and give her time to respond (Lotan 2007a). It is necessary to communicate this information to her therapist, school staff, and her care providers. Participation in daily activities, being able to express needs, ideas, and emotions should be considered in providing opportunities for expression (Djukic et al. 2012), and cognitive development (Fabio et al. 2013).Various ways to encourage expression are through understanding her eye blinks, facial expressions, intense eye gaze, and using symbols for yes/no. There are a variety of AAC devices such flash cards, picture exchange communication systems, communication boards, head pointers, switch activated systems, voice output devices, computers with touch screens, and eye tracking technology (Lotan 2007a).

MUSIC THERAPY

Many individuals with neurodevelopmental disorders respond well to music and those with RTT also show a very positive response to music therapy. Music definitely calms agitated behavior, improves attention, eye gaze, and responses. Most girls prefer certain types of music, will express their likes and dislikes, and demonstrate an ability to learn and retain it over time (Elefant 2011; Wigram and Lawrence 2001). Unfortunately, music programs are not being used consistently in school curricula because of a lack of experienced therapists and the costs involved.

EDUCATIONAL CURRICULUM

Current educational systems in the USA and other parts of the world require that each person with a developmental disorder have an Individualized Educational Plan (IEP).

This is developed in conjunction with the therapist providing treatment and the special educational teacher, will take into account the resources that particular school has, and will have the approval of the parent or care provider. Teachers' aides assist in carrying out the individualized program and access to the child's environment through various therapies. A coordinated effort is made to facilitate and maintain an individual's skills and the IEP is reviewed frequently. At the request of the parent, the IEP is incorporated into the curriculum. In some countries, school programs for children with developmental disorders are provided until 21 years of age. Mainstreaming of children with special educational needs for certain social activities such as recess, lunch breaks, music, and gym are included, and the curriculum is modified to provide services such as a life skills program, in classroom settings, resource rooms, and learning centers.

Many school districts have nursing support to monitor the effect of health related issues that may impact on the person's curriculum and also assist in coordinating with health care providers and community services.

Transportation of individuals with RTT is a necessary aspect that needs attention and assistance of the physical therapist to ensure safety and comfort.

PSYCHOSOCIAL SUPPORT

A team approach in caring for individuals with RTT provides parents and caregivers reassurance and support, in that they can access any member of the team familiar with their daughter and who is able to answer their questions, or access required medical services. An important member of the team is either a nurse or social worker who is familiar with the family, is well informed about RTT, and is knowledgeable about how to access community services, respite care, and financial support, as well as being available to counsel parents, siblings, grandparents, close friends, and neighbors. Each family has individual needs and it is important that family strengths and their support systems be identified. Medical management requires access to several different subspecialists that are best coordinated through a team approach; sharing information between the therapists providing treatment and the school is crucial to coordinated, continued management. Parent support groups in most US states as well as internationally, have been of tremendous support to many families.

Care for adult individuals with Rett syndrome

There are a variety of ways adults with developmental disorders, including RTT, are cared for internationally. The majority of young women live in small group homes or foster care. On rare occasions, families have made provisions for continued care in their own homes and have planned for the future when they are unable to carry on doing so. Parents of young adults with RTT relate that some young women start to use simple two or three word sentences in making requests (author's personal experience) and others have started to walk or showed improved hand use (Jacobsen et al. 2001); this provides evidence that RTT is not a degenerative condition. Hence, it is essential that living in enriched environments, the provision of adult therapy services, and the ability to access activity centers are made available to enable access opportunities and allow adults with RTT to become assimilated within society. Continuity of good medical and therapeutic involvement remains a major challenge for all.

Conclusion

In sum, a comprehensive and multidisciplinary approach to the care of individuals with RTT seems to be the most successful. This is particularly the case for non-pharmacological, rehabilitative interventions, such as those reviewed here and in the literature (Lotan and Hanks 2006; Lotan 2007a, b; Downs et al. 2014).

REFERENCES

Aron M (1990) The use and effectiveness of elbow splints in the Rett syndrome. *Brain Dev* 12: 162–163.

Amir RE, Van den Veyver IB, Wan M, Tran CQ, Franke U, Zoghbi H (1999) Rett syndrome caused by mutations in X-linked MECP2, encoding methyl CpG binding protein 2. *Nat Genet* 23: 185–188.

Anderson A, Long K, Jacoby P, Downs J, Leonard H (2014) Twenty years of surveillance in Rett syndrome: What does this tell us? *Orphanet J Rare Dis* 9: 87.

Armstrong DD (1992) The neuropathology of Rett syndrome. *Brain Dev* 14(Suppl): 747–753.

Armstrong DD, Dunn JK, Antalffy B, Trivedi R (1995) Selective dendritic alterations in the cortex of Rett syndrome. *J Neuropathol Exp Neurol* 54: 195–201.

Banerjee A, Castro J, Sur M (2012) Rett syndrome: Genes, synapses, circuits, therapeutics. *Front Psychiatry* 3: Article 34, 1–13.

Belichenko PV, Oldorfs A, Hagberg B, Dahlstrom A (1994) Rett syndrome 3-D confocal microscopy of cortical pyramidal dendrites and afferents. *Neuro Report* 5: 1509–1513.

Blue ME, Naidu S, Johnston MV (1999) Altered development of glutamate and GABA receptors in basal ganglia of girls with Rett syndrome. *Exp Neurol* 156(2): 345–352.

Budden SS, Gunness ME (2003) Possible mechanisms of osteopenia in Rett syndrome. Bone histomorphometric studies. *J Child Neurol* 18(10): 698–702.

Budden SS, Myer EC, Butler IJ (1990a) Cerebrospinal fluid studies in Rett syndrome: Biogenic amines and beta-endorphins *Brain Dev* 12(1): 81–84.

Budden SS, Meek M, Henighan C (1990b) Communication and oral motor function in Rett syndrome. *Dev Med Child Neurol* 32(1): 51–55.

Budden SS, Dorsey H, Steiner R (2005) Clinical profile of a male with Rett syndrome. *Brain Dev* (Suppl 1): S69–S71.

Bumin G, Uyanik M, Yilmaz I, Kayihan H, Topcu M (2003) Hydrotherapy for Rett syndrome. *J Rehab Med* 35(1): 44–45.

Byard RW (2006) Forensic issues and possible mechanisms of sudden death in Rett syndrome. *J Clin Forensic Med* 13: 96–99.

Djukic A, McDermott MV, Mavrommatis K, Martins CL (2012) Rett syndrome: Basic features of visual processing – a pilot study. *Pediatr Neurol* 47: 25–29.

Downs J, Bergman A, Carter P et al. (2009) Guidelines for management of scoliosis in Rett syndrome patients based on expert consensus and clinical evidence. *Spine* 1: 34(17): E607–E617.

Downs J, Parkinson S, Ranelli S, Leonard H, Diener P, Lotan M (2014) Perspectives on hand function in girls and women with Rett syndrome. *Dev Neurorehabil* 17(3): 210–217.

Duncan JR, Patterson DS, Hoffman JM et al. (2010) Brain stem serotonergic deficiency in sudden infant death syndrome. *JAMA* 303(5): 430–437.

Elefant C (2011) Music therapy for individuals with Rett syndrome. *Int J Disab Human Dev* 8(4): 359–368.

Elian M, Rudolf N de M (1996) Observations on hand movements in Rett Syndrome: A pilot study. *Acta Neurol Scand* 94: 212–214.

Ellaway CJ, Peat J, Williams K, Leonard H, Christodoulou J (2001) Medium term open label trial of L-carnitine in Rett syndrome. *Brain Dev* 1: S85–S89.

Fabio RA, Castelli I, Marchetti A, Antonietti A (2013) Training communication abilities in Rett syndrome through reading and writing. *Front Psychol* 4: 911.

Guideri F, Acampa M, Hayek G, Zappella M, Di Perri T (1999) Reduced heart rate variability in patients affected with Rett syndrome. A possible explanation for sudden death. *Neuropediatrics* 30: 146–148.

Guideri F, Acampa M, Hayek Y, Zappella M (2005) Effects of acetyl-L-carnitine on cardiac dysautonomia in Rett syndrome: Prevention of death? *Pediatr Cardiol* 26(5): 574–577.

Hagberg B, Aicardi J, Dias K, Ramos O (1983) A progressive syndrome of autism, dementia, ataxia and loss of purposeful hand use in girls: Rett's syndrome: Report on 35 cases. *Ann Neurol* 14: 471–479.

Hagberg B, Berg M, Steffenberg U (2001) Three decades of socio-medical experiences from West Swedish Rett Females 4–60 years of age. *Brain Dev* 23: S28–S31.

Hanks SB (1990) Motor disabilities in Rett syndrome and physical therapy strategies. *Brain Dev* 1: 157–161.

Hass RH, Dixon SD, Sartoris DJ, Hennesy MJ (1997) Osteopenia in Rett syndrome. *J Pediatr* 131(5): 771–774.

Hodges MR, Wehner M, Aungst J, Smith JC, Richerson GB (2009) Transgenic mice lacking serotonin neurons have severe apnea and high mortality during development. *J Neurosci* 29: 10341–10349.

Jacobsen K, Viken A, von Tetzchner S (2001) Rett syndrome and aging. A case study. *Disabl Rehab* 23(3–4): 160–166.

Katz MD, Dutschmann, MT, Ramirez JM, Hilaire G (2009) Breathing disorders in Rett syndrome: progressive neurochemical dysfunction in the respiratory network after birth. *Respir Physiol Neurobiol* 168: 101–108.

Kerr AM, Julu PO (1999) Recent insights into hyperventilation from the study of Rett syndrome. *Arch Dis Child* 80: 384–387.

Kerr AM, Belichenko PV, Woodcock T, Woodcock M (2001) Mind and brain in Rett disorder. *Brain Dev* 23(Suppl 1): S44–S49.

Kirby RS, Lane JB, Childres J et al. (2010) Longevity in Rett syndrome analysis of North American Database. *J Pediatr* 56: 135–138.

Kondo M, Gray LJ, Pelka GJ, Christodoulou J, Tam PPL, Hannan AJ (2005) Environmental enrichment ameliorates a motor coordination deficit in mouse model of Rett syndrome – Mecp2 gene dose effects and BDNF exposure. *Euro J Neurosci* 27: 3342–3350.

Kondo MA, Gray LJ, Pelka GJ, et al. (2015) Affective dysfunction in a mouse model of Rett syndrome: Therapeutic effects of environmental stimulation and physical activity. *Dev Neurobiol* 76(2): 209–224.

Kosai K, Kusaga A, Isagai T, et al. (2005) Rett syndrome is reversible and treatable by MeCP2 gene therapy into the striatum in mice. *Mol Ther* 11(Suppl 1): S24.

Lappalainen R, Riikonen RS (1996) High levels of cerebrospinal fluid glutamate in Rett syndrome. *Pediatr Neurol* 15: 213–216.

Leonard H, Thomson MR, Glasson EJ et al. (1999) A population-based approach to the investigation of osteopenia in Rett syndrome. *Dev Med Child Neurol* 41(5): 323–328.

Lotan M (2007a) Alternative therapeutic intervention for individuals with Rett syndrome. *ScientificWorldJournal* 7: 698–714.

Lotan M (2007b) Assistive technology and supplementary treatment for individuals with Rett syndrome. *Sci World J* 12(7): 903–948.

Lotan M, Hanks SB (2006) Physical therapy interventions for individuals with Ret syndrome. *ScientificWorldJournal* 6: 1314–1338.

Lotan M, Isakov E, Merrick J (2004) Improving functional skills and physical fitness in children with Rett syndrome. *J Intellec Disabil Res* 48(8): 730–735.

McArthur AJ, Budden SS (1998) Sleep dysfunction in Rett syndrome. A trial of exogenous melatonin treatment. *Dev Med Child Neurol* 40(3): 186–192.

McClure MK, Battaglia C, McClure R (1998) The relationship of cumulative motor asymmetries in Rett syndrome. *Am J Occ Ther* 54(3): 196–204.

McGill BE, Bundle SF, Yaylaoglu MB, Carson JP, Thaller C, Zoghbi HY (2006) Enhanced anxiety and stress-induced corticosterone release are associated with increased Crh expression in a mouse model of Rett syndrome. *Proc Natl Acad Sci* 103: 18267–18272.

Motil KJ, Shultz RJ, Glaze DG, Armstrong D (2001) Oropharyngeal dysfunction and upper gastrointestinal dysmotility, a reflection of disturbances in the autonomic nervous system in Rett syndrome. In: Kerr A. and Witt-Engerstrom I, editors. *Rett Disorder and the Developing Brain*, p. 259. Oxford: Oxford University Press.

Motil KJ, Morrissey M, Caeg E, Barrish JO, Glaze DG (2009) Gastrostomy placement improves height and weight in girls with Rett syndrome. *J Pediatr Gastroenterol Nutr* 49(2): 237–242.

Naganuma GM, Bellingsley FE (1998) Effect of hand splints on stereotypic hand behavior of three girls with Rett syndrome. *Phys Ther* 68(5): 664–666.

Naidu S (1997) Rett syndrome: A disorder affecting early brain growth. *Ann Neurol* 42(1): 3–10.

Naidu S, Kauffmann WE, Abrams MT et al. (2001) Neuroimaging studies in Rett syndrome. *Brain Dev* 23 (Suppl 1): S62–S71.

Nomura Y, Segawa M (1990) Clinical features of early stage Rett syndrome. *Brain Dev* 12: 16–19.

Nomura Y, Segawa M (2001) The monoamine hypothesis in Rett syndrome. In: Rett disorder and the developing brain. Kerr A, Witt Engerström I (Eds). Oxford University Press. New York.

Nomura Y, Segawa M, Hasegawa M (1984) Rett syndrome-clinical studies and pathophysiological considerations. *Brain Dev* 6: 475–486.

O'Haire ME (2013) Animal-assisted intervention for autism spectrum disorder: a systematic literature review. J Autism Dev Disord 43: 1606–22.

Pelson RO, Budden SS (1987) Auditory brain stem response findings in Rett syndrome. *Brain Dev* 9(5): 514–516.

Philippart M (1992) Hand ringing in Rett syndrome. A normal developmental stage. *Pediatr Neurol* 8: 1977–1999.

Ronnett GV, Leopold D, Cai X, Hoffbeur K, Moses L, Hoffman E, Naidu S (2003) Olfactory biopsies demonstrate defect in neuronal development in Rett syndrome. *Ann Neurol* 54: 206–218.

Schanen NC, Kurczynski TW, Brunelle D (1998) Neonatal encephalopathy in two boys in families with recurrent Rett syndrome. *J Child Neurol* 13: 229–231.

Shapiro JR, Bibat G, Hiremath G et al. (2010) Bone mass in Rett syndrome: Association with clinical parameters and MECP2 mutations. *Pediatr Res* 68(5): 446–451.

Sharpe PA, Ottenbacher KJ (1990) Use of elbow restraint to improve finger-feeding skills in a child with Rett syndrome. *Am J Occup Ther* 44: 328–332.

Villard L, Cardoso AK, Chelly PJ (2000) Two affected boys in a Rett syndrome family: Clinical and molecular findings. *Neurology* 55: 1183–1193.

Weese-Mayer DE, Lieske SP, Boothy CM, Kenny AS, Bennett, HL, Ramirez JM (2008) Autonomic dysregulation in young girls with Rett syndrome during nighttime in-home recordings. *Pediatr Pulmonol* 43(11): 1045–1060.

Whalen CN, Case-Smith J (2012) Therapeutic effects of horseback riding on gross motor function of children with cerebral palsy: a systematic review. Phys Occup Ther Pediatr 32: 229–32.

Wigram T, Lawrence M (2005) Music therapy as a tool for assessing hand use and communicativeness in children with Rett syndrome. *Brain Devel* 27(1): S95–S96.

Zoghbi H, Percy AK, Glaze DG, Butler IJ, Riccardi VM (1985) Reduction in biogenic amine levels in Rett syndrome. *N Engl J Med* 313: 921–924.

16
PERSPECTIVES IN RETT SYNDROME: WHERE WE ARE AND WHERE WE SHOULD GO

Walter E Kaufmann, Alan K Percy, Angus Clarke, Helen Leonard and SakkuBai Naidu

Rett syndrome (RTT) became known worldwide following the landmark paper of Hagberg and colleagues (Hagberg et al. 1983). They had made independent assessments of girls or women who had the same profile as those described by Andreas Rett in 1966 (Rett 1966). Based on the work of these eminent clinicians, the understanding of RTT has advanced in clinical and laboratory studies, guided by the important identification of the gene, *MECP2*, which is modified in most girls and women with features of this disorder. This remarkable progress, only 16 years after the worldwide reporting of this disorder has led to critical laboratory progress in understanding and correcting abnormalities in MeCP2-deficient animal and human cells. Looking back on this progress, it is informative to understand the perspective of three individuals who devoted much of their lives to improving our understanding of this unique neurodevelopmental disorder: Bengt Hagberg, Kathy Hunter, and Alison Kerr. Their viewpoints can guide researchers and clinicians in the next 50 years and beyond. Taking inspiration from the aforementioned foundational work, here we provide perspectives on *where we are* and *where we should go*.

The diagnostic challenge

From the clinical side, important progress resulted from the establishment of firm criteria for both classic and atypical RTT. When carefully followed, these criteria allow the clinician to establish the diagnosis accurately in most cases. Diagnostic criteria have evolved successively as clinical experience has provided clearer discrimination of the key features in RTT, and are the result of international expertise that should provide clarity in establishing and comparing diagnoses across the world. Inasmuch as some affected individuals do not have *MECP2* mutations, the importance of providing strict diagnostic criteria is paramount. Despite the marked improvement in accuracy of diagnosis and prognosis, a laboratory-based diagnostic test has remained an important but elusive goal. Improving diagnosis is particularly important for those individuals with an atypical presentation or with some features of RTT but not sufficient to make a firm clinical diagnosis. Nonetheless, the established fidelity of diagnostic features has led to the development of critical natural history studies, pioneered in the United States by Hugo Moser and currently exemplified by the Natural History Study (RNHS), which now has longitudinal data on more than 1500 individuals (Percy 2016). These data and that of other databases in Europe (Nissenkorn et al. 2015), Australia (Anderson et al. 2014), and internationally (Bebbington et al. 2008) through large *MECP2* genotype-phenotype correlative studies, have been instrumental in demonstrating the prognostic value of specific mutations. Natural history studies also play a critical role, as recruitment sites and reference data, in developing improved treatment options arising from the increasing number of multi-site clinical trials. Although natural history studies indicate that over their lifetime clinical severity increases in females with RTT, they also reveal that both the length and probably also the quality of life have improved in recent years (Freilinger et al. 2010; Tarquinio et al. 2015). The evolution of RTT diagnostic criteria and disorder profiles has altered the diagnostic landscape, especially the differential diagnoses, of several categories of neurological disease. It has led to the suggestion that we should recognise the broader categories of MECP2- and RTT-related disorders. As expected from any taxonomy, the implementation of these categories has multiple advantages and disadvantages. The future diagnostic and taxonomic location of some disorders, such as those associated with CDKL5 mutations and MECP2 duplications, remain uncertain (Fehr et al. 2013; Lim et al. 2017).

Genetic bases of Rett syndrome: some surprises and a promising future

What we thought we knew about RTT before its relation to *MECP2* mutation was established has been shown to be correct only in part. The more interesting finding to emerge has been that *MECP2* mutations in males are not lethal *in utero* but arise much more frequently in girls because the mutation is much more common in spermatogenesis than oogenesis. In addition, MeCP2 deficiency not only affects neurodevelopment but also mature neurologic function as demonstrated in mice in which the gene is switched off later in life (Guy et al. 2007). Although general profiles emerge in genotype-phenotype correlations in RTT, the relationship is inevitably obscured by the vagaries of X chromosome inactivation. This makes it harder to identify the genetic and non-genetic modifiers of disease severity.

The link between RTT and *MECP2* mutations has opened a new era of mechanistic and therapeutic research. While neurobiology and pathophysiology research on RTT began shortly after the initial clinical reports in the 1980's, the more recent availability of mouse and other genetic models has had a profound impact upon our understanding of the disorder. It has confirmed and expanded our view of RTT as a disorder of the synapses, with unique features as well as commonalities with other neurodevelopmental disorders. Effective treatments will come from neurobiologically-based interventions applied to a variety of neurodevelopmental disorders, but are more likely to emerge from therapies targeting the molecular and neurologic consequences of *MECP2* mutations (Kaufmann et al. 2016). Management of systemic complications, such as prolonged QT and osteopenia (Herrera et al. 2015; Shapiro et al. 2017), has now a stronger foundation thanks to work on mouse models. Targeted treatments, covering a wide range of symptoms of the disorder and based on preclinical trials in Mecp2-deficient mice, have taken the shape of controlled drug trials re-purposing existing medications or requiring approval for new, more RTT-specific drugs. Although reporting encouraging results, it is too early to draw definitive conclusions about initial MeCP2 neurobiology-based drug trials, particularly considering the recent disappointing experience with fragile X syndrome. The 'reversal' of 'murine RTT' by Guy and Bird (2007) has raised both hopes and expectations. Those experiments do not provide a clear route to developing human therapies but they do provide enormous motivation for treatment beyond early childhood. They show that the potential benefits from any effective treatments could be vast. Nonetheless, genetic therapies are in the initial planning phase after recent promising preclinical studies and only time will tell how safe and effective they will be.

Treating Rett syndrome today

There is considerable variation in what we know about the clinical manifestations of each of the RTT comorbidities described in this book. Equally, there is variation in both the existence and the accessibility of effective treatments and in the existence of evidence-based management guidelines. This information is vital for clinicians caring for these girls and women as we await the advent of new therapeutic strategies. Scoliosis is the most common orthopaedic abnormality in RTT but, despite its severity and impact, up until almost a decade ago little was known about the factors predicting its onset, its clinical progression or the optimal management strategies. However, in the last decade, a wealth of information has been published relating to clinical and genetic predictors, population data on the natural history of scoliosis progression, evaluation of spinal fusion as a surgical treatment, and guidelines for management (Downs et al. 2009, 2016). A second area where significant progress has been made is in the management of growth and gastro-intestinal problems in RTT (Leonard et al. 2013; Baikie et al. 2014). Several clinical studies, undertaken at Baylor College of Medicine by Dr. Kay Motil (Motil et al. 2012; Tarquinio et al. 2012), have contributed to this collective knowledge as has population-based research in Australia (Downs et al. 2014). Once again, guidelines have been assembled with the input of a multinational expert panel, published and disseminated in a variety of formats for the consumption of both clinicians and families (Leonard et al. 2013; Baikie et al. 2014). Gastrostomy placement is one option being taken up by one quarter to a third of families in countries such as Australia and the United States and evaluations of its impact on growth have been positive (Leonard et al. 2013; Baikie et al. 2014). Bone health is another area where knowledge has increased dramatically over the last two decades (Shapiro et al. 2010; Jefferson et al. 2011). Prior to this, little was known about the susceptibility of these girls and women to fractures and what strategies could be used for prevention. Once again guidelines have been published by an international group, providing relevant information for the frontline clinician (Jefferson et al. 2016).

Epilepsy has been a particularly challenging area to study in RTT. Although the EEG is uniformly abnormal from about 18 months of age, this does not necessarily indicate seizure activity while reported seizures may actually reflect autonomic or motor events rather than true epilepsy (Glaze et al. 1998). The first study to examine epilepsy in RTT suggested a prevalence of 95% (Steffenburg et al. 2001); however, subsequent studies have provided lower estimates (Jian et al. 2006; Glaze et al. 2010). Recent research originates from many different regions and countries, including Europe, North America, Israel, Italy and Australia as well as an international data collection (Bao et al. 2013; Nissenkorn et al. 2015; Tarquinio et al. 2017). It has been difficult to establish any consistent genotype–phenotype relationships partly because of methodological differences among studies and lack of representativeness in some. Current antiepileptic management will often still depend on clinicians' preferences since no published guidelines are available. As for other neurodevelopmental disorders, sleep disturbances are a particularly burdensome attribute of RTT and have been studied intermittently since the 1990s (Piazza et al. 1990; Wong et al. 2015). There is still much to learn especially in relation to the optimal medication regime to use when response to sleep hygiene measures is inadequate, and possible genotype–phenotype correlations. It is almost thirty years since breathing abnormalities were first described as a potentially treatable component of RTT. Three decades on, we still have no treatment for this symptom or other associated autonomic abnormalities that affect girls and women with RTT. Despite the impact of these abnormal breathing patterns the literature on their characteristics, prevalence, and natural history is relatively sparse and limited to a handful of papers (Julu et al. 2001; Weese-Mayer et al. 2006; Mackay et al. 2017). In contrast, work on mouse models has been much more prolific and already provided the underlying rationale for a clinical trial using a serotoninergic 5HT1a agonist (Abdala et al. 2014). There is an increasing consensus that rehabilitation treatments, such as speech and language, occupational, and physical therapy, play an important role in promoting and preserving skills. Another current view is that novel, neurobiologically targeted drug-based, and perhaps also genetic, treatments need to be developed and implemented in association with therapies or learning interventions (Kaufmann et al. 2016).

Working together towards transformational research

Although there is yet a way to go, progress has been made in the clinical understanding and management of the comorbidities affecting girls and women with RTT and new treatments are under development. The important roles played by research infrastructures, international collaborations and parent advocacy groups in facilitating this progress cannot be underestimated (Kaufmann et al. 2016; Percy 2016) and nor can the value of the Internet in connecting families previously geographically isolated because of the rarity of their child's disorder (Leonard et al. 2017). The sense of promise brought by the recent drug and genetic experimental trials has motivated different people in different ways. One consequence, which contrasts with the collaborative approach regarding natural history and consensus guidelines, perhaps, has been the unhelpful fragmentation of the RTT community's efforts to make research progress towards effective treatments. While eagerness to test new treatments or develop new measures in the most expedited way is understood, transformational outcomes will only be obtained through large-scale, collaborative studies. As with other rare disorders, RTT faces logistical challenges, including subject recruitment and availability of resources. Thus, strategic partnerships involving clinicians, researchers, funding agencies, industry, and advocacy groups are essential in order to establish research priorities.

Treatments are undoubtedly coming. Some, such as neurotransmitter modulators, may mitigate some of the effects of the condition without being transformational while the potential "cures" may also emerge before long, although their effectiveness in stabilising or even reversing the disease will remain unclear until they have been tried in clinical practice. Development, implementation, and long-term surveillance of new interventions will also require education of caregivers and other stakeholders. While the Internet and social media may create barriers by raising unreasonable expectations and promoting misconceptions; nevertheless, they remain as powerful tools for dissemination of information and research participation. Clinicians, researchers and advocacy groups will have again to collaborate in tempering hope with realism in a compassionate way.

This volume intends to educate anyone who is interested or curious about RTT. We hope it will serve as a foundation for obtaining more in-depth and up-to-date information about the disorder, and ultimately it will encourage more clinicians and researchers to consider RTT as a career focus. The next 50 years of RTT progress will require an even larger group of enthusiastic clinicians and researchers.

REFERENCES

Abdala AP, Bissonnette JM, Newman-Tancredi A (2014) Pinpointing brainstem mechanisms responsible for autonomic dysfunction in Rett syndrome: therapeutic perspectives for 5-HT1A agonists. *Front Physiol* 5: 205.

Ager S, Fyfe S, Christodoulou J, et al. (2006) Predictors of scoliosis in Rett syndrome. *J Child Neurol* 21(9): 809–813.

Anderson A, Wong K, Jacoby P, Downs J, Leonard H (2014) Twenty years of surveillance in Rett syndrome: what does this tell us? *Orphanet J Rare Dis* 9: 87.

Baikie G, Ravikumara M, Downs J, et al. (2014) Gastrointestinal dysmotility in Rett syndrome. *J Pediatr Gastroenterol Nutr* 58(2): 237–244.

Bao X, Downs J, Wong K, Williams S, Leonard H (2013) Using a large international sample to investigate epilepsy in Rett syndrome. *Dev Med Child Neurol* 55(6): 553–558.

Bebbington A, Anderson A, Ravine D, et al. (2008) Investigating genotype-phenotype relationships in Rett syndrome using an international data set. *Neurology* 70(11): 868–875.

Downs J, Bergman A, Carter P, et al. (2009) Guidelines for management of scoliosis in Rett syndrome patients based on expert consensus and clinical evidence. *Spine (Phila Pa 1976)* 34(17): E607–E617.

Downs J, Wong K, Ravikumara M, et al. (2014) Experience of gastrostomy using a quality care framework: the example of rett syndrome. *Medicine (Baltimore)* 93(28): e328.

Downs J, Torode I, Wong K, et al. (2016) Surgical fusion of early onset severe scoliosis increases survival in Rett syndrome: a cohorts *Dev Med Child Neurol* 58(6): 632–638.

Fehr S, Wilson M, Downs J, et al. (2013) The CDKL5 disorder is an independent clinical entity associated with early-onset encephalopathy. *Eur J Hum Genet* 21(3): 266–273.

Freilinger M, Bebbington A, Lanator I, et al. (2010) Survival with Rett syndrome: comparing Rett's original sample with data from the Australian Rett Syndrome Database. *Dev Med Child Neurol* 52(10): 962–965.

Glaze DG, Schultz RJ, Frost JD (1998) Rett syndrome: characterization of seizures versus non-seizures. *Electroencephalogr Clin Neurophysiol* 106(1): 79–83.

Glaze DG, Percy AK, Skinner S, et al. (2010) Epilepsy and the natural history of Rett syndrome. *Neurology* 74(11): 909–912.

Guy J, Gan J, Selfridge J, Cobb S, Bird A (2007) Reversal of neurological defects in a mouse model of Rett syndrome. *Science* 315(5815): 1143–1147.

Hagberg B, Aicardi J, Dias K, Ramos O (1983) A progressive syndrome of autism, dementia, ataxia, and loss of purposeful hand use in girls: Rett's syndrome: report of 35 cases. *Ann Neurol* 14(4): 471–479.

Herrera JA, Ward CS, Pitcher MR, et al. (2015) Treatment of cardiac arrhythmias in a mouse model of Rett syndrome with Na+-channel-blocking antiepileptic drugs. *Dis Model Mech* 8(4): 363–371.

Jefferson AL, Woodhead HJ, Fyfe S, et al. (2011) Bone mineral content and density in Rett syndrome and their contributing factors. *Pediatr Res* 69(4): 293–298.

Jefferson A, Leonard H, Siafarikas A, et al. (2016) Clinical Guidelines for Management of Bone Health in Rett Syndrome Based on Expert Consensus and Available Evidence. *PLoS One* 11(2): e0146824.

Jian L, Nagarajan L, de Klerk N, et al. (2006) Predictors of seizure onset in Rett syndrome. *J Pediatr* 149(4): 542–547.

Julu PO, Kerr AM, Apartopoulos F, et al. (2001) Characterisation of breathing and associated central autonomic dysfunction in the Rett disorder. *Arch Dis Child* 85(1): 29–37.

Kaufmann WE, Stallworth JL, Everman DB, Skinner SA (2016) Neurobiologically-based treatments in Rett syndrome: Opportunities and challenges. *Expert Opin Orphan Drugs* 4(10): 1043–1055.

Leonard H, Ravikumara M, Baikie G, et al. (2013) Assessment and management of nutrition and growth in Rett syndrome. *J Pediatr Gastroenterol Nutr* 57(4): 451–460.

Leonard H, Cobb S, Downs J (2017) Clinical and biological progress over 50 years in Rett syndrome. *Nat Rev Neurol* 13(1): 37–51.

Lim Z, Downs J, Wong K, Ellaway C, Leonard H (2017) Expanding the clinical picture of the MECP2 Duplication syndrome. *Clin Genet* 91(4): 557–563.

Mackay J, Downs J, Wong K, Heyworth J, Epstein A, Leonard H (2017) Autonomic breathing abnormalities in Rett syndrome: caregiver perspectives in an international database study. *J Neurodev Disord* 9: 15.

Motil KJ, Morrissey M, Caeg E, Barrish JO, Glaze DG (2009) Gastrostomy placement improves height and weight gain in girls with Rett syndrome. *J Pediatr Gastroenterol Nutr* 49(2): 237–242.

Motil KJ, Caeg E, Barrish JO et al. (2012) Gastrointestinal and nutritional problems occur frequently throughout life in girls and women with Rett syndrome. *J Pediatr Gastroenterol Nutr* 55(3): 292–298.

Nissenkorn A, Levy-Drummer RS, Bondi O, et al. (2015) Epilepsy in Rett syndrome--lessons from the Rett networked database. *Epilepsia* 56(4): 569–576.

Percy AK (2016) Progress in Rett syndrome: From discovery to clinical trials. *Wien Med Wochenschr* 166(11–12): 325–332.

Piazza CC, Fisher W, Kiesewetter K, Bowman L, Moser H (1990) Aberrant sleep patterns in children with the Rett syndrome. *Brain Dev* 12(5): 488–493.

Rett A (1966) On an unusual brain atrophy syndrome in hyperammonemia in childhood. *Wien Med Wochenschr* 116(37): 723–726.

Shapiro JR, Bibat G, Hiremath G, et al. (2010) Bone mass in Rett syndrome: association with clinical parameters and MECP2 mutations. *Pediatr Res* 68(5): 446–451.

Shapiro JR, Boskey AL, Doty SB, Lukashova L, Blue ME (2017) Zoledronic acid improves bone histomorphometry in a murine model of Rett syndrome. *Bone* 99: 1–7.

Steffenburg U, Hagberg G, Hagberg B (2001) Epilepsy in a representative series of Rett syndrome. *Acta Paediatr* 90(1): 34–39.

Tarquinio DC, Motil KJ, Hou WE et al. (2012) Reference growth standards in Rett syndrome. *Neurology* 79(16): 1653–1661.

Tarquinio DC, Hou W, Neul JL, et al. (2015) The Changing Face of Survival in Rett Syndrome and MECP2-Related Disorders. *Pediatr Neurol* 53(5): 402–411.

Tarquinio DC, Hou W, Berg A, et al. (2017) Longitudinal course of epilepsy in Rett syndrome and related disorders. *Brain* 140(Pt 2): 306–318.

Weese-Mayer DE, Lieske SP, Boothby CM, et al. (2006) Autonomic nervous system dysregulation: breathing and heart rate perturbation during wakefulness in young girls with Rett syndrome. *Pediatr Res* 60(4): 443–449.

Wong K, Leonard H, Jacoby P, Ellaway C, Downs J (2015) The trajectories of sleep disturbances in Rett syndrome. *J Sleep Res* 24(2): 223–233.

INDEX

b = boxed section; *f* = figure; *t* = table.